Table of Contents

PDR® Pharmacopoeia Pocket Dosing Guide 2007

Foreword

Welcome to the *PDR Pharmacopoeia Pocket Dosing Guide*, now in its seventh edition. This convenient little book is designed to be at your fingertips whenever you need to double-check dosage recommendations, review available forms and strengths, or confirm a pregnancy rating. For the 2007 edition, it has been completely updated to include all the latest new drugs, forms, strengths, and indications.

To aid quick lookups and comparisons, *PDR Pharmacopoeia* is organized by major drug category and specific indication. Under each indication, you'll find applicable drugs sorted by class and listed alphabetically by generic name. For combination products, generic ingredients are listed alphabetically, with the strengths of the ingredients presented in the same order.

The book's major sections are listed on the Contents Page. The location of entries for specific brands, generics, and indications can be found in the index at the end of the book. For drugs with multiple uses, the index lists the page of each indication separately.

The *PDR Pharmacopoeia* also offers you a variety of quick-reference tables listing frequently used formulas and comparative prescribing information. For the exact location of these convenient resources, check the index at the end of the book.

Unlike other dosing guides, the *PDR Pharmacopoeia* is drawn almost exclusively from the FDA-approved drug labeling published in *Physicians' Desk Reference®*. Although diligent efforts have been made to ensure the accuracy of this information, please remember that this book is sold without warranties, express or implied, and that the publisher and editors disclaim all liability in connection with its use.

Remember, too, that this book deals only with dosage for the typical patient, and includes little information on usage in special populations and circumstances. The need for dosage adjustments in the presence of hepatic or renal insufficiency is signaled in the Comments column of the entries. For details regarding these adjustments, as well as complete pediatric and geriatric dosage guidelines, consult the latest edition of *PDR®*. Be sure to check *PDR*, too, whenever contraindications, warnings, or precautions may be an issue.

Throughout the book, you will find a drug's Controlled Substances Category (if any) immediately following its name. The drug's pregnancy rating and breastfeeding status appear in the Comments column of the entry. Keys to the symbols can be found below:

Controlled Substances Categories

CII. High potential for abuse, leading to severe psychological or physical dependence. **CIII.** Abuse may lead to moderate or low physical dependence or high psychological dependence. **CIV.** Abuse may lead to limited physical dependence or psychological dependence. **CV.** Consequences of abuse are more limited than those of drugs in Category CIV.

Use-In-Pregnancy Ratings

A. Controlled studies shown no risk. **B.** No evidence of risk in humans. **C.** Risk cannot be ruled out. **D.** Positive evidence of risk: Use only when no safer alternative exists for a serious problem. **X.** Contraindicated in pregnancy. **N.** Not rated.

Breastfeeding Safety

^ May be used in breastfeeding. > Caution advised or effect undetermined. v Contraindicated or not recommended.

H Dosage adjustment required for hepatic insufficiency.
R Dosage adjustment required for renal insufficiency.

Dosage Forms

A key to the abbreviations may be found on page 4.

PDR® PHARMACOPOEIA POCKET DOSING GUIDE 2007

Manager, Professional Services: Michael DeLuca, PharmD
Managing Editor: Greg Tallis, RPh
Associate Editor: Majid Kerolous, PharmD, Nermin Shenouda, PharmD
Senior Electronic Publishing Designer: Livio Udina
Production Editor: Elise Philippi
Project Managers: John Castro, Edward Guerra, Don Pond

Executive Vice President, PDR: Kevin Sanborn
Vice President, PDR Services: Brian Holland
Vice President, Product Management: William T. Hicks
Senior Director, Brand and Product Management: Valerie Berger
Director of Product Management: Swan Oey
Director of Operations: Robert Klein
Director, Editorial Services: Bette LaGow

Chief Medical Officer: Rich Klasco, MD, FACEP

THOMSON PDR

2007.1

ABBREVIATIONS

ABBREVIATIONS & DESCRIPTIONS

CAP	community-aquired pneumonia
Cap	capsule
Cap,ER	extended release capsule
CI	contraindicated
Cnt	concentrate
conc	concentration
Cre	cream
d	day
D/C	discontinue
Eli	elixir
Foa	foam
Gel	gel/jelly
gm	gram
h	hour
hs	at bedtime
IM	intramuscular
inj	injection
IU	international units
IV	intravenous

ABBREVIATIONS & DESCRIPTIONS

ml	milliliter
mth	month
NTE	not to exceed
Oint	ointment
Pkt	packet
PO	by mouth
Pow	powder
prn	as needed
q	every
qd	once daily
qid	four times daily
qod	every other day
qow	every other week
SC	subcutaneous
Sl	sublingual
Sol	solution
Sol,Neb	solution, nebulized
Spr	spray(s)
Sup	suppository

Kg	kilogram
Liq	liquid
Lot	lotion
Loz	lozenge
mcg	microgram
MDI	metered dose inhaler
mEq	milli-equivalent
mg	milligram
min	minute
MIU	million international units
Susp	suspension
Syr	syrup
Tab	tablet
Tab,ER	extended release tablet
tid	3 times daily
tiw	3 times weekly
U	units
w/a	while awake
wk	week
yo	years old

WEIGHTS & MEASURES; CONVERSIONS & FORMULAS

METRIC WEIGHT

1 kilogram (kg)	=	1,000 gram
1 gram (g)	=	1,000 mg
1 milligram (mg)	=	0.001 gm

U.S. FLUID MEASURE

1 fluidrachm	=	60 minim (min)
1 fluidounce	=	8 fld drachm
	=	480 min

METRIC WEIGHT

1 microgram (mcg)	=	0.001 mg
1 gamma	=	1 mcg

U.S. FLUID MEASURE

1 pint (pt)	=	16 fl oz
	=	7,680 min
1 quart (qt)	=	2 pt
	=	32 fl oz
1 gallon (gal)	=	4 qts
	=	128 fl oz

APOTHECARY WEIGHT

1 scruple	=	20 grains (gr)
1 drachm	=	3 scruples
	=	60 gr
1 ounce (oz)	=	8 drachms
	=	24 scruples
	=	480 gr
1 pound (lb)	=	12 oz
	=	96 drachms
	=	288 scruples
	=	5,760 gr

AVOIRDUPOIS WEIGHT

1 ounce	=	437.5 gr
1 pound	=	16 oz

CONVERSION FACTORS

1 gram	=	15.4 gr
1 grain	=	64.8 mg
1 ounce (AV)	=	28.35 gm
	=	437.5 gr
1 ounce (Ap)	=	31.1 gm
	=	480 gr
1 pound (Av)	=	453.6 gm
1 kilogram	=	2.68 pound Ap
	=	2.2 lbs Av
1 fluidounce	=	29.57 ml
1 fluidrachm	=	3.697 ml
1 minim	=	0.06 ml

COMMON MEASURES

1 teaspoonful	=	5 ml
	=	1/6 fl oz
1 tablespoonful	=	15 ml
	=	1/2 fl oz
1 wineglassful	=	60 ml
	=	2 fl oz
1 teacupful	=	120 ml
	=	4 fl oz

TEMPERATURE

For °F to °C, the formula is: 5/9 (°F minus 32) = °C
For °C to °F, the formula is: 9/5 °C plus 32 = °F
1 kelvin (K) = 9/5 °F

COCKCROFT/GAULT CREATININE CLEARANCE FORMULA

$$Cl_{Cr\ (males^{*}\ ml/min)} = \frac{(140 - Age)(Body\ Weight\ in\ kg)}{(SrCr)(72\ kg)}$$

*For females multiply result by 0.85

BODY SURFACE AREA [BSA (M^2)]

$BSA = ([Ht (cm) \bullet Wt (kg)] / 3600)^{1/2}$

ANION GAP (AG)

$AG = (Na^+ + K^+) - (Cl^- + HCO_3^-)$ or $AG = Na^+ - (Cl^- + HCO_3^-)$

NEUTROPENIA CALCULATION

ANC = (% segs + % bands) X total WBC

ANALGESICS

Arthritis Therapy

SEE ALSO NSAIDS

NAME	FORM/STRENGTH	DOSAGE	COMMENTS
Abatacept (Orencia)	**Inj:** 250 mg	**Adults: IV: Initial: <60 kg:** 500 mg; **60-100 kg:** 750 mg; **>100 kg:** 1 gm. Infuse over 30 min. **Maint:** Give at 2 & 4 wks after initial infusion, then q4wks thereafter.	◙C ❃v
Adalimumab (Humira)	**Inj:** 40 mg/0.8 ml	**RA/Psoriatic Arthritis: Adults:** 40 mg SC qowk. Patients w/ RA not taking MTX may derive additional benefit by increasing to 40 mg qwk.	◙B ❃v TB & other opportunistic infections reported.
Anakinra (Kineret)	**Inj:** 100 mg/0.67 ml	**RA: Adults: ≥18 yo:** 100 mg SC qd.	◙B ❃>
Auranofin (Ridaura)	**Cap:** 3 mg	**RA: Adults: Usual:** 3 mg bid or 6 mg qd. **Max:** 9 mg/d.	◙C ❃v May cause gold toxicity.
Aurothioglucose (Solganal)	**Inj:** 50 mg/ml	**RA: Adults: Initial:** 1st wk 10 mg IM. **Titrate:** 2nd & 3rd wk 25 mg IM, 4th & subsequent wks 50 mg IM until 0.8-1 gm given; continue 50 mg IM q3-4wks. **JRA: Peds: 6-12 yo:** 1/4 of adult dose IM. **Max:** 25 mg/dose.	◙C ❃v Possible toxic reactions.
Azathioprine (Imuran, Azasan)	**Tab:** (Imuran) 50mg; **Tab:** (Azasan) 25 mg, 50 mg, 75 mg, 100 mg	**RA: Adults: Initial:** 1 mg/kg/d given qd-bid. **Titrate:** Increase by 0.5 mg/kg/d after 6-8 wks & then q4wks. **Max:** 2.5 mg/kg/d. **Maint:** Decrease by 0.5 mg/kg/d or 25 mg/d q4wks until lowest effective dose.	◙D ❃v **R** Neoplasia. Mutagenesis. Hematologic toxicity.
Celecoxib (Celebrex)	**Cap:** 100 mg, 200 mg, 400 mg	**Adults: OA:** 200 mg qd or 100 mg bid. **RA:** 100-200 mg bid. **AS: Initial** 200 mg qd or 100 mg bid. **Titrate:** May increase to 400 mg/d after 6 wks.	◙C ❃v **H** 66, 67

Cyclosporine (Neoral)	**Cap:** 25 mg, 100 mg; **Sol:** 100 mg/ml	**RA: Adults ≥18 yo: Initial:** 2.5 mg/kg/d, taken bid. **Titrate:** Increase by 0.5-0.75 mg/kg/d after 8 wks & again after 12 wks. **Max:** 4 mg/kg/d. Decrease by 25-50% to control adverse events. **Combo w/ MTX: Maint:** 3 mg/kg/d or less. **Max:** 15 mg/wk.	C v Infection. Neoplasia. HTN. Nephrotoxicity. Malignancy risk w/certain psoriasis therapies.
Etanercept (Enbrel)	**Inj:** 25 mg, 50 mg/ml	**RA/Psoriatic Arthritis/Ankylosing Spondylitis: Adults:** 50 mg/wk SC. **JRA: Peds: 4-17 yo:** 0.8 mg/kg/wk SC. **Max:** 50 mg/wk & 25 mg/inj site. **≥63 kg:** Give dose as one SC inj. **31-62 kg:** Give dose as two SC inj on same day or 3-4 days apart. **≤31 kg:** Give dose as one SC inj once wkly.	B v
Gold Sodium Thiomalate (Aurolate)	**Inj:** 50 mg/ml	**RA: Adults: Usual:** 10 mg IM 1st wk, 20 mg 2nd wk, 25-50 mg IM wkly until cumulative dose of 1 gm, toxicity, or clinical improvement. **Maint:** 25-50 mg every other wk. **JRA: Peds: Initial:** Test dose of 10 mg. **Maint:** 1 mg/kg IM wkly. **Max:** 50 mg/single inj.	C v Possible toxic reactions.
Hydroxychloroquine Sulfate (Plaquenil)	**Tab:** 200 mg	**RA: Adults: Initial:** 400-600 mg/d w/ food or glass of milk. Increase dose in 5-10d until optimum response. **Maint:** After 4-12 wks, 200-400 mg/d.	N >

66 NSAIDs may cause an increased risk of serious CV thrombotic events, MI, stroke and serious GI adverse events including bleeding, ulceration, and perforation of the stomach or intestines.

67 Contraindicated for treatment of peri-operative pain in CABG surgery.

NAME	FORM/STRENGTH	DOSAGE	COMMENTS
Infliximab (Remicade)	**Inj:** 100 mg	**Adults: RA (Combo w/ MTX):** 3 mg/kg IV, repeat at 2 & 6 wks. **Maint:** Give q8wks thereafter. **Incomplete Response:** Increase to 10mg/kg or give q4wks. **Ankylosing Spondylitis:** 5 mg/kg IV, repeat at 2 & 6 wks. **Maint:** Give q6wks thereafter. **Psoriatic Arthritis:** 5 mg/kg IV, repeat at 2 & 6 wks. **Maint:** Give q8wks thereafter.	◉B ❋v TB, fungal, & other opportunistic infections reported.
Leflunomide (Arava)	**Tab:** 10 mg, 20 mg	**RA: Adults: LD:**100 mg qd x 3 d. **Maint:** 20 mg qd. **Max:** 20 mg/d. **If dose not tolerated or ALT elevations >2 but ≤3X ULN:** Reduce dose to 10 mg/d. If elevations persist or ALT >3X UNL, d/c.	◉X ❋v **H** CI in pregnancy. Hepatotoxicity. Immunosuppression.
Meloxicam (Mobic)	**Susp:** 7.5 mg/5 ml; **Tab:** 7.5 mg, 15 mg	**OA/RA: Adults: ≥18 yo: Initial/Maint:** 7.5 mg qd. **Max:** 15 mg/d. **JRA: Peds: ≥2 yo:** 0.125 mg/kg qd. **Max:** 7.5 mg/d.	◉C ❋v [66, 67]
Methotrexate Sodium (Rheumatrex)	**Tab:** 2.5 mg, 5 mg, 7.5 mg, 15 mg	**RA: Adults: Initial:** 7.5 mg once weekly or 2.5 mg q12h x 3 doses once weekly. **Max:** 20 mg/wk. Reduce to lowest effective dose. **JRA: Peds 2-16 yo:** 10 mg/m² once weekly. Adjust dose to optimal response.	◉X ❋v CI in pregnancy & nursing. [19]
Penicillamine (Cuprimine)	**Cap:** 125 mg, 250 mg	**RA: Adults: Initial:** 125 mg-250 mg qd; increase q1-3mths by 125 mg-250 mg/d. **Maint:** 500-750 mg/d.	◉D ❋v CI in pregnancy, renal insufficiency & agranulocytosis.
Penicillamine (Depen)	**Tab:** 250 mg	**RA: Adults: Initial:** 125 mg-250 mg qd; increase q1-3mths by 125 mg-250 mg/d. **Maint:** 500-750 mg/d.	◉N ❋v CI in pregnancy, renal insufficiency & agranulocytosis.

Rituximab (Rituxan)	**Inj:** 10 mg/ml	**RA: Adults:** Give w/ methotrexate. Give two-1000 mg IV infusions separated by 2 wks. Administer methylprednisolone 100 mg IV (or equivalent) 30 min prior to each infusion to reduce the incidence & severity of infusion reactions.	◙C ❃v [65]
Sulfasalazine (Azulfidine EN-tabs)	**Tab,Delay:** 500 mg	**RA: Adults: Initial:** 0.5-1 gm qd. **Usual:** 1 gm bid. **Max:** 3 gm/d. **JRA: Peds: 6-16 yo:** 30-50 mg/kg/d given bid. **Max:** 2 gm/d.	◙B ❃>

Narcotics

Codeine CII	(Phosphate) **Inj:** 15 mg/ml, 30 mg/ml; **Sol:** 15 mg/5 ml; **Tab:** 30 mg, 60 mg; (Sulfate) **Tab:** 15 mg, 30 mg, 60 mg	**Adults:** 15-60 mg PO/IM/SC q4-6h. **Peds: ≥1 yo:** 0.5 mg/kg PO q4-6h or 0.5 mg/kg IM/SC q4h, up to 3 mg/kg/d IM/SC in divided doses.	◙C ❃>
Codeine Phosphate/ APAP CIII (Tab) CV (Eli) (Tylenol w/ Codeine)	**Eli:** 12-120 mg/5 ml; **Tab:** (#3) 30-300 mg, (#4) 60-300 mg	**Tab: Adults:** 15 mg-60 mg codeine/dose & 300 mg-1 gm APAP/dose up to q4h prn. **Max:** 360 mg codeine & 4 gm APAP per 24h. **Peds:** 0.5 mg/kg of codeine. **Eli: Adults:** 15 ml q4h prn. **Peds: 3-6 yo:** 5 ml tid-qid. **7-12 yo:** 10 ml tid-qid.	◙C ❃>

[19] Monitor for bone marrow, lung, liver & kidney toxicities. Serious toxic reactions.
[65] Fatal infusion reactions, tumor lysis syndrome & severe mucocutaneous reactions reported.
[66] NSAIDs may cause an increased risk of serious CV thrombotic events, MI, stroke and serious GI adverse events including bleeding, ulceration, and perforation of the stomach or intestines.
[67] Contraindicated for treatment of peri-operative pain in CABG surgery.

NAME	FORM/STRENGTH	DOSAGE	COMMENTS
Fentanyl CII (Duragesic)	**Patch:** 12.5 mcg/h, 25 mcg/h, 50 mcg/h, 5 mcg/h, 100 mcg/h	**Adults & Peds: ≥2 yo: Opioid Tolerant:** Individualize dose based on opioid tolerance. **Initial:** Base on daily oral morphine dose (see PI). **Titrate:** Adjust dose after 3d based on daily supplemental opioid analgesic dose; use ratio of 45 mg/24h of oral morphine to a 12.5 mcg/h increase in Duragesic dose. May take 6d to reach equilibrium after dose change.	C v
Fentanyl Citrate CII (Actiq)	**Loz:** 0.2 mg, 0.4 mg, 0.6 mg, 0.8 mg, 1.2 mg, 1.6 mg	**Breakthrough Pain: Adults & Peds: ≥16 yo: Initial:** 0.2 mg for pain (consume over 15 min). **Titrate:** Increase to next strength if pain episodes require >1 unit/pain episode. **Maint:** 1 unit/pain episode. **Max:** 2 units/pain episode or 4 units/d.	C v CI in acute or post-op pain, non-opioid tolerant patients.
Hydrocodone Bitartrate/ APAP CIII (Lortab, Maxidone, Vicodin, Vicodin ES, Vicodin HP)	**Sol:** (Lortab) 7.5-500 mg/ 15 ml; **Tab:** (Lortab) 2.5-500 mg, 5-500 mg, 7.5-500 mg, 10-500 mg; **Tab:** (Maxidone) 10-750 mg, (Vicodin) 5-500 mg, (Vicodin ES) 7.5-750 mg, (Vicodin HP) 10-660 mg	**Pain: Adults: Vicodin:** 1-2 tabs q4-6h prn. **Max:** 8 tabs/d. **Vicodin HP:** 1 tab q4-6h prn. **Max:** 6 tabs/d. **Vicodin ES/Maxidone:** 1 tab q4-6h prn. **Max:** 5 tabs/d. **Lortab:** (2.5-500 mg tab, 5-500 mg tab) 1-2 tabs q4-6h prn. **Max:** 8 tabs/d. (7.5-500 mg tab, 10-500 mg tab) 1 tab q4-6h prn. **Max:** 6 tabs/d. (Sol) 15 ml q4-6h prn. **Max:** 90 ml/d. **Peds: ≥2 yrs: Lortab: Sol: 12-15 kg:** 3.75 ml. **16-22 kg:** 5 ml. **23-31 kg:** 7.5 ml. **32-45 kg:** 10 ml. **≥46 kg:** 15 ml. May repeat q4-6h prn.	C v
Hydrocodone Bitartrate/ Ibuprofen CIII (Reprexain, Vicoprofen)	**Tab:** (Reprexain) 5-200 mg, (Vicoprofen) 7.5-200 mg	**Adults & Peds: ≥16 yo: Usual:** 1 tab q4-6h prn. **Max:** 5 tabs/d.	C v

Hydromorphone HCl CII (Dilaudid, Dilaudid HP)	**Inj:** 1 mg/ml, 2 mg/ml, 4 mg/ml, (HP form) 10 mg/ml; **Liq:** 1 mg/ml; **Sup:** 3 mg; **Tab:** 2 mg, 4 mg, 8 mg	**Adults: Usual: Inj:** 1-2 mg IM/IV/SC q4-6h prn. **HP Inj:** 1-14 mg IM/SQ. **Liq:** 2.5-10 mg PO q3-6h prn. **Tab:** 2-4 mg q4-6h PO prn. **Sup:** 1 sup PR q6-8h prn.	◉C ✿v
Meperidine HCl CII (Demerol)	**Inj:** 25 mg/ml, 50 mg/ml, 75 mg/ml, 100 mg/ml; **Syr:** 50 mg/5 ml; **Tab:** 50 mg, 100 mg	**Adults: Usual:** 50-150 mg PO/IM/SC q3-4h prn. **Peds: Usual:** 0.5 mg/lb-0.8 mg/lb PO/IM/SC, up to adult dose, q3-4h prn. Mix syrup in 1/2 glass of water to prevent topical anesthetic effect on mucous membranes.	◉N ✿> **H R** CI with MAOI use within 14 days.
Meperidine/ Promethazine CII	**Cap:** 50-25 mg	**Adults:** 1 cap q4-6h prn.	◉N ✿> **H R** CI with MAOI use within 14 days.
Methadone HCl CII (Dolophine)	**Tab:** 5 mg, 10 mg	**Pain: Adults: Usual**: 2.5-10 mg PO/IM/SC q3-4h prn. Special dosing for detox/maintenance treatment.	◉N ✿>
Morphine Sulfate CII	**Sol:** 10 mg/5 ml, 20 mg/5 ml; **Tab:** 15 mg, 30 mg	**Adults: Sol:** 10-20 mg q4h. **Tab:** 15-30mg q4h.	◉C ✿v
Morphine Sulfate CII (Astramorph/PF, Duramorph)	**Inj:** 0.5 mg/ml, 1 mg/ml, 5 mg/ml	**Adults: IV: Initial:** 2-10 mg/70 kg. **Epidural: Initial:** 5 mg in lumbar region, increase by 1-2 mg if needed. **Max:** 10 mg/24h. **Continuous Epidural: Initial:** 2-4 mg/24h, give additional 1-2 mg if needed. **Max:** 10 mg/24h. **Intrathecal:** 0.2-1 mg single inj.	◉C ✿>

NAME	FORM/STRENGTH	DOSAGE	COMMENTS
Morphine Sulfate CII (Avinza)	**Cap,ER:** 30 mg, 60 mg, 90 mg, 120 mg	**Adults: ≥18 yo: Conversion from PO Morphine:** Give total daily morphine dose as a single dose q24h. **Conversion from Parenteral Morphine: Initial:** Give about 3x previous daily parenteral morphine requirement. **Conversion from Other Parenteral or PO Non-Morphine Opioids: Initial:** Give 1/2 of estimated daily morphine requirement q24h. May supplement w/ immediate-release morphine or short-acting analgesics. **Titrate:** Adjust as frequently as qod. **Non-Opioid Tolerant:** 30 mg q24h. **Titrate:** Increase by no more than 30 mg q4d. **Max:** 1600 mg/d. The 60, 90, & 120 mg caps are for opioid-tolerant patients.	●C ✿v [51]
Morphine Sulfate CII (Kadian, MS Contin, Oramorph SR)	**Cap,ER:** (Kadian) 20 mg, 30 mg, 50 mg, 60 mg, 100 mg; **Tab,ER:** (MS Contin, Oramorph SR) 15 mg, 30 mg, 60 mg, 100 mg, (MS Contin) 200 mg	**Adults: Conversion to MS Contin/Oramorph SR:** Give 1/2 of the 24h immediate-release oral morphine dose q12h. May give 1/3 of daily oral morphine dose q8h w/ MS Contin. **Conversion to Kadian:** Give 1/2 of the total daily oral morphine dose as Kadian q12h or total daily oral morphine dose as q24h.	●C ✿v Swallow whole. MS Contin 200 mg tab is only for opioid-tolerant patients.
Morphine Sulfate CII (Roxanol, Roxanol-T)	**Sol, Concentrate:** 20 mg/ml	**Adults: Usual:** 10-30 mg q4h. During first effective pain relief, dose should be maintained for at least 3 days before any dose reduction, if respiratory activity & other vital signs are adequate.	●C ✿> **H R** [57]

Oxycodone HCl CII (Oxycontin)	**Tab,ER:** 10 mg, 20 mg, 40 mg, 80 mg, 160 mg	**Adults: ≥18 yrs: Opioid Naive:** 10 mg q12h. **Titrate:** Increase to 20 mg q12h, then increase total daily dose by 25-50% of current dose. Increase q1-2d. **Conversion from Oxycodone:** Divide 24h oxycodone dose by 50% to obtain q12h dose. Round down to appropriate strength. **Opioid Tolerant:** May use 80 mg or 160 mg tabs. D/C other around-the-clock opioids. High-fat meals increase peak levels of 160 mg tab. **With CNS Depressants:** Reduce by 1/3 or 1/2.	◙B ❉v For continuous analgesia. Abuse potential. 80 mg & 160 mg tabs are only for opioid-tolerant patients. Swallow whole.
Oxycodone HCl CII (OxyFast, OxyIR, Roxicodone)	(OxyFast) **Sol:** 20 mg/ml; (OxyIR) **Cap:** 5 mg; (Roxicodone) **Sol:** 5 mg/5 ml, 20 mg/ml; **Tab:** 5 mg, 15 mg, 30 mg	**Pain: Adults:** (OxyFast, OxyIR) 5 mg q6h prn. (Roxicodone) 5-30 mg q4-6h prn.	◙B ❉v
Oxycodone HCl/APAP CII (Percocet, Roxicet, Tylox)	(Percocet) **Tab:** 2.5-325 mg, 5-325 mg, 7.5-325 mg, 7.5-500 mg, 10-325 mg, 10-650 mg; (Roxicet) **Sol:** 5-325 mg/5 ml; **Tab:** 5-325 mg; 5-500 mg; (Tylox) **Cap:** 5-500 mg	**Pain: Adults: Percocet** (2.5-325 mg tab) 1-2 tabs q6h prn. (5-325 mg tab) 1 tab q6h prn. (7.5-500 mg tab) 1 tab q6h. (10-650 mg tab) 1 tab q6h. (7.5-325 mg tab) 1 tab q6h prn. **Max:** 8 tabs/d. (10-325 mg tab) 1 tab q6h prn. **Max:** 6 tabs/d. Do not exceed 4 gm APAP/d. **Roxicet:** (5-325 mg tab or 5-500 mg tab) 1 tab q6h prn. (5-325 mg/5 ml) 5 ml q6h prn. **Tylox:** 1 cap q6h prn.	◙C ❉>
Oxycodone HCl/Ibuprofen CII (Combunox)	**Tab:** 5-400 mg	**Adults:** 1 tab/dose. Do not exceed 4 tabs/d & 7 days.	◙C ❉>

51 Swallow caps whole or sprinkle contents on applesauce. Do not crush, chew, or dissolve cap beads. Avoid alcohol or any alcohol-containing medications; may result in rapid absorption of potentially fatal dose of morphine.

57 Highly Concentrated. Check dose carefully.

NAME	FORM/STRENGTH	DOSAGE	COMMENTS
Oxycodone HCl/Oxycodone Terephthalate/ASA CII (Percodan, Endodan)	**Tab:** 4.5-0.38-325 mg	**Pain: Adults: Usual:** 1 tab q6h prn. **Max:** 12 tabs/d.	●N ❀>
Pentazocine HCl/ASA CIV (Talwin Compound)	**Tab:** 12.5-325 mg	**Pain: Adults & Peds: ≥12 yo: Usual:** 2 tabs tid-qid.	●N ❀>
Pentazocine/Naloxone HCl CIV (Talwin NX)	**Tab:** 50-0.5 mg	**Pain: Adults & Peds: ≥12 yo: Initial:** 1 tab q3-4h. **Titrate:** Increase to 2 tabs prn when needed. **Max:** 12 tabs/d.	●C ❀> Not for injection.
Propoxyphene HCl/ Caffeine/ASA CIV (Darvon Compound 65)	**Cap:** 65-32.4-389 mg	**Adults:** 1 cap q4h prn. **Max:** 390 mg propoxyphene HCl/d. **Elderly:** Increase dose interval.	●N ❀> **H R**
Propoxyphene Napsylate CIV (Darvon-N)	**Tab:** 100 mg	**Pain: Adults: Usual:** 100 mg q4h prn. **Max:** 600 mg/d.	●N ❀> **H R**
Propoxyphene Napsylate/ APAP CIV (Darvocet A500)	**Tab:** 100-500 mg	**Adults: Usual:** 1 tab q4h prn. **Max:** 6 tabs/24 h. **Elderly:** Increase dosing interval.	●N ❀> **H R**
Propoxyphene Napsylate/ APAP CIV (Darvocet-N 50, Darvocet-N 100)	**Tab:** 50-325 mg, 100-650 mg	**Pain: Adults: Usual:** 100 mg propoxyphene & 650 mg APAP q4h prn. **Max:** 600 mg/d of propoxyphene.	●N ❀> **H R**

NSAIDs

NAME	FORM/STRENGTH	DOSAGE	COMMENTS
Celecoxib (Celebrex)	**Cap:** 100 mg, 200 mg, 400 mg	**Adults: Acute Pain: Day 1:** 400 mg, then 200 mg if needed. **Maint:** 200 mg bid prn. **OA:** 200 mg qd or 100 mg bid. **RA:** 100-200 mg bid. **FAP:** 400 mg bid.	●C ❀v **H** [66, 67]

Diclofenac Potassium (Cataflam)	**Tab:** 50 mg	**Adults: Pain:** 50 mg tid or 100 mg x 1 dose, then 50 mg tid. **Max:** 150 mg/d (200 mg/d on Day 1). **OA:** 50 mg bid-tid. **Max:** 200 mg/d. **RA:** 50 mg tid-qid. **Max:** 225 mg/d.	C v [66, 67]
Diclofenac Sodium (Voltaren, Voltaren-XR)	**Tab,Delay:** 25 mg, 50 mg, 75 mg; **Tab,ER:** 100 mg	**Adults: OA: Voltaren:** 50 mg bid-tid or 75 mg bid. **Voltaren-XR:** 100 mg qd. **RA: Voltaren:** 50 mg tid-qid or 75 mg bid. **Voltaren-XR:** 100 mg qd-bid. **Max:** 225 mg/d.	C v [66, 67]
Diclofenac Sodium/ Misoprostol (Arthrotec)	**Tab,Delay:** 50-0.2 mg, 75-0.2 mg	**Adults: OA:** 50 mg tid. **RA:** 50 mg tid-qid. If intolerable, give 50-75 mg bid for OA or RA.	X v [66, 67] Misoprostol is an abortifacient.
Diflunisal (Dolobid)	**Tab:** 250 mg, 500 mg	**Adults & Peds: ≥12 yo: Pain: Initial:** 1 gm, then 500 mg q8-12h. **OA/RA: Usual:** 250-500 mg bid. **Max:** 1500 mg/d.	C v [66, 67]
Etodolac (Lodine, Lodine XL)	**Cap:** 200 mg, 300 mg; **Tab,ER:** 400 mg, 500 mg, 600 mg	**Adults: Lodine: Pain: Usual:** 200-400 mg q6-8h. **Max:** 1200 mg/d. **OA/RA: Usual:** 300 mg bid-tid, or 400-500 mg bid. **Max:** 1200 mg/d. **Lodine XL: OA/RA: Usual:** 400-1000 mg qd. **Max:** 1200 mg/d.	C v [66, 67]
Flurbiprofen (Ansaid)	**Tab:** 50 mg, 100 mg	**OA/RA: Adults:** 200-300 mg/d given as bid, tid, or qid. **Max:** 300 mg/d or 100 mg/dose.	C v **R** [66, 67]

66 NSAIDs may cause an increased risk of serious CV thrombotic events, MI, stroke and serious GI adverse events including bleeding, ulceration, and perforation of the stomach or intestines.
67 Contraindicated for treatment of peri-operative pain in CABG surgery.

NAME	FORM/STRENGTH	DOSAGE	COMMENTS
Ibuprofen (Infants' Motrin, Children's Motrin, Junior Strength Motrin, Motrin IB)	**Drops:** (Infants') 50 mg/1.25 ml; **Susp:** (Children's) 100 mg/ 5 ml; **Tab:** (Junior) 100 mg; **Tab, Chew:** (Children's) 50 mg, (Junior) 100 mg; **Tab:** (Motrin IB) 200 mg	**Infants: 12-23 mths (18-23 lbs):** 1.875 ml (75 mg) q6-8h prn. **6-11 mths (12-17 lbs):** 1.25 ml (50 mg) q6-8h prn. **Children's/Junior: 11 yo (72-95 lbs)**: 300 mg q6-8h prn. **9-10 yo (60-71 lbs):** 250 mg q6-8h prn. **6-8 yo (48-59 lbs):** 200 mg q6-8h prn. **4-5 yo (36-47 lbs):** 150 mg q6-8h prn. **2-3 yo (24-35 lbs):** 100 mg q6-8h prn. **Max: 6 mths-11 yo:** 4 doses/d. **Motrin IB: ≥12 yo:** 200 mg q4-6h while symptoms persist, may increase to 400 mg q4-6h. **Max:** 1200 mg/24h.	N >
Ibuprofen (Motrin)	**Susp:** 100 mg/5 ml; **Tab:** 400 mg, 600 mg, 800 mg	**Adults: OA/RA:** 300 mg qid or 400-800 mg tid-qid. **Pain:** 400 mg q4-6h. **≥6 mths: JRA:** 30-40 mg/kg/d given tid-qid. 20 mg/kg/d w/ milder disease. **6 mths-12 yo: Pain:** 10 mg/kg q6-8h. **Max:** 40 mg/kg/d.	C v **R** 66, 67
Indomethacin (Indocin, Indocin SR)	(Indocin) **Cap:** 25 mg; **Susp:** 25 mg/5 ml; (IndocinSR) **Cap,ER:** 75 mg; (Generic) **Cap:** 25 mg,50 mg; **Cap,ER:** 75 mg; **Susp:**25 mg/5 ml	**Adults & Peds: ≥14 yo: Indocin: RA/OA: Initial:** 25 mg PO bid-tid. **Titrate:** Increase by 25-50 mg/d wkly. **Max:** 200 mg/d. **Bursitis/Tendinitis:** 75-150 mg/d given tid-qid x 7-14d. **Acute Gouty Arthritis:** 50 mg PO tid until tolerable, then d/c. **Indocin SR: RA/OA: Initial:** 75 mg qd. **Maint:** 75 mg bid. Take w/ food.	C v 66, 67
Ketoprofen (Oruvail)	**Cap:** (Generic) 50 mg, 75 mg; **Cap,ER:** (Oruvail) 200 mg	**Adults: Cap: Pain:** 25-50 mg q6-8h prn. **Max:** 300 mg/d. **OA/RA:** 75 mg tid or 50 mg qid. **Max:** 300 mg/d. **Oruvail: OA/RA:** 200 mg qd.	C v **H R** 66, 67

Ketorolac Tromethamine (Toradol)	(Generic) **Inj:** 15 mg/ml, 30 mg/ml; **Tab:** 10 mg; (Toradol) **Tab:** 10 mg	**Adults: 16 to <65 yo: Single Dose:** 60 mg IM or 30 mg IV. **Multiple Dose:** 30 mg IV/IM q6h. **Max:** 120 mg/d. **Transition from IV/IM to PO:** 20 mg PO, then 10 mg PO q4-6h. **Max:** 40 mg/24h. **≥65 yo or <50 kg: Single Dose:** 30 mg IM or 15 mg IV. **Multiple Dose:** 15 mg IV/IM q6h. **Max:** 60 mg/d. **Transition from IV/IM to PO:** 10 mg PO q4-6h. **Max:** 40 mg/24h. Max duration is 5d.	C v **R** Short-term use only (≤5d).
Mefenamic Acid (Ponstel)	**Cap:** 250 mg	**Pain: Adults & Peds: ≥14 yo:** 500 mg, then 250 mg q6h prn, up to 1 wk.	C v [66, 67]
Meloxicam (Mobic)	**Susp:** 7.5 mg/5 ml; **Tab:** 7.5 mg, 15 mg	**OA/RA: Adults: ≥18 yo: Initial/Maint:** 7.5 mg qd. **Max:** 15 mg/d. **JRA: Peds: ≥2 yo:** 0.125 mg/kg qd. **Max:** 7.5 mg/d.	C v [66, 67]
Nabumetone (Relafen)	**Tab:** 500 mg, 750 mg	**OA/RA: Adults: Initial:** 1 gm qd. **Usual:** 1.5-2 gm/d as qd-bid. **Max:** 2 gm/d.	C v [66, 67]
Naproxen (Naprosyn, EC-Naprosyn)	(Naprosyn) **Susp:** 25 mg/ml; **Tab:** 250 mg, 375 mg, 500 mg; (EC-Naprosyn) **Tab,Delay:** 375 mg, 500 mg	**Adults: RA/OA/Ankylosing Spondylitis: Naprosyn:** 250-500 mg bid. **EC-Naprosyn:** 375-500 mg bid. **Acute Gout: Naprosyn: Initial:** 750 mg, then 250 mg q8h. **JRA: Peds: ≥2 yo:** 5 mg/kg of naproxen bid.	C v [66, 67]

66 NSAIDs may cause an increased risk of serious CV thrombotic events, MI, stroke and serious GI adverse events including bleeding, ulceration, and perforation of the stomach or intestines.

67 Contraindicated for treatment of peri-operative pain in CABG surgery.

NAME	FORM/STRENGTH	DOSAGE	COMMENTS
Naproxen Sodium (Anaprox, Anaprox DS, Naprelan)	**Tab:** (Anaprox) 275 mg, (Anaprox DS) 550 mg; **Tab,ER:** (Naprelan) 375 mg, 500 mg	**Adults: RA/OA/Ankylosing Spondylitis: Tab:** 275 mg-550 mg bid. **Tab,ER:** 750-1000 mg qd. **Max:** 1500 mg/d. **Pain/Tendinitis/Bursitis: Tab: Initial:** 550 mg, then 550 mg q12h or 275 mg q6-8h prn. **Max:** 1100 mg/d for maint. **Tab,ER: Intial:** 1000-1500 mg qd. **Max:** 1000 mg/d for maint. **Acute Gout: Tab:** 825 mg, then 275 mg q8h. **Tab,ER:** 1000-1500 gm on day 1, then 1000 mg qd. **JRA: Peds: ≥2 yo: Tab:** 5 mg/kg of naproxen bid.	◉C ❁v [66, 67]
Oxaprozin (Daypro)	**Tab:** 600 mg	**Adults: OA:** 600-1200 mg qd. **Max:** 1800 mg/d. **RA:** 1200 mg qd. **Max:** 1800 mg/d. **Peds: 6-16 yo: JRA: ≥55 kg:** 1200 mg qd. **32-54 kg:** 900 mg qd. **22-31 kg:** 600 mg qd.	◉C ❁v **R** [66, 67]
Sulindac (Clinoril)	**Tab:** (Clinoril) 200 mg, (Generic) 150 mg, 200 mg	**Adults: Pain/Gouty Arthritis:** 200 mg bid. **OA/RA:** 150 mg bid. **Max:** 400 mg/d.	◉C ❁v [66, 67]

Salicylates

Aspirin (Bayer Aspirin)	**Chewtab:** 81 mg; **Tab:** 81 mg, 325 mg, 500 mg; **Tab,Delay:** 81 mg, 325 mg	**Pain: Adults & Peds: ≥12 yo:** 325-1000 mg q4-6h prn. **Max:** 4 gm/d.	◉N ❁> **H R** Avoid use during 3rd trimester.

Miscellaneous

Acetaminophen (Tylenol Children's, Tylenol Extra Strength, Tylenol Infants', Tylenol Junior, Tylenol Regular Strength)	**Drops:** (Infants') 80 mg/0.8 ml; **Sol:** (Extra Strength) 500 mg/15 ml; **Susp:** (Children's) 160 mg/5 ml; **Tab:** (Regular Strength) 325 mg, (Extra Strength) 500 mg; **Tab, Chewable:** (Children's) 80 mg, (Junior) 160 mg	**Peds: Max:** 5 doses/d. **0-3 mths (6-11 lbs):** 40 mg q4h prn. **4-11 mths (12-17 lbs):** 80 mg q4h prn. **12-23 mths (18-23 lbs):** 120 mg q4h prn. **2-3 yo (24-35 lbs):** 160 mg q4h prn. **4-5 yo (36-47 lbs):** 240 mg q4h prn. **6-8 yo (48-59 lbs):** 320 mg q4h prn. **9-10 yo (60-71 lbs):** 400 mg q4h prn. **11 yo (72-95 lbs):** 480 mg q4h prn. **12 yo:** 640 mg q4h prn. **Older Children/Adults: Regular Strength:6-11 yo:** 325 mg q4-6h prn. **Max:** 1625 mg/d. **≥12 yo:** 650 mg q4-6h prn **Max:** 3900 mg/d. **Extra Strength: ≥12 yo:** 1000 mg q4-6h prn. **Max:** 4000 mg/d.	■N ❊>
Duloxetine (Cymbalta)	**Cap,Delay:** 20 mg, 30 mg, 60 mg	**Diabetic Peripheral Neuropathic Pain: Adults: Usual:** 60 mg/d given once daily. **Max:** 120 mg/d. May lower starting dose if tolerability is a concern. Do not chew or crush.	■C ❊v **H R** [29]
Gabapentin (Neurontin)	**Cap:** 100 mg, 300 mg, 400 mg; **Sol:** 250 mg/ 5 ml; **Tab:** 600 mg, 800 mg	**Postherpetic Neuralgia: Adults:** 300 mg single dose on Day 1, then 300 mg bid on Day 2, & 300 mg tid on Day 3. Increase further prn pain. **Max:** 600 mg tid.	■C ❊> **R**

[29] Antidepressants may increase the risk of suicidality in children and adolescents.

[66] NSAIDs may cause an increased risk of serious CV thrombotic events, MI, stroke and serious GI adverse events including bleeding, ulceration, and perforation of the stomach or intestines.

[67] Contraindicated for treatment of peri-operative pain in CABG surgery.

NAME	FORM/STRENGTH	DOSAGE	COMMENTS
Lidocaine (Lidoderm Patch)	**Patch:** 5%	**Postherpetic Neuralgia: Adults:** Apply to intact skin, cover most painful area. Apply up to 3 patches, once for up to 12 h within 24-h period. May cut patches into smaller sizes before removal of the release liner. **Debilitated/Impaired Elimination:** Treat smaller areas. Remove if irritation or burning occurs; may re-apply when irritation subsides.	◙B ❋>
Lidocaine/Tetracaine (Synera)	**Patch:** 70-70 mg	**Adults & Peds: ≥ 3 yo: Venipuncture or IV Cannulation:** Apply to intact skin for 20-30 min prior to procedure. **Superficial Dermatological Procedure:** Apply to intact skin for 30 min prior to procedure.	◙B ❋>
Pregabalin CV (Lyrica)	**Cap:** 25 mg, 50 mg, 75 mg, 100 mg, 150 mg, 200 mg, 225 mg, 300 mg	**Adults: Neuropathic Pain: Initial:** 50 mg tid (150 mg/d). **Titrate:** May increase to 300 mg/d within 1 wk. **Max:** 100 mg tid (300 mg/d). **Postherpetic Neuralgia: Initial:** 150 mg/d divided bid or tid. **Max:** 600 mg/d divided bid or tid.	◙C ❋v **R**
Tramadol HCl (Ultram, Ultram ER)	**Tab:** 50 mg; **Tab,ER:** 100 mg, 200 mg, 300 mg	**Moderate to Moderately Severe Pain: Adults: ≥17 yo: Tab: Initial:** 25 mg qam. **Titrate:** Increase by 25 mg/d q3d to 25 mg qid, then by 50 mg/d q3d to 50 mg qid. **Maint:** 50-100 mg q4-6h prn. **Max:** 400 mg/d. **Tab,ER: Adults: ≥18 yo: Initial:** 100 mg qd. **Titrate:** Increase by 100-mg increments q5d. **Max:** 300 mg/d.	◙C ❋v **H R**
Tramadol HCl/APAP (Ultracet)	**Tab:** 37.5-325 mg	**Acute Pain: Adults:** 2 tabs q4-6h, up to 5d. **Max:** 8 tabs/d.	◙C ❋v **H R**
Ziconotide (Prialt)	**Sol:** 25 mcg/ml, 100 mcg/ml	**Adults: Initial:** No more than 2.4 mcg/d IT (0.1 mcg/hr). **Titrate:** 2.4 mcg/d no more than 2-3x/wk. **Max:** 19.2 mcg/d (0.8 mcg/h) by Day 21.	◙C ❋>

AIDS Therapy

FUSION INHIBITORS

Enfuvirtide (Fuzeon)	**Inj:** 90 mg/ml	**Adults:** 90 mg SC bid. **Peds: 6-16 yo:** 2 mg/kg SC bid. **Max:** 90 mg bid. Inject into upper arm, anterior thigh, or abdomen.	B v

NON-NUCLEOSIDE REVERSE TRANSCRIPTASE INHIBITORS

Delavirdine Mesylate (Rescriptor)	**Tab:** 100 mg, 200 mg	**Adults & Peds: ≥16 yo:** 400 mg tid.	C v
Efavirenz (Sustiva)	**Cap:** 50 mg, 100 mg, 200 mg; **Tab:** 600 mg	**Adults:** 600 mg qd. **Peds: ≥3 yo: 10-40 kg:** 200-400 mg qd. **≥40 kg:** 600 mg qd. Take on empty stomach, preferably hs.	D v Avoid high fat meals.
Nevirapine (Viramune)	**Tab:** 200 mg; **Susp:** 50 mg/5 ml	**Adults: Initial:** 200 mg qd x 14d. **Maint:** 200 mg bid. **Peds: ≥8 yo: Initial:** 4 mg/kg qd x 14d. **Maint:** 4 mg/kg bid. **2 mths-8 yo: Initial:** 4 mg/kg qd x 14d. **Maint:** 7 mg/kg bid.	C v **H** Severe hypersensitivity & skin reactions. Hepatotoxicity.

NUCLEOSIDE REVERSE TRANSCRIPTASE INHIBITORS

Abacavir Sulfate (Ziagen)	**Sol:** 20 mg/ml; **Tab:** 300 mg	**Adults:** 300 mg bid or 600 mg qd. **Peds: 3 mths-16 yo: Usual:** 8 mg/kg bid. **Max:** 300 mg bid.	C v [31, 33]
Abacavir/Lamivudine (Epzicom)	**Tab:** 600-300 mg	**Adults: ≥18 yo: CrCl >50 ml/min:** 1 tab qd.	C v **R** [31, 33]

[31] Lactic acidosis and severe hepatomegaly with steatosis reported.
[33] Fatal hypersensitivity reactions reported.

NAME	FORM/STRENGTH	DOSAGE	COMMENTS
Abacavir/Lamivudine/ Zidovudine (Trizivir)	**Tab:** 300-150-300 mg	**Adults & Adolescents: >40 kg:** 1 tab bid. Avoid in patients <40 kg.	C v **R** 31, 33, 34
Didanosine (Videx, Videx EC)	**Cap,Delay:** (Videx EC) 125 mg,200 mg, 250 mg,400 mg; **Sol:** (Videx) 2 gm, 4 gm	**Adults: ≥60 kg: Cap,Delay:** (Videx EC) 400 mg qd. **≤60 kg: Cap,Delay:** (Videx EC) 250 mg qd. **Peds: >8 mths: Sol:** (Videx) 120 mg/m² bid. **2 wks-8 mths: Sol:** (Videx) 100 mg/m² bid. Take on empty stomach.	B v **R** 31, 35
Emtricitabine (Emtriva)	**Cap:** 200 mg; **Sol:** 10mg/ml	**Adults: ≥18 yrs: Cap:** 200 mg qd.**Sol:**240 mg qd. **Peds: 3 mths-17 yrs: >33 kg: Cap:** 200 mg qd.**Sol:** 6 mg/kg qd.**Max:** 240 mg.	B v **R** 31, 32
Emtricitabine/Tenofovir Disoproxil (Truvada)	**Tab:** 200-300 mg	**Adults: ≥18 yo: CrCl: ≥50 ml/min:** 1 tab qd. **CrCl: 30-49 ml/min:** 1 tab q48h.	B v **R** 31, 32
Lamivudine (Epivir)	**Sol:** 10 mg/ml; **Tab:** 150 mg, 300 mg	**HIV: Adults:** 150 mg bid or 300 mg qd. **Peds: 3 mths-16 yo: Usual:** 4 mg/kg bid. **Max:** 150 mg bid.	B v **R** 31, 32
Lamivudine/Zidovudine (Combivir)	**Tab:** 150-300 mg	**Adults & Peds: ≥12 yo:** 1 tab bid.	C v **H R** 31, 32, 34
Stavudine (Zerit)	**Cap:** 15 mg, 20 mg, 30 mg, 40 mg; **Sol:** 1 mg/ml	**Adults: <60 kg:** 30 mg bid. **≥60 kg:** 40 mg bid. **Peds: Birth-13d:** 0.5 mg/kg q12h. **≥14d & <30 kg:** 1 mg/kg q12h. **>30 kg:** Adult dose. Adjust dose based on peripheral neuropathy.	C v **R** 31, 35

Zalcitabine (Hivid)	**Tab:** 0.375 mg, 0.75 mg	**Adults & Peds:** **≥13 yo:** 0.75 mg q8h.	C v **H R** 31, 35, 36
Zidovudine (Retrovir)	**Cap:** 100 mg; **Inj:** 10 mg/ml; **Syr:** 50 mg/5 ml; **Tab:** 300 mg	**Adults:** 600 mg/d PO in divided doses or 1 mg/kg IV 5-6x/d. **Peds: 6 wks-12 yo:** 160 mg/m^2 PO q8h. **Maternal-Fetal Transmission:** 100 mg PO 5x/d until labor, then 2 mg/kg IV, then 1 mg/kg/h until umbilical cord clamped. **Neonatal:** 2 mg/kg PO or 1.5 mg/kg IV q6h until 6 wks old. Start 12h after birth.	C v **H R** 31, 34

NUCLEOTIDE REVERSE TRANSCRIPTASE INHIBITORS

Tenofovir Disoproxil (Viread)	**Tab:** 300 mg	**Adults:** 300 mg qd w/ a meal.	B v 31, 32

PROTEASE INHIBITORS

Amprenavir (Agenerase)	**Cap:** 50 mg; **Sol:** 15 mg/ml	**Adults & Peds: ≥13 yo or ≥50 kg: Cap** 1200 mg bid. **Sol:** 1400 mg bid. **4-12 yo or <50 kg: Cap:** 20 mg/kg bid or 15 mg/kg tid. **Max:** 2400 mg/d. **Sol:** 22.5 mg/kg bid or 17 mg/kg tid. **Max:** 2800 mg/d. Sol & cap are not interchangeable. Avoid high fat meals & vitamin E.	C (Cap) Sol CI in pregnancy. v **H R** (Sol) Sol contains propylene glycol.

31 Lactic acidosis and severe hepatomegaly with steatosis reported.

32 Severe acute exacerbations of hepatitis B reported in patients who have discontinued anti-hepatitis B therapy; monitor hepatic function closely.

33 Fatal hypersensitivity reactions reported.

34 Associated with hematologic toxicity. Prolonged use associated with myopathy.

35 Fatal and nonfatal pancreatitis reported.

36 May cause severe peripheral neuropathy.

NAME	FORM/STRENGTH	DOSAGE	COMMENTS
Atazanavir Sulfate (Reyataz)	**Cap:** 100 mg, 150 mg, 200 mg	**Adults: Therapy-naive:** 400 mg qd. **Therapy-experienced:** 300 mg w/ ritonavir 100 mg qd. **Concomitant Efavirenz:** Give atazanavir 300 mg & ritonavir 100 mg w/ efavirenz 600 mg qd w/ food. **Concomitant Buffered Didanosine:** Give atazanavir 2 h before or 1 h after didanosine. **Concomitant Tenofovir:** Give atazanavir 300 mg w/ ritonavir 100 mg & tenofovir 300 mg.	B v **H**
Fosamprenavir Calcium (Lexiva)	**Tab:** 700 mg	**Adults: Therapy-naive:** 1400 mg bid OR 1400 mg qd + ritonavir 200 mg qd OR 700 mg bid + ritonavir 100 mg bid. **PI-Experienced:** 700 mg bid + ritonavir 100 mg bid.	C v **H**
Indinavir Sulfate (Crixivan)	**Cap:** 100 mg, 200 mg, 333 mg, 400 mg	**Adults:** 800 mg q8h w/ water. Hydrate to prevent nephrolithiasis/urolithiasis.	C v **H**
Lopinavir/Ritonavir (Kaletra)	**Tab** 200-50 mg; **Sol:** 80-20 mg/ml	**Adults & Peds: >12 yo: Therapy-Naive:** 400/100 mg (2 tabs or 5 ml) bid or 800/200 mg qd (4 tabs or 10 ml). **Therapy-Experienced:** 400/100 mg (2 tabs or 5ml) bid. Once daily administration not recommended. **Concomitant Efavirenz/Nevirapine/Fosamprenavir/ Nelfinavir: Therapy-Naive:** (Tab) 400/100 mg (2 tabs) bid. **Concomitant Efavirenz/Nevirapine/Amprenavir/ Nelfinavir:** (Sol) 533/133 mg (6.5 ml) bid. **Concomitant Efavirenz/Nevirapine/ Fosamprenavir without Ritonavir/ Nelfinavir: Treatment-Experienced w/ Decreased Susceptibility to Lopinavir:** 600/150 mg (3 tabs) bid. **6 mths-12 yo: >40 kg:** 400/100 mg (2 tabs or 5 ml) bid. **15-40 kg:** (Sol) 10/2.5 mg/kg bid. **7 to <15kg:** (Sol)	C v

		12/3 mg/kg bid. **Concomitant Efavirenz/Nevirapine/ Amprenavir: >45 kg:** 533/133 mg (2 tabs or 6.5 ml) bid. **15-45kg:** (Sol) 11/2.75 mg/kg bid. **7 to <15kg:** (Sol) 13/3.25 mg/kg bid. Tablets can be taken w/ or w/o food. Oral solution must be taken w/ food.	
Nelfinavir Mesylate (Viracept)	**Pow (susp):** 50 mg/gm; **Tab:** 250 mg, 625 mg	**Adults:** 1250 mg bid or 750 mg tid. **Peds: 2-13 yo:** 20-30 mg/kg tid. Take w/ food.	B v
Ritonavir (Norvir)	**Cap:** 100 mg; **Sol:** 80 mg/ml	**Adults: Initial:** 300 mg bid & increase q2-3d by 100 mg bid. **Maint:** 600 mg bid. **Concomitant Saquinavir:** Better tolerated w/ 400 mg bid. **Peds: >1 month: Initial:** 250 mg/m^2 po bid. **Titrate:** Increase by 50 mg/m^2 bid q2-3d. **Maint:** 350-400 mg/m^2 po bid or highest tolerated dose. **Max:** 600 mg bid.	B v Avoid certain antihistamines, sedative hypnotics, antiarrhythmics, or ergot alkaloids.
Saquinavir (Fortovase)	**Cap:** 200 mg	**Adults: ≥16 yo:** 1200 mg tid w/ food or up to 2h after a meal.	B v
Saquinavir Mesylate (Invirase)	**Cap:** 200 mg; **Tab:** 500 mg	**Adults: >16 yo:** 1000 mg bid w/ ritonavir 100 mg bid. Take within 2h after full meal.	B v Invirase and Fortovase are not bioequivalent.
Tipranavir (Aptivus)	**Cap:** 250 mg	**Adults:** 500 mg, w/ 200 mg of ritonavir, bid. Take w/ food.	C v **H** [45]

45 Hepatitis and hepatic decompensation reported with ritonavir co-administration. Monitor closely with chronic hepatitis B or C co-infection.

Antiviral Agents

ANTI-CYTOMEGALOVIRUS AGENTS

NAME	FORM/STRENGTH	DOSAGE	COMMENTS
Cidofovir (Vistide)	**Inj:** 75 mg/ml	**CMV Retinitis: Adults & Peds: Induction:** 5 mg/kg qwk x 2wks. **Maint:** 5 mg/kg q2wks. Patients must receive hydration & probenecid w/ each dose.	◉C ❋v **R**[59]
Fomivirsen Sodium (Vitravene)	**Inj:** 6.6 mg/ml	**CMV Retinitis: Adults: Induction:** 330 mcg (0.05 ml) intravitreal every other wk x 2 doses. **Maint:** 330 mcg (0.05 ml) intravitreal q4wks.	◉C ❋v
Foscarnet Sodium (Foscavir)	**Inj:** 24 mg/ml	**CMV Retinitis: Adults & Peds: Induction:** 90 mg/kg q12h or 60 mg/kg q8h. **Maint:** 90-120 mg/kg/d. Should hydrate patient.	◉C ❋> **R** Renal impairment. Seizures.
Ganciclovir (Cytovene)	**Cap:** 250 mg, 500 mg	**Adults & Peds: CMV Disease Prevention in Advanced HIV (at risk) or Transplant Patients:** 1000 mg tid. **Alternative to IV for CMV Retinitis Treatment in Immunocompromised Patients:** 1000 mg tid or 500 mg 6x/d q3h. Take w/food.	◉C ❋v **R**[12]
Ganciclovir Sodium (Cytovene-IV)	**Inj:** 500 mg/10 ml	**Adults & Peds: Treatment of CMV Retinitis in Immunocompromised Patients: Induction:** 5 mg/kg q12h x 14-21d. **Maint:** 5 mg/kg qd x 7d/wk or 6 mg/kg qd x 5d/wk. **Prevention of CMV Disease in Transplant Patients (at risk): Initial:** 5 mg/kg q12h x 7-14d. **Maint:** 5 mg/kg qd x 7d/wk or 6 mg/kg qd x 5d/wk.	◉C ❋v **R**[12]
Ganciclovir (Vitrasert)	**Implant:** 4.5 mg	**CMV Retinitis: Treatment: Adults & Peds: ≥9 yo:** Each implant releases the drug over 5-8 mths; may remove or replace after depletion.	◉C ❋v

Valganciclovir (Valcyte)	**Tab:** 450 mg	**Adults: CMV Retinitis: Induction:** 900 mg bid x 21d. **Maint:** 900 mg qd. **Prevention of CMV Disease in High-Risk Kidney, Heart, & Kidney-Pancreas Transplant Patients:** 900 mg qd within 10 days of transplant until 100 days post-transplant. Take w/ food.	◙C ❁v **R** 12 Follow exact dosing guidelines.

HEPATITIS

Adefovir Dipivoxil (Hepsera)	**Tab:** 10 mg	**HBV: Adults:** 10 mg qd.	◙C ❁v **R** 31, 32, 37, 38
Entecavir (Baraclude)	**Sol:** 0.05 mg/ml; **Tab:** 0.5 mg, 1 mg	**HBV: Adults/Peds: ≥16 yo: Nucleoside-Treatment-Naïve:** 0.5 mg qd. **Receiving Lamivudine or Known Lamivudine Resistance Mutation:** 1 mg qd. Take on empty stomach.	◙C ❁v **R** 31, 32
Hepatitis A Inactivated/Hepatitis B Recombinant (Twinrix)	**Inj:** 720 U-20 mcg	**Adults:** 1 ml IM at 0-, 1- & 6-mth schedule.	◙C ❁>

12 Granulocytopenia. Anemia. Thrombocytopenia. Carcinogenic, teratogenic & aspermatogenic in animal studies.
31 Lactic acidosis and severe hepatomegaly with steatosis reported.
32 Severe acute exacerbations of hepatitis B reported in patients who have discontinued anti-hepatitis B therapy; monitor hepatic function closely.
37 Chronic administration may result in nephrotoxicity; monitor renal function with, or if at risk of, renal dysfunction.
38 HIV resistance may emerge.
59 Renal impairment is major toxicity. CI w/nephrotoxic agents. Neutropenia reported. Carcinogenic, teratogenic, and hypospermatic in animal studies.

NAME	FORM/STRENGTH	DOSAGE	COMMENTS
Hepatitis B Vaccine, Recombinant (Engerix-B, Recombivax HB)	**Inj:** (Engerix-ped) 10 mcg/0.5 ml, (Recombivax HB-ped) 5 mcg/0.5 ml, (Engerix-adult) 20 mcg/ml, (Recombivax HB adult) 10 mcg/ml	**Engerix: Adults: >19 yo:** 20 mcg/ml IM at 0, 1, 6 mths. **Peds: ≤19 yo:** 10 mcg/0.5 ml IM at 0, 1, 6 mths. **Booster: Adults & Peds: ≥11 yo:** 20 mcg IM. **≤10 yo:** 10 mcg IM. **Recombivax: Adults: ≥20 yo:** 10 mcg IM at 0, 1, 6 mths. **Peds: 0-19 yo:** 5 mcg IM at 0, 1, 6 mths.	●C ❋>
Interferon alfa-2a (Roferon-A)	**Inj:** 3 MIU, 6 MIU, 9 MIU, 36 MIU	**HCV: Adults: ≥18 yo: SC:** 3 MIU TIW x 12 mths or 6 MIU TIW x 3 mths, then 3 MIU TIW x 9 mths.	●C ❋v [13]
Interferon alfa-2b (Intron-A)	**Inj:** 10 MIU, 18 MIU, 50 MIU, 10 MIU/ml, 3 MIU/0.2 ml, 5 MIU/0.2 ml, 10 MIU/0.2 ml	**HCV: Adults: ≥18 yo:** 3 MIU IM/SC TIW x 18-24 mths. **HBV: Adults:** 5 MIU IM/SC qd or 10 MIU TIW x 16 wks. **Peds:** 3 MIU/m² IM/SC TIW x 1 wk, then 6 MIU/m² TIW x 15-23 wks. **Max:** 10 MIU/m² TIW. Adjust based on WBC, granulocyte, and/or platelet counts.	●C ❋v [13]
Interferon alphacon-1 (Infergen)	**Inj:** 30 mcg/ml	**HCV: Adults: ≥18 yo:** 9 mcg SC TIW x 24 wks, then 15 mcg SC TIW x 6 mths if needed.	●C ❋>
Lamivudine (Epivir-HBV)	**Sol:** 5 mg/ml; **Tab:** 100 mg	**HBV: Adults:** 100 mg qd. **Peds: 2-17 yo:** 3 mg/kg qd. **Max:** 100 mg/d.	●C ❋v **R** [31, 32]
Peginterferon alfa-2a (Pegasys)	**Inj:** 180 mcg/0.5 ml, 180 mcg/ml	**HCV & HCV/HIV: Adults: ≥18 yo: Monotherapy:** 180 mcg SC once wkly x 48 wks. Adjust dose by neutrophils, platelets, severity of depression, & renal/hepatic function.**HCV: With Copegus: Adults: ≥18 yo:** 180 mcg SC once wkly x 48 wks for genotypes 1, 4; x 24 wks for genotypes 2, 3. **HCV/HIV: With Copegus: Adults: ≥18 yo:** 180 mcg SC once wkly x 48 wks regardless of genotype. **HBV: Monotherapy:** 180 mcg SC once wkly x 48 wks.	●C (monotherapy) ●X (with ribavirin) ❋v **H R** [13]

Peginterferon alfa-2b (Peg-Intron)	**Inj:** 100 mcg/ml, 160 mcg/ml, 240 mcg/ml, 300 mcg/ml	**HCV: Adults: ≥18 yo:** Administer SC once wkly x 1 yr. **Monotherapy: 50 mcg/0.5 ml vial: ≤45 kg:** 40 mcg (0.4 ml); **46-56 kg:** 50 mcg (0.5 ml). **80 mcg/0.5 ml vial: 57-72 kg:** 64 mcg (0.4 ml); **73-88 kg:** 80 mcg (0.5 ml). **120 mcg/0.5 ml vial: 89-106 kg:** 96 mcg (0.4 ml); **107-136 kg:** 120 mcg (0.5 ml). **150 mcg/0.5 ml vial: 137-160 kg:** 150 mcg (0.5 ml). **With Rebetol: 50 mcg/0.5 ml vial: <40 kg:** 50 mcg (0.5 ml). **80 mcg/0.5 ml vial: 40-50 kg:** 64 mcg (0.4 ml); **51-60 kg:** 80 mcg (0.5 ml). **120 mcg/0.5 ml vial: 61-75 kg:** 96 mcg (0.4 mll); **76-85 kg:** 120 mcg (0.5 ml). **150 mcg/0.5 ml vial: >85 kg:** 150 mcg (0.5 ml). Dose varies based on wt, WBC, platelets, neutrophils and/or severity of depression.	◉C ❋v [13]
Ribavirin (Copegus)	**Tab:** 200 mg	**HCV: Adults: ≥18 yo w/ PEGASYS: Genotypes 1,4: <75 kg:** 500 mg bid x 48 wks. **≥75 kg:** 600 mg bid x 48 wks. **Genotypes 2,3:** 400 mg bid x 24 wks. **HCV/HIV: Adults: ≥18 yo w/ PEGASYS:** 800 mg qd x 48 wks. Dosage adjustment or d/c based on CV status, Hgb, renal function.	◉X ❋v **R** CI in pregnancy, male partners of pregnant females, & significant cardiac disease. Hemolytic anemia.

[13] May cause or aggravate neuropsychiatric, autoimmune, ischemic, & infectious disorders; monitor closely.
[31] Lactic acidosis and severe hepatomegaly with steatosis reported.
[32] Severe acute exacerbations of hepatitis B reported in patients who have discontinued anti-hepatitis B therapy; monitor hepatic function closely.

NAME	FORM/STRENGTH	DOSAGE	COMMENTS
Ribavirin (Rebetol)	**Cap:** 200 mg; **Sol:** 40 mg/ml	**HCV: Adults: With INTRON A: ≤75 kg:** 400 mg qam & 600 mg qpm. **>75 kg:** 600 mg qam & 600 mg qpm. Treat x 24-48 wks if no prior interferon (IFN) therapy & x 24 wks if prior IFN therapy. **With PEG-INTRON:** 400 mg bid, qam & qpm w/ food. Dose based on Hgb & cardiac history. **Peds: ≥3 yrs:** 15 mg/kg/day in divided doses qam & qpm. Use sol if =25 kg or cannot swallow caps. **With INTRON A: 25-36 kg:** 200 mg bid, qam & qpm. **37-49 kg:** 200 mg qam & 400 mg qpm. **50-61kg:** 400 mg bid, qam & qpm. **>61kg:** Dose as adult. **Genotype 1:** Treat x 48 wks. **Genotype 2/3:** Treat x 24 wks.	X v **R** CI in pregnancy, male partners of pregnant females, & significant cardiac disease. Hemolytic anemia.
Ribavirin/Interferon alfa-2b (Rebetron)	**Kit (Inj-Cap):** 200 mg-3 MIU/0.2 ml, 200 mg-3 MIU/0.5 ml	**HCV: Adults: ≥18 yo: ≤75 kg:** 3 MIU SC TIW w/ 400 mg PO qam & 600 mg PO qpm. **>75 kg:** 3 MIU SC TIW w/ 600 mg PO bid. Adjust based on cardiac history, Hgb, neutrophil, platelet and/or WBC count.	X v **R** CI in pregnancy & male partners of pregnant females.
HERPES INFECTION			
Acyclovir Sodium (Zovirax)	**Inj:** 25 mg/ml, 50 mg/ml	**Herpes Simplex: Adults & Peds: >12 yo:** 5 mg/kg IV q8h x 7d. **<12 yo:** 10 mg/kg IV q8h x 7d. **Birth-3 mths:** 10 mg/kg q8h IV x 10d. **Genital Herpes: Adults & Peds: >12 yo:** 5 mg/kg IV q8h x 5d. **Encephalitis: Adults & Peds: >12 yo:** 10 mg/kg IV q8h x 10d. **<12 yo:** 20 mg/kg IV q8h x 10d. **Zoster: Adults & Peds: >12 yo:** 10 mg/kg IV q8h x 7d. **<12 yo:** 20 mg/kg IV q8h x 7d.	B > **R**

Acyclovir (Zovirax)	**Cap**: 200 mg; **Susp:** 200 mg/5 ml; **Tab:** 400 mg, 800 mg	**Zoster:** 800 mg 5x/d x 7-10d. **Genital Herpes: Initial:** 200 mg 5x/d x 10d. **Maint:** 400 mg bid x 1yr or 200 mg 3-5x/d x 1yr. **Recurrent:** 200 mg 5x/d x 5d. **Varicella: ≥2 yo: <40 kg:** 20 mg/kg qid x 5d. **>40 kg:** 800 mg qid x 5d.	◙B ❊> **R**
Acyclovir (Zovirax)	**Oint:** 5%	**Adults: Herpes Genitalis/Herpes Labialis:** Apply q3h, 6x/d x 7d. Initiate w/ 1st sign/symptom.	◙B ❊>
Famciclovir (Famvir)	**Tab:** 125 mg, 250 mg, 500 mg	**Adults: ≥18 yo: Zoster:** 500 mg q8h x 7d. **Genital Herpes: Recurrent:** 125 mg bid x 5d. **Suppression:** 250 mg bid up to 1yr. **Recurrent Orolabial or Genital Herpes in HIV Patients:** 500 mg bid x 7d.	◙B ❊> **R**
Valacyclovir HCl (Valtrex)	**Tab:** 500 mg, 1 gm	**Adults & Post-Pubertal Peds: Zoster:** 1 gm tid x 7d. **Genital Herpes: Initial:** 1 gm bid x 10d. **Recurrent:** 500 mg bid x 3d. **Suppressive:** (≤9 episodes/yr) 500 mg or (>9 episodes/yr) 1000 mg qd, up to 1yr. **Suppressive Therapy with HIV & CD4 ≥100 cells/mm³**: 500 mg bid, up to 6 mths. **Labialis:** 2 g q12h x 1d. Start at earliest symptom.	◙B ❊> **R**

INFLUENZA

Amantadine HCl (Symmetrel)	**Tab:** 100 mg; **Syr:** 50 mg/5 ml	**Influenza A Prophylaxis & Treatment: Adults** 200 mg qd or 100 mg bid. **≥65 yo:** 100 mg qd. **Peds: 9-12 yo:** 100 mg bid. **1-9 yo:** 4.4-8.8 mg/kg/d. **Max:** 150 mg/d.	◙C ❊v **R**

NAME	FORM/STRENGTH	DOSAGE	COMMENTS
Oseltamivir Phosphate (Tamiflu)	**Cap:** 75 mg; **Susp:** 12 mg/ml	**Treatment: Adults & Peds: ≥13 yo: Cap/Susp:** 75 mg bid x 5d, begin within 2d of symptom onset. **≥1 yo: Susp: ≤15 kg:** 30 mg bid x 5d. **>15-23 kg:** 45 mg bid x 5d. **>23-40 kg:** 60 mg bid x 5d. **>40 kg:** 75 mg bid x 5d. **Prophylaxis: Adults & Peds: ≥13 yrs: Cap/Susp:** Begin within 2d of exposure. 75 mg qd for at least 10d, up to 6 wks with community outbreak. **≥1 yo: Susp: ≤15 kg:** 30 mg qd x 10d. **>15-23 kg:** 45 mg qd x 10d. **>23-40 kg:** 60 mg qd x 10d. **>40 kg:** 75 mg qd x 10d.	C > R
Rimantadine HCl (Flumadine)	**Tab:** 100 mg; **Syr:** 50 mg/5 ml	**Influenza A: Prophylaxis: Adults & Peds: ≥10 yo:** 100 mg bid. **<10 yo:** 5 mg/kg qd. **Max:** 150 mg/d. **Treatment: Adults:** 100 mg bid; begin within 48h of symptom onset & treat x 7d from initial symptom onset.	C v H R
Zanamivir (Relenza)	**Disk:** 5 mg/inh	**Adults & Peds: ≥7 yo: Treatment:** 2 inh (10 mg) q12h x 5d. **≥5 yo: Prophylaxis: Household Setting:** 2 inh (10 mg) qd x 10d. **Community Setting:** 2 inh (10 mg) qd x 28d. Administer at same time every day.	C >

Bone and Joint Infection

AMINOGLYCOSIDES

Amikacin Sulfate (Amikin)	**Inj:** 50 mg/ml, 250 mg/ml	**IM/IV: Adults, Children & Older Infants:** 7.5 mg/kg q12h or 5 mg/kg IM/IV q8h. **Max:** 1.5 gm/d **Newborns: LD:** 10 mg/kg. **Maint:** 7.5 mg/kg q12h.	D v R [1]

Gentamicin Sulfate (Garamycin)	**Inj:** 40 mg/ml	**IM/IV: Adults:** 3 mg/kg/d given q8h. **Max:** 5 mg/kg/d in 3-4 doses. Reduce to 3 mg/kg/d as soon as clinically indicated. **Peds:** 2-2.5 mg/kg q8h. **Infants/Neonates:** 2.5 mg/kg q8h. ≤**1 wk:** 2.5 mg/kg q12h.	N > **R** [1]
Tobramycin Sulfate (Nebcin)	**Inj:** 10 mg/ml, 40 mg/ml, 1.2 gm	**IM/IV: Adults:** 3 mg/kg/d given q8h. **Max:** 5 mg/kg/d in 3-4 doses. Reduce to 3 mg/kg/d as soon as clinically indicated. **Peds: >1 wk:** 2-2.5 mg/kg q8h or 1.5-1.89 mg/kg q6h. ≤**1 wk:** Up to 2 mg/kg q12h.	D > **R** [1]

CEPHALOSPORINS

Cefazolin (Ancef, Kefzol)	**Inj:** 500 mg/50 ml, 1 gm/50 ml, 500 mg, 1 gm, 10 gm, 20 gm	**IM/IV: Adults: Usual:** 500 mg-1 gm q6-8h. **Peds: Usual:** 25-50 mg/kg/d given as tid-qid. **Max:** 100 mg/kg/d.	B > **R** Safety in prematures & neonates not known.
Cefotaxime Sodium (Claforan)	**Inj:** 500 mg, 1 gm, 2 gm, 10 gm	**IM/IV: Adults & Peds: ≥ 50kg:** 1-2 gm q8h. **Max:** 12 gm/d. **1 mth-12 yo: <50 kg:** 50-180 mg/kg/d divided into 4-6 doses. **1-4 wks:** 50 mg/kg IV q8h. **0-1 wk:** 50 mg/kg IV q12h.	B > **R**
Cefoxitin (Mefoxin)	**Inj:** (Generic) 1 gm, 1 gm/50 ml, 2 gm, 2 gm/50 ml, 10 gm, (Mefoxin) 1 gm/50 ml, 2 gm/ 50 ml	**IV: Adults:** 1 gm q4h or 2 gm q6-8h. **Peds: ≥3 mths:** 80-160 mg/kg/d given as q4-6h. **Max:** 12 gm/d.	B > **R**

[1] Potential neurotoxicity, ototoxicity & neuromuscular blockade. Avoid concurrent use with neurotoxic/nephrotoxic agents & diuretics.

NAME	FORM/STRENGTH	DOSAGE	COMMENTS
Ceftazidime (Ceptaz, Fortaz, Tazicef)	**Inj:** 500 mg, 1 gm, 2 gm, 6 gm, 10 gm	**IV: Fortaz/Tazicef: Adults:** 2 gm q12h. **Peds: 1 mth-12 yo:** 30-50 mg/kg q8h, up to 6 gm/d. **0-4 wks:** 30 mg/kg q12h. **Ceptaz: Adults & Peds: ≥12 yo:** 2 gm q12h.	◉B ✻> (Fortaz, Tazicef) ✻v (Ceptaz) **R**
Ceftizoxime (Cefizox)	**Inj:** 500 mg, 1 gm, 2 gm, 10 gm	**IM/IV: Adults:** 1-2 gm q8-12h. **Max:** 6 gm/d. **Peds: ≥6 mths:** 50 mg/kg q6-8h, not to exceed adult dose.	◉B ✻> **R**
Ceftriaxone Sodium (Rocephin)	**Inj:** 1 gm/50 ml, 2 gm/ 50 ml, 250 mg, 500 mg, 1 gm, 2 gm, 10 gm	**Adults: IM/IV: Usual:** 1-2 gm qd (or in equally divided doses bid.) **Max:** 4 gm/d.	◉B ✻>
Cefuroxime (Kefurox, Zinacef)	**Inj:** 750 mg, 1.5 gm, 7.5 gm	**IM/IV: Adults:** 1.5 gm q8h. **Peds: >3 mths:** 50 mg/kg q8h. **Max:** 4.5 gm/d.	◉B ✻> **R**
Cephalexin (Keflex, Panixine DisperDose)	**Cap:** (Keflex) 250 mg, 333 mg, 500 mg, 750 mg; **Tab, Dispersible:** (Panixine DisperDose) 125 mg, 250 mg.	**Adults: Usual:** 250 mg q6h. **Max:** 4 gm/d. **Peds: Usual:** 25-50 mg/kg/d in divided doses.	◉B ✻>

PENICILLINS

NAME	FORM/STRENGTH	DOSAGE	COMMENTS
Piperacillin Sodium	**Inj:** 2 gm, 3 gm, 4 gm	**Adults & Peds: ≥12 yo: IM/IV:** 3-4 gm q4-6h. **Max:** 24 gm/d.	◉B ✻> **R**
Ticarcillin Disodium/ Clavulanate Potassium (Timentin)	**Inj:** 3 gm-100 mg, 3 gm-100 mg/100 ml, 30 gm-1 gm	**IV: Adults: ≥60 kg:** 300 mg/kg/d ticarcillin given q4h. **<60 kg:** 200-300 mg/kg/d ticarcillin given q4-6h. **Peds: ≥3 mths & <60 kg:** 50 mg/kg/d ticarcillin given q4-6h. **≥3 mths & ≥60 kg:** 3.1 gm q4-6h.	◉B ✻> **R**

QUINOLONES

Ciprofloxacin (Cipro)	**Inj:** 10 mg/ml, 200 mg/100 ml, 400 mg/200 ml; **Susp:** 250 mg/5 ml, 500 mg/5 ml; **Tab:** 250 mg, 500 mg, 750 mg	**Adults: ≥18 yo: Mild/Moderate:** 500 mg PO q12h or 400 mg IV q12h x ≥4-6 wks. **Severe/Complicated:** 750 mg PO q12h or 400 mg IV q8h x ≥4-6 wks.	◙C ❊v **R** CI with tizanidine

MISCELLANEOUS

Clindamycin (Cleocin)	**Cap:** 75 mg, 150 mg, 300 mg; **Inj:** 150 mg/ml, 300 mg/50 ml, 600 mg/50 ml, 900 mg/50 ml; **Susp:** 75 mg/5 ml	**IM/IV: Adults:** 600-2700 mg/d in 2-4 doses. **Max:** 600 mg IM single dose. **Peds: 1 mth-16 yo:** 20-40 mg/kg/d in 3-4 doses. **<1 mth:** 15-20 mg/kg/d in 3-4 doses. **PO: Adults:** 150-450 mg q6h. **Peds:** 8-20 mg/kg/d given 3-4 doses.	◙B ❊v (IV) ❊> (PO) Associated with severe, fatal colitis.
Imipenem/Cilastatin Sodium (Primaxin IV)	**Inj:** 250-250 mg, 500-500 mg	**IV: Adults: ≥70 kg: Mild:** 250-500 mg q6h. **Moderate:** 500 mg q6-8h or 1 gm q8h. **Severe:** 500 mg q6h or 1 gm q6-8h. **Max:** 50 mg/kg/d or 4 gm/d, whichever is lower. **Peds: ≥3 mths:** 15-25 mg/kg q6h. **Max:** 4 gm/d. **4 wks-3 mths & ≥1500 gm:** 25 mg/kg q6h. **1-4 wks & ≥1500 gm:** 25 mg/kg q8h. **<1 wk & ≥1500 gm:** 25 mg/kg q12h.	◙C ❊> **R**
Metronidazole (Flagyl)	**Cap:** 375 mg; **Inj:** 500 mg/100 ml; **Tab:** 250 mg, 500 mg	**Adults: PO:** 7.5 mg/kg q6h. **IV: LD:** 15 mg/kg. **Maint:** After 6h, 7.5 mg/kg q6h. **Max:** 4 gm/d.	◙B ❊v **H** CI in 1st trimester.

Fungal Infection

NAME	FORM/STRENGTH	DOSAGE	COMMENTS
Amphotericin B Lipid Complex (Abelcet)	**Inj:** 5 mg/ml	**Invasive Fungal Infections: Adults & Peds:** 5 mg/kg as a single IV infusion at 2.5 mg/kg/h. If infusion time >2h, mix contents by shaking infusion bag q2h.	B v **R**
Amphotericin B Liposome (Ambisome)	**Inj:** 50 mg; **Susp:** 100 mg/ml	**Adult & Peds:** Give over 120 min & reduce to 60 min if well tolerated. **Emperic Therapy in Febrile, Neutropenic Patients:** 3 mg/kg/d IV. ***Aspergillosis/Candida/Cryptococcus:*** 3-5 mg/kg/d IV. **Visceral Leishmaniasis:** (Immunocompetent) 3 mg/kg/d IV for days 1-5, 14, 21. (Immunocompromised) 4 mg/kg/d IV for days 1-5, 10, 17, 24, 31, 38. **Cryptococcal Meningitis in HIV Patients:** 6 mg/kg/d IV.	B v
Amphotericin B (Amphocin, Fungizone)	**Inj:** 50 mg	**Life-Threatening Fungal Infections: Adults:** 0.25-1 mg/kg/d IV. **Peds:** Limit to smallest effective dose.	B v **R** Not for noninvasive disease.
Anidulafungin (Eraxis)	**Inj:** 50 mg	**Adults: Candidemia/*Candida* Infections (Intra-Abdominal Abscess & Peritonitis): Loading Dose:** 200 mg on Day 1. Follow w/ 100 mg qd thereafter. Continue therapy for at least 14d after last positive culture. **Esophageal Candidiasis: Loading Dose:** 100 mg on Day 1. Follow w/ 50 mg qd thereafter. Treat for minimum of 14d and for at least 7d after symptoms resolve.	C >

Caspofungin Acetate (Cancidas)	**Inj:** 50 mg, 70 mg	**Adults: Invasive Aspergillosis/Empirical Therapy: LD:** 70 mg IV on Day 1. **Maint:** 50 mg/d IV. **Esophageal Candidiasis:** 50 mg/d IV. **Candidemia/*Candida* Infections (intra-abdomnial abscesses, peritonitis, & pleural space infection): LD:** 70 mg IV on Day 1. **Maint:** 50 mg/d IV.	C > **H**
Fluconazole (Diflucan)	**Inj:** 200 mg/100 ml, 400 mg/200 ml; **Susp:** 50 mg/5 ml, 200 mg/5 ml; **Tab:** 50 mg, 100 mg, 150 mg, 200 mg	**Adults: PO: Vaginal Candidiasis:** 150 mg single dose. **IV/PO: Oropharyngeal Candidiasis:** 200 mg on d1, then 100 mg qd x min 2 wks. **Esophageal Candidiasis:** 200 mg on d1, then 100 mg qd x min 3 wks & 2 wks after symptoms resolve. **Max:** 400 mg/d. **Systemic *Candida* Infections:** 400 mg/d. **UTI & Peritonitis:** 50-200 mg/d. **Cryptococcal Meningitis:** 400 mg on d1, then 200 mg qd x 10-12 wks after negative CSF culture. **Relapse Suppression in AIDS:** 200 mg qd. **Prophylaxis in BMT:** 400 mg qd. **Peds: IV/PO: Oropharyngeal Candidiasis:** 6 mg/kg on d1, then 3 mg/kg/d x min 2 wks. **Esophageal Candidiasis:** 6 mg/kg on d1, then 3 mg/kg/d x min 3 wks & 2 wks after symptoms resolve. **Max:** 12 mg/kg/d. **Systemic *Candida* Infections:** 6-12 mg/kg/d. **Cryptococcal Meningitis:** 12 mg/kg on d1, then 6 mg/kg/d x 10-12 wks after negative CSF culture. **Relapse Suppression in AIDS:** 6 mg/kg/d.	C v **R**
Flucytosine (Ancobon)	**Cap**: 250 mg, 500 mg	**Adults: *Candida/Cryptococcus:*** 50-150 mg/kg/d in divided doses at 6h intervals.	C v **R** [60]

[60] Extreme caution with renal dysfunction. Monitor hematologic, renal and hepatic status.

NAME	FORM/STRENGTH	DOSAGE	COMMENTS
Griseofulvin, Microcrystalline (Grifulvin V)	**Susp:** 125 mg/5 ml; **Tab:** 500 mg	**Adults: Tinea Corporis, Cruris & Capitis:** 500 mg qd; **Tinea Pedis, Unguium:** 1 gm qd. **Peds: 30-50 lbs:** 125-250 mg qd. **>50 lbs:** 250-500 mg qd. Treat capitis x 4-6 wks, corporis x 2-4 wks, pedis x 4-8 wks, unguium x min 4 mths (fingernails) or 6 mths (toenails).	●N ❋> CI in pregnancy.
Griseofulvin, Ultramicrocrystalline (Gris-Peg)	**Tab:** 125 mg, 250 mg	**Adults: Tinea Corporis, Cruris & Capitis:** 375 mg/d as single or divided doses. **Tinea Pedis, Unguium:** 375 mg bid. **>2 yo: Usual:** 3.3 mg/lb/d. **35-60 lb:** 125-187.5 mg qd. **>60 lb:** 187.5-375 mg qd. Treat capitis x 4-6 wks, corporis x 2-4 wks, pedis x 4-8 wks, unguium x min 4 mths (fingernails) or 6 mths (toenails).	●N ❋> CI in pregnancy.
Itraconazole (Sporanox)	**Cap:** 100 mg; **Inj:** 10 mg/ml; **Sol:** 10 mg/ml	**Adults: Cap:** Take w/full meal. **Blastomycosis/Histoplasmosis:** 200 mg qd. Increase by 100 mg if no improvement. **Max:** 400 mg/d. **Aspergillosis:** 200-400 mg/d. **Life-threatening Infection: LD:** 200 mg tid x 1st 3d. Continue x min 3 mths & until infection subsides. **Onychomycosis: Toenails:** 200 mg qd x 12 wks. **Fingernails:** 200 mg bid x 1 wk, stop therapy x 3 wks, then repeat. **Inj: Emperic Therapy in Febrile, Neutropenic Patients:** 200 mg IV bid x 4 doses, then 200 mg IV qd up to 14d. Continue w/sol 200 mg PO bid up to 28d. **Blastomycosis/Histoplasmosis/Aspergillosis:** 200 mg bid x 4 doses, then 200 mg qd, up to 14d. Continue w/caps for min 3 mths & until infection subsides. **Sol:** Take on empty stomach. Swish 10 ml at a time for several sec, then swallow. **Oropharyngeal Candidiasis:** 200 mg/d x 1-2 wks. **Esophageal Candidiasis:** 100-200 mg qd x min 3 wks. Continue x 2 wks after symptoms resolve.	●C ❋v CI w/cisapride, pimozide, quinidine, dofetilide. Serious cardiovascular events reported w/ CYP450 3A4 inhibitors. Avoid inj w/CrCl <30 ml/min. Do not interchange cap & sol.

Ketoconazole (Nizoral)	**Tab:** 200 mg	**Adults: Initial:** 200 mg qd. **Titrate:** May increase to 400 mg qd. **Peds:** **≥2 yo:** 3.3-6.6 mg/kg qd. For topical, see under Dermatology Antifungals.	◙C ❉v [61]
Nystatin (Mycostatin)	**Loz:** 200,000 U; **Susp:** 100,000 U/ml; **Tab:** 500,000 U	**Oral Candidiasis: Adults & Peds: Loz:** 200,000-400,000 U 4-5x/d up to 14d. **Susp:** 4-6 ml qid. Continue x 48h after relief of symptoms. **Infants: Susp:** 2 ml qid. **GI Candidiasis: Tab:** 500,000-1,000,000 U tid. Continue x min 48h after cure.	◙C ❉>
Terbinafine HCl (Lamisil)	**Tab:** 250 mg	**Adults: Fingernail Onychomycosis:** 250 mg qd x 6 wks. **Toenail Onychomycosis:** 250 mg qd x 12 wks.	◙B ❉v
Voriconazole (Vfend)	**Inj:** 200 mg/30 ml; **Susp:** 40 mg/ml; **Tab:** 50 mg, 200 mg	**Adults & Peds: ≥12 yo: Invasive Apergillosis/ *Scedosporium apiospermum* or *Fusarium* Infection: LD:** 6 mg/kg IV q12h x 2 doses. **Maint:** 4 mg/kg IV q12h. Switch to PO when appropriate. **Maint: >40 kg:** 200 mg PO q12h; increase to 300 mg PO q12h if needed. **<40 kg:** 100 mg PO q12h; increase to 150 mg PO q12h if needed. **Esophageal Candidiasis: (Tab) >40 kg:** 200 mg PO q12h. **<40 kg:** 100 mg PO q12h. Treat for minimum of 14d & at least 7d following resolution of symptoms. **Candidemia Nonneutropenic Patients/Deep Tissue *Candida* Infections**: 6 mg/kg IV q12h x 2 doses. **Maint:** 3-4 mg/kg IV q12h or 200 mg PO q12h. **Intolerant to Treatment:** Decrease IV maint dose to 3 mg/kg q12h, & PO maint dose by 50 mg steps to 200 mg q12h (or 100 mg q12h for <40 kg). Take PO 1h before or after a meal.	◙D ❉v **H R**

[61] Risk of fatal hepatotoxicity. CI w/terfenadine, astemizole, cisapride, oral triazolam.

Lower Respiratory Tract Infection

AMINOGLYCOSIDES

NAME	FORM/STRENGTH	DOSAGE	COMMENTS
Amikacin Sulfate (Amikin)	**Inj:** 50 mg/ml, 250 mg/ml	**IV: Adults, Children & Older Infants:** 7.5 mg/kg q12h or 5 mg/kg IM/IV q8h. **Max:** 1.5 gm/d **Newborns: LD:** 10 mg/kg. **Maint:** 7.5 mg/kg q12h.	◉D ✽v **R** [1]
Gentamicin Sulfate (Garamycin)	**Inj:** 40 mg/ml	**IV: Adults:** 3 mg/kg/d given q8h. **Max:** 5 mg/kg/d in 3-4 doses. Reduce to 3 mg/kg/d as soon as clinically indicated. **Peds:** 2-2.5 mg/kg q8h. **Infants/Neonates:** 2.5 mg/kg q8h. **≤1 wk:** 2.5 mg/kg q12h.	◉N ✽> **R** [1]
Tobramycin Sulfate (Nebcin)	**Inj:** 10 mg/ml, 40 mg/ml, 1.2 gm	**IV: Adults:** 3 mg/kg/d given q8h. **Max:** 5 mg/kg/d in 3-4 doses. Reduce to 3 mg/kg/d as soon as clinically indicated. **Peds: >1 wk:** 2-2.5 mg/kg q8h or 1.5-1.89 mg/kg q6h. **<1 wk:** Up to 2 mg/kg q12h.	◉D ✽> **R** [1]

CARBAPENEM

NAME	FORM/STRENGTH	DOSAGE	COMMENTS
Ertapenem Sodium (Invanz)	**Inj:** 1 gm	**Adults:** 1 gm qd x 10-14d. May give IV up to 14d; IM up to 7d.	◉B ✽> **R**

CEPHALOSPORINS

NAME	FORM/STRENGTH	DOSAGE	COMMENTS
Cefaclor (Ceclor, Ceclor CD)	**Cap:** 250 mg, 500 mg; **Susp:** 125 mg/5 ml, 187 mg/5 ml, 250 mg/5 ml,375 mg/5 ml; **Tab,ER:** (CD) 375 mg, 500 mg	**Adults: Cap/Susp:** 500 mg q8h. **Tab,ER:** 500 mg q12h x 7d. **Peds: ≥1 mth: Cap/Susp:** 40 mg/kg/d given q8h. **Max:** 1 gm/d.	◉B ✽>

Cefdinir (Omnicef)	**Cap:** 300 mg	**Adults & Peds: ≥13 yo: CAP:** 300 mg q12h x 10d. **ABECB:** 300 mg q12h x 5-10d or 600 mg q24h x 10d.	B > R
Cefditoren Pivoxil (Spectracef)	**Tab:** 200 mg	**Adults & Peds: ≥12 yo: ABECB:** 400 mg bid x 10d. **Pneumonia:** 400 mg bid x 14d.	B > R
Cefepime HCl (Maxipime)	**Inj:** 500 mg, 1 gm, 2 gm	**Adults: Moderate-Severe:** 1-2 gm IV q12h x 10d. **Peds: 2 mths-16 yo: ≤40 kg:** 50 mg/kg IV q12h. **Max:** Do not exceed adult dose.	B > R
Cefixime (Suprax)	**Susp:** 100 mg/5 ml	**Pharyngitis/Tonsillitis: Adults & Peds: >12 yo or >50 kg: Tab/Susp:** 400 mg qd or 200 mg bid. **≤50 kg or ≥6 mths: Susp:** 8 mg/kg qd or 4 mg/kg bid.	B v R
Cefpodoxime Proxetil (Vantin)	**Susp:** 50 mg/5 ml, 100 mg/5 ml; **Tab:** 100 mg, 200 mg	**Adults & Peds: ≥12 yo:** 200 mg q12h x 10-14d.	B v R
Cefprozil (Cefzil)	**Susp:** 125 mg/5 ml, 250 mg/5 ml; **Tab:** 250 mg, 500 mg	**Acute Bronchitis/ABECB: Adults & Peds: ≥13 yo:** 500 mg q12h x 10d.	B > R
Ceftibuten (Cedax)	**Cap:** 400 mg; **Susp:** 90 mg/5 ml	**Adults & Peds: ≥12 yo:** 400 mg qd x 10d. **≥6 mths:** 9 mg/kg qd x 10d. **Max:** 400 mg/d.	B > R
Ceftriaxone Sodium (Rocephin)	**Inj:** 1 gm/50 ml, 2 gm/50 ml, 250 mg, 500 mg, 1 gm, 2 gm, 10 gm	**Adults: IM/IV: Usual:** 1-2 gm qd (or in equally divided doses bid). **Max:** 4 gm/d.	B >
Cefuroxime Axetil (Ceftin)	**Tab:** 125 mg, 250 mg, 500 mg	**Adults & Peds: ≥13 yo:** 250-500 mg bid x 5-10d.	B v R

[1] Potential neurotoxicity, ototoxicity & neuromuscular blockade. Avoid concurrent use with neurotoxic/nephrotoxic agents & diuretics.

NAME	FORM/STRENGTH	DOSAGE	COMMENTS
Cephalexin (Keflex)	**Cap:** 250 mg, 333 mg, 500 mg, 750 mg	**Adults: Usual:** 250 mg q6h. **Max:** 4 gm/d. **Peds: Usual:** 25-50 mg/kg/d in divided doses.	◙B ✿>
Cephradine (Velosef)	**Cap:** 250 mg, 500 mg; **Susp:** 250 mg/5 ml	**Pneumonia: Adults:** 500 mg q6h or 1 gm q12h. **Peds: >9 mths:** 25-50 mg/kg/d given q6h or q12h (up to adult dose).	◙B ✿> **R**
KETOLIDES			
Telithromycin (Ketek)	**Tab:** 300 mg, 400 mg,	**Adults:** 800 mg qd x 5d (ABECB) or 7-10d (CAP).	◙C ✿> **H R**
MACROLIDES			
Azithromycin (Zithromax, Zmax)	(Zithromax) **Inj:** 500 mg; **Susp:** 100 mg/5 ml, 200 mg/5 ml, 1 gm/pkt; **Tab:** 250 mg, 500 mg, 600 mg. (Zmax) **Susp,ER:** 2 gm	**CAP: Zithromax: Adults: ≥16 yo: PO:** 500 mg qd x 1d, then 250 mg qd on Days 2-5. **IV:** 500 mg qd x 2d, then 250 mg bid x 5-8d. **Peds: ≥6 mths: Susp:** 10 mg/kg qd x 1d, then 5 mg/kg on Days 2-5. **Zmax: Adults:** 2 gm single dose. **COPD: Zithromax: Adults: PO:** 500 mg qd x 3d or 500 mg qd x 1d, then 250 mg qd on Days 2-5.	◙B ✿>
Clarithromycin (Biaxin)	**Susp:** 125 mg/5 ml, 250 mg/5 ml; **Tab:** 250 mg, 500 mg; **Tab,ER:** 500 mg	**Adults: ABECB: Susp/Tab:** 250-500 mg q12h x 7-14d. **Tab,ER:** 1 gm qd x 7d. **CAP: Susp/Tab:** 250 mg q12h x 7-14d. **Tab,ER:** 1 gm qd x7d. **Peds: ≥6 mths: CAP: Susp/Tab:** 7.5 mg/kg q12h x 10d.	◙C ✿> **R**
Dirithromycin (Dynabac)	**Tab,Delay:** 250 mg	**Adults & Peds: ≥12 yo:** 500 mg qd x 7-14d.	◙C ✿>
Erythromycin Base	**Tab:** 250 mg	**Adults: Usual:** 250 mg q6h or 500 mg q12h. **Peds: Usual:** 30-50 mg/kg/d in divided doses. **Max:** 4 gm/d.	◙B ✿>

Erythromycin (Ery-Tab, PCE)	**Tab,Delay:** (Ery-Tab) 250 mg, 333 mg, 500 mg; **Tab,ER:** (PCE) 333 mg, 500 mg	**Adults: Usual:** 250 mg qid, 333 mg q8h, or 500 mg q12h. **Peds: Usual:** 30-50 mg/kg/d in divided doses. **Max:** 4 gm/d.	B >
Erythromycin Ethylsuccinate (E.E.S., EryPed)	**Chewtab:** (EryPed) 200 mg; **Susp:** (EryPed) 100 mg/2.5 ml, 200 mg/5 ml, 400 mg/5 ml, (E.E.S.) 200 mg/5 ml, 400 mg/5 ml; **Tab:** (E.E.S.) 400 mg	**Adults: Usual:** 1600 mg/d given q6h, q8h, or q12h. **Max:** 4 gm/d. **Peds: Usual:** 30-50 mg/kg/d in divided doses q6h, q8h, or q12h. Double dose for more severe infections.	B >
Erythromycin Stearate (Erythrocin)	**Tab:** 250 mg, 500 mg	**Adults: Usual:** 250 mg q6h or 500 mg q12h. **Peds: Usual:** 30-50 mg/kg/d in divided doses. **Max:** 4 gm/d.	B >

MONOBACTAMS

Loracarbef (Lorabid)	**Cap:** 200 mg, 400 mg; **Susp:** 100 mg/5 ml, 200 mg/5 ml	**Adults & Peds: ≥13 yo: Bronchitis:** 200-400 mg q12h x 7d. **Pneumonia:** 400mg q12h x 14d.	B > R

OXAZOLIDINONE

Linezolid (Zyvox)	**Inj:** 2 mg/ml; **Susp:** 100 mg/5 ml; **Tab:** 600 mg	**Usual:** Treat x 10-14d. **Adults & Peds ≥12 yo:** 600 mg IV/PO q12h. **Birth-11 yo:** 10 mg/kg IV/PO q8h.	C >

NAME	FORM/STRENGTH	DOSAGE	COMMENTS
PENICILLINS			
Amoxicillin (Amoxil, DisperMox, Trimox)	**Cap:** (Amoxil, Trimox) 250 mg, 500 mg; **Chewtab:** (Amoxil) 200 mg, 400 mg; **Susp:** (Amoxil) 50 mg/ml, 125 mg/5 ml, 200 mg/5 ml, 250 mg/5 ml, 400 mg/5 ml, (Trimox) 125 mg/5 ml, 250 mg/ 5 ml; **Tab:** (Amoxil) 500 mg, 875 mg; **Tab, Dispersible:** (DisperMox) 200 mg, 400 mg, 600 mg	**Adults & Peds: >40 kg:** 875 mg q12h or 500 mg q8h. **>3 mths & <40 kg:** 45 mg/kg/d given q12h or 40 mg/kg/d given q8h. **≤3 mths: Usual/Max:** 15 mg/kg q12h.	◙B ❁> **R**
Amoxicillin/Clavulanate (Augmentin)	**Chewtab:** 125-31.25 mg, 200-28.5 mg, 250-62.5 mg, 400-57 mg; **Susp:** (per 5 ml) 125-31.25 mg, 200-28.5 mg, 250-62.5 mg, 400-57 mg; **Tab:** 250-125 mg, 500-125 mg, 875-125 mg	Dose based on amoxicillin component. **Adults & Peds: ≥40 kg: Tab:** 875 mg q12h or 500 mg q8h. May use 125 mg/5 ml or 250 mg/5 ml susp in place of 500 mg tab & 200 mg/5 ml susp or 400 mg/5 ml susp in place of 875 mg tab. **Chewtab/Susp: ≥12 wks:** 45 mg/kg/d given q12h or 40 mg/kg/d given q8h. **<12 wks:** 15 mg/kg q12h (use 125 mg/5 ml susp).	◙B ❁> **H R** 2- 250 mg tabs are not equivalent to 1- 500 mg tab. Only use 250 mg tab if peds ≥40 kg. Chewtab & tab not interchangeable.
Amoxicillin/Clavulanate (Augmentin XR)	**Tab,ER:** 1000-62.5 mg	**Adults & Peds: ≥16 yo:** 2 tabs q12h x 7-10d.	◙ B ❁>

Ampicillin (Principen)	**Cap:** 250 mg, 500 mg; **Susp:** 125 mg/5ml, 250 mg/5ml	**Adults & Peds: >20 kg:** 250 mg qid. **≤20 kg:** 50 mg/kg/d given tid-qid.	B ❀v
Dicloxacillin Sodium (Dynapen)	**Cap:** 250 mg, 500 mg; **Susp:** 62.5 mg/5 ml	**Adults & Peds: ≥40 kg: Mild-Moderate:** 125 mg q6h. **Severe:** 250 mg q6h. **<40 kg: Mild-Moderate:** 3.125 mg/kg q6h. **Severe:** 6.25 mg/kg q6h.	B ❀>
Penicillin V Potassium (Penicillin VK, Veetids)	**Susp:** 125 mg/5 ml, 250 mg/5 ml; **Tab:** 250 mg, 500 mg	**Adults & Peds: ≥12 yo: Pneumococcal:** 250-500 mg q6h until afebrile x 2d.	B ❀>
Piperacillin Sodium/ Tazobactam (Zosyn)	**Inj:** 40-5 mg/ml, 60-7.5 mg/ml, 2-0.25 gm, 3-0.375 gm, 4-0.5 gm, 4-0.5 gm/ 100 ml, 36-4.5 gm	**Adults: Usual:** 3.375 gm IV q6h x 7-10d. **Nosocomial Pneumonia:** 4.5 gm IV q6h x 7-14d plus aminoglycoside.	B ❀> **R**

QUINOLONES

Ciprofloxacin (Cipro)	**Inj:** 10 mg/ml, 200 mg/100 ml, 400 mg/200 ml; **Susp:** 250 mg/5 ml, 500 mg/5 ml; **Tab:** 250 mg, 500 mg, 750 mg	**Adults: ≥18 yo: Mild/Moderate:** 500 mg PO q12h or 400 mg IV q12h x 7-14d. **Severe/Complicated:** 750 mg PO q12h or 400 mg IV q8h x 7-14d. **Nosocomial Pneumonia:** 400 mg IV q8h x 10-14d. **Inhalation Anthrax (Post-Exposure): Adults:** 500 mg PO q12h or 400 mg IV q12h x 60d. **Peds:** 15 mg/kg PO q12h or 10 mg/kg IV q12h x 60d. **Max:** 500 mg PO or 400 mg IV per dose.	C ❀v **R** CI with tizanidine
Gemifloxacin Mesylate (Factive)	**Tab:** 320 mg	**Adults: ≥18 yo:** 320 mg qd x 5d (ABECB) or 7d (CAP).	C ❀v **R**

NAME	FORM/STRENGTH	DOSAGE	COMMENTS
Levofloxacin (Levaquin)	**Inj:** 5 mg/ml, 25 mg/ml; **Sol:** 25 mg/ml; **Tab:** 250 mg, 500 mg, 750 mg	**Adults: ≥18 yo: CAP:** 500 mg IV/PO qd x 7-14d or 750 mg IV/PO qd x 5d. **Nosocomial Pneumonia:** 750mg IV/PO qd x 7-14d. **ABECB:** 500 mg IV/PO x 7d. **Inhalation Anthrax (Post-Exposure):** 500 mg IV/PO qd x 60d.	C v **R**
Lomefloxacin (Maxaquin)	**Tab:** 400 mg	**ABECB: Adults: ≥18 yo:** 400 mg qd x 10d.	C v **R**
Moxifloxacin HCl (Avelox)	**Inj:** 400 mg/250 ml; **Tab:** 400 mg	**Adults: ≥18 yo:** 400 mg IV/PO qd x 5d (ABECB) or 7-14d (CAP).	C v
Ofloxacin (Floxin)	**Tab:** 200 mg, 300 mg, 400 mg	**ABECB/CAP: Adults: ≥18 yo:** 400 mg q12h x 10d.	C v **H R**
Sparfloxacin (Zagam)	**Tab:** 200 mg	**Adults: ≥18 yo: LD:** 400 mg on Day 1. **Maint:** 200 mg q24h x 9d.	C v **R**
Trovafloxacin Mesylate (Trovan)	**Inj:** (Alatrofloxacin Mesylate) 5 mg/ml; **Tab:** 100 mg, 200 mg	**Adults: Nosocomial Pneumonia:** 300 mg IV q24h, then 200 mg qd PO x 10-14d. **CAP:** 200 mg PO qd or 200 mg IV q24h, then 200 mg PO qd x 7-14d.	C v **H** Serious liver injury reported.
SULFONAMIDES AND COMBINATIONS			
Sulfamethoxazole/ Trimethoprim (Bactrim, Bactrim DS, Septra, Septra DS, Sulfatrim Pediatric)	**Susp:** 200-40 mg/5 ml; **Tab:** (SS) 400-80 mg, (DS) 800-160 mg	**Adults:** 800 mg SMX & 160 mg TMP (1 DS tab, 2 SS tabs, or 20 ml) q12h x 14d.	C v **R** CI in pregnancy & nursing.

Doxycycline Hyclate (Doryx, Vibramycin, Vibra-Tabs)	**Cap:** (Vibramycin) 100 mg; **Cap,Delay:** (Doryx) 75 mg, 100 mg; **Tab:** (Vibra-Tabs) 100 mg	**Adults:** 100 mg q12h on Day 1, then 100 mg qd or 50 mg q12h. **Severe:** 100 mg q12h. **Peds: >8 yo & ≤100 lbs:** 1 mg/lb bid on Day 1, then 1 mg/lb qd or 0.5 mg/lb bid. **Severe:** 2 mg/lb. **>100 lbs:** Adult dose. **Inhalation Anthrax (Post-Exposure): Adults:** 100 mg bid x 60d. **Peds: >8 yo & <100 lbs:** 1 mg/lb bid x 60d. **≥100 lbs:** Adult dose.	D v
Doxycycline Monohydrate (Monodox, Vibramycin)	**Cap:** (Monodox) 50 mg, 100 mg; **Susp:** (Vibramycin) 25 mg/5 ml	**Adults:** 100 mg q12h or 50 mg q6h on Day 1, then 100 mg qd or 50 mg q12h. **Severe:** 100 mg q12h. **Peds: >8 yo & ≤100 lbs:** 1 mg/lb bid on Day 1, then 1 mg/lb qd or 0.5 mg/lb bid. **Severe:** 2 mg/lb. **>100 lbs:** Adult dose. **Inhalation Anthrax (Post-Exposure): Adults:** 100 mg bid x 60d. **Peds: >8 yo & <100 lbs:** 1 mg/lb bid x 60d. **≥100 lbs:** Adult dose.	D v
Minocycline HCl (Dynacin, Minocin)	**Cap:** (Dynacin) 50 mg, 75 mg, 100 mg, (Minocin) 50 mg, 100 mg; **Inj:** (Minocin) 100 mg; **Tab:** (Dynacin) 50 mg, 75 mg, 100 mg	**Adults:** 200 mg PO/IV, then 100 mg q12h or 50 mg qid. **Peds: >8 yo:** 4 mg/kg PO/IV, then 2 mg/kg q12h.	D v **R**
Tetracycline HCl (Sumycin)	**Cap:** 250 mg, 500 mg; **Susp:** 125 mg/5 ml	**Adults:** 250 mg qid or 500 mg bid. **Peds: >8 yo:** 25-50 mg/kg divided bid-qid.	D v **R**

NAME	FORM/STRENGTH	DOSAGE	COMMENTS
MISCELLANEOUS			
Clindamycin (Cleocin)	**Cap:** 75 mg, 150 mg, 300 mg; **Inj:** 150 mg/ml, 300 mg/50 ml, 600 mg/ 50 ml, 900 mg/50 ml; **Susp:** 75 mg/5 ml	**IM/IV: Adults:** 600-2700 mg/d in 2-4 doses. **Max:** 600 mg IM single dose. **Peds: 1 mth-16 yo:** 20-40 mg/kg/d in 3-4 doses. **<1 mth:** 15-20 mg/kg/d in 3-4 doses. **PO: Adults:** 150-450 mg q6h. **Peds:** 8-20 mg/kg/d given 3-4 doses.	◙B ❋v (IV) ❋> (PO) Associated with severe, fatal colitis.

Meningitis, Bacterial

NAME	FORM/STRENGTH	DOSAGE	COMMENTS
AMINOGLYCOSIDES			
Amikacin Sulfate (Amikin)	**Inj:** 50 mg/ml, 250 mg/ml	**IV: Adults, Children & Older Infants:** 7.5 mg/kg q12h or 5 mg/kg IM/IV q8h. **Max:** 1.5 gm/d. **Newborns: LD:** 10 mg/kg. **Maint:** 7.5 mg/kg q12h.	◙D ❋v **R**[1]
Gentamicin Sulfate (Garamycin)	**Inj:** 40 mg/ml	**IV: Adults:** 3 mg/kg/d given q8h. **Max:** 5 mg/kg/d in 3-4 doses. Reduce to 3 mg/kg/d as soon as clinically indicated. **Peds:** 2-2.5 mg/kg q8h. **Infants/Neonates:** 2.5 mg/kg q8h. **≤1 wk:** 2.5 mg/kg q12h.	◙N ❋> **R**[1]
Tobramycin Sulfate (Nebcin)	**Inj:** 10 mg/ml, 40 mg/ml, 1.2 gm	**IV: Adults:** 3 mg/kg/d given q8h. **Max:** 5 mg/kg/d in 3-4 doses. Reduce to 3 mg/kg/d as soon as clinically indicated. **Peds: >1 wk:** 2-2.5 mg/kg q8h or 1.5-1.89 mg/kg q6h. **<1 wk:** Up to 2 mg/kg q12h.	◙D ❋> **R**[1]
CARBAPENEM			
Meropenem (Merrem)	**Inj:** 500 mg, 1 gm	**IV: Adults & Peds: ≥3 mths: >50 kg:** 1 gm q8h. **≤50 kg:** 40 mg/kg q8h. **Max:** 2 gm q8h.	◙B ❋> **R**

CEPHALOSPORINS

Cefotaxime Sodium (Claforan)	**Inj:** 500 mg, 1 gm, 2 gm, 10 gm	**IV: Adults or >50 kg:** 2 gm q6-8h. **Max:** 12 gm/d. **1 mth-12 yo: <50 kg:** 50-180 mg/kg/d divided into 4-6 doses. **1-4 wks:** 50 mg/kg IV q8h. **0-1 wk:** 50 mg/kg IV q12h.	◙B ❁> **R**
Ceftazidime (Ceptaz, Fortaz, Tazicef)	**Inj:** 500 mg, 1 gm, 2 gm, 6 gm, 10 gm	**IV: Fortaz/Tazicef: Adults:** 2 gm q8h. **Peds: 1 mth-12 yo:** 30-50 mg/kg q8h, up to 6 gm/d. **0-4 wks:** 30 mg/kg q12h. **Ceptaz: Adults & Peds: ≥12 yo:** 2 gm q8h.	◙B ❁> (Fortaz, Tazicef) ❁v (Ceptaz) **R**
Ceftizoxime (Cefizox)	**Inj:** 500 mg, 1 gm, 2 gm, 10 gm	**IV: Adults:** 3-4 gm q8h. **Peds: ≥6 mths:** 50 mg/kg q6-8h, not to exceed adult dose.	◙B ❁> **R**
Ceftriaxone Sodium (Rocephin)	**Inj:** 1 gm/50 ml, 2 gm/50 ml, 250 mg, 500 mg, 1 gm, 2 gm, 10 gm	**IV: Adults:** 1-2 gm qd (or in equally divided doses bid). **Max:** 4 gm/d. **Peds:** Initial of 100 mg/kg (NTE 4 gm), then 100 mg/kg qd or (in equally divided doses q12h) x 7-14d. **Max:** 4 gm/d.	◙B ❁>
Cefuroxime (Kefurox, Zinacef)	**Inj:** 750 mg, 1.5 gm, 7.5 gm	**IV: Adults:** 1.5 gm q6h. **Max:** 3 gm q8h. **Peds: >3 mths:** 200-240 mg/kg/d divided q6-8h.	◙B ❁> **R**

PENICILLINS

Ampicillin Sodium	**Inj:** 125 mg, 250 mg, 500 mg, 1 gm, 2 gm, 10 gm	**IV: Adults & Peds:** 150-200 mg/kg/day given q3-4h.	◙B ❁>

[1] Potential neurotoxicity, ototoxicity & neuromuscular blockade. Avoid concurrent use with neurotoxic/nephrotoxic agents & diuretics.

NAME	FORM/STRENGTH	DOSAGE	COMMENTS
Penicillin G Potassium (Pfizerpen)	**Inj:** 5 MU, 20 MU	**IV: Adults: *Listeria:*** 15-20 MU/d x 2 wks. ***Pasteurella:*** 4-6 MU/d x 2 wks. ***Meningococcus:*** 1-2 MU IM q2h or 20-30 MU/d continuous IV.	■B ❋>

Mycobacterium Avium Complex

NAME	FORM/STRENGTH	DOSAGE	COMMENTS
Azithromycin (Zithromax)	**Susp:** 100 mg/5 ml, 200 mg/5 ml, 1 gm/pkt; **Tab:** 600 mg	**Adults: Prevention:** 1200 mg qwk. **Treatment:** 600 mg qd w/ ethambutol 15 mg/kg/d.	■B ❋>
Clarithromycin (Biaxin)	**Susp:** 125 mg/5 ml, 250 mg/5 ml; **Tab:** 250 mg, 500 mg	**Prevention & Treatment: Adults:** 500 mg bid. **Peds: ≥20 mths:** 7.5 mg/kg bid. **Max:** 500 mg bid.	■C ❋> **R**
Rifabutin (Mycobutin)	**Cap:** 150 mg	**Adults:** 300 mg qd or 150 mg bid w/ food. Reduce dose w/ nelfinavir or indinavir.	■B ❋v **R**

Otitis Media, Acute

CEPHALOSPORINS

NAME	FORM/STRENGTH	DOSAGE	COMMENTS
Cefaclor (Ceclor)	**Cap:** 250 mg, 500 mg; **Susp:** 125 mg/5 ml, 187 mg/5 ml, 250 mg/5 ml, 375 mg/5 ml	**Peds: ≥1 mth:** 40 mg/kg/d given in divided doses. **Max:** 1 gm/d.	■B ❋>
Cefdinir (Omnicef)	**Susp:** 125 mg/5 ml; 250 mg/5 ml	**Peds: 6 mths-12 yo:** 7 mg/kg q12h x 5-10d or 14 mg/kg q24h x 10d.	■B ❋> **R**
Cefixime (Suprax)	**Susp:** 100 mg/5 ml	**Adults & Peds: >12 yo or >50 kg: Tab/Susp:** 400 mg qd or 200 mg bid. **≤50 kg or >6 mths: Susp:** 8 mg/kg qd or 4 mg/kg bid.	■B ❋v **R**

Cefpodoxime Proxetil (Vantin)	**Susp:** 50 mg/5 ml, 100 mg/5 ml; **Tab:** 100 mg, 200 mg	**Peds: 2 mths-11 yo:** 5 mg/kg q12h x 5d.	B v **R**
Cefprozil (Cefzil)	**Susp:** 125 mg/5 ml, 250 mg/5 ml; **Tab:** 250 mg, 500 mg	**Peds: 6 mths-12 yo:** 15 mg/kg q12h x 10d.	B > **R**
Ceftibuten (Cedax)	**Cap:** 400 mg; **Susp:** 90 mg/5 ml	**Adults & Peds: ≥6 mths:** 9 mg/kg qd x 10d. **Max:** 400 mg/d.	B > **R**
Ceftriaxone Sodium (Rocephin)	**Inj:** 1 gm/50 ml, 2 gm/ 50 ml, 250 mg, 500 mg, 1 gm, 2 gm, 10 gm	**Peds:** 50 mg/kg IM single dose. **Max:** 1 gm/dose.	B >
Cefuroxime Axetil (Ceftin)	**Susp:** 125 mg/5 ml, 250 mg/5 ml; **Tab:** 125 mg, 250 mg, 500 mg	**Peds: 3 mths-12 yo: Susp:** 15 mg/kg bid x 10d. **Max:** 1 gm/d. **Tab:** 250 mg bid x 10d.	B v **R** Tabs & susp not bioequivalent.
Cephalexin (Keflex, Panixine DisperDose)	**Cap:** (Keflex) 250 mg, 333 mg,500 mg, 750 mg; **Tab, Dispersible:** (Panixine DisperDose) 125 mg, 250 mg.	**Peds:** 75-100 mg/kg/d in divided doses.	B >
Cephradine (Velosef)	**Cap:** 250 mg, 500 mg; **Susp:** 250 mg/5 ml	***H.influenzae*: Peds: >9 mths:** 75-100 mg/kg/d given q6h or q12h. **Max:** 4 gm/d.	B > **R**
MACROLIDES			
Azithromycin (Zithromax)	**Susp:** 100 mg/5 ml, 200 mg/5 ml; 1 gm/pkt	**Peds: ≥6 mths:** 30 mg/kg x 1 dose; 10 mg/kg qd x 3d; or 10 mg/kg qd x 1d, then 5 mg/kg qd on Days 2-5.	B >

NAME	FORM/STRENGTH	DOSAGE	COMMENTS
Clarithromycin (Biaxin)	**Susp:** 125 mg/5 ml, 250 mg/5 ml; **Tab:** 250 mg, 500 mg	**Peds: ≥6 mths:** 7.5 mg/kg q12h x 10d.	◙C ❃> **R**
MACROLIDES AND COMBINATIONS			
Erythromycin Ethylsuccinate/ Sulfisoxazole Acetyl (Pediazole)	**Susp:** 200-600 mg/5 ml	**Peds: ≥2 mths:** Dose based on 50 mg/kg/d erythromycin or 150 mg/kg/d sulfisoxazole given tid-qid x 10d. **Max:** 6 gm/d sulfisoxazole.	◙C ❃v
MONOBACTAMS			
Loracarbef (Lorabid)	**Susp:** 100 mg/5 ml, 200 mg/5 ml	**Peds: 6 mths-12 yo:** 15 mg/kg q12h x 10d.	◙B ❃> **R**
PENICILLINS			
Amoxicillin (Amoxil, DisperMox, Trimox)	**Cap:** (Amoxil, Trimox) 250 mg, 500 mg; **Chewtab:** (Amoxil) 200 mg, 400 mg; **Susp:** (Amoxil) 50 mg/ml, 125 mg/5 ml, 200 mg/5 ml, 250 mg/5 ml, 400 mg/5 ml, (Trimox) 125 mg/5 ml, 250 mg/5 ml; **Tab:** (Amoxil) 500 mg, 875 mg; **Tab, Dispersible:** (DisperMox) 200 mg, 400 mg, 600 mg	**Peds: >40 kg:** 500-875 mg q12h or 250-500 mg q8h, depending on severity. **>3 mths:** 25-45 mg/kg/d divided q12h or 20-40 mg/kg/d divided q8h, depending on severity. **≤3 mths: Usual/Max:** 15 mg/kg q12h.	◙B ❃> **R**

Amoxicillin/Clavulanate (Augmentin)	**Chewtab:** 125-31.25 mg, 200-28.5 mg, 250-62.5 mg, 400-57 mg; **Susp:** (per 5 ml) 125-31.25 mg, 200-28.5 mg, 250-62.5 mg, 400-57 mg; **Tab:** 250-125 mg, 500-125 mg, 875-125 mg	Dose based on amoxicillin component. **Peds: ≥40 kg: Tab:** 500 mg q12h or 250 mg q8h. May use 125 mg/5 ml or 250 mg/5 ml susp in place of 500 mg tab & 200 mg/5 ml or 400 mg/5 ml susp in place of 875 mg tab. **≥12 wks: Susp/Chewtab:** 45 mg/kg/d given q12h or 40 mg/kg/d given q8h. **<12 wks: Susp:** 15 mg/kg q12h (use 125 mg/5 ml susp).	B > **H R** 2- 250 mg tabs are not equivalent to 1- 500 mg tab. Only use 250 mg tab if peds ≥40 kg. Chewtab & tab not interchangeable.
Amoxicillin/Clavulanate (Augmentin ES-600)	**Susp:** 600-42.9 mg/5 ml	**Peds: 3 mths-12 yo: <40 kg:** 45 mg/kg q12h based on amoxicillin component x 10d. Not interchangeable w/ other Augmentin susp.	B > **H R**

SULFONAMIDES AND COMBINATIONS

Sulfamethoxazole/ Trimethoprim (Bactrim, Bactrim DS, Septra, Septra DS, Sulfatrim Pediatric)	**Susp:** 200-40 mg/5 ml; **Tab:** (SS) 400-80 mg, (DS) 800-160 mg	**Peds: ≥2 mths:** 4 mg/kg TMP & 20 mg/kg SMX q12h x 10d.	C v **R** CI in pregnancy & nursing.

Pneumocystis Carinii **Pneumonia**

Atovaquone (Mepron)	**Susp:** 750 mg/5 ml	**Adults & Peds: ≥13 yrs:** Take w/ food. **Prevention:** 1500 mg qd. **Treatment:** 750 mg bid x 21d.	C >
Pentamidine Isethionate (Pentam, Nebupent)	**Inj:** (Pentam) 300 mg; **Sol,Neb:** (Nebupent) 300 mg	**Adults/Peds: Pentam: ≥4 mths: Treatment:** 4 mg/kg IM/IV qd x 14-21d. **Nebupent: ≥16 yo: Prevention:** 300 mg q4wks via nebulizer.	C v

NAME	FORM/STRENGTH	DOSAGE	COMMENTS
Sulfamethoxazole/ Trimethoprim (Bactrim, Bactrim DS, Septra, Septra DS, Sulfatrim Pediatric)	**Susp:** 200-40 mg/5 ml; **Tab:** (SS) 400-80 mg, (DS) 800-160 mg	**Treatment: Adults & Peds:** 15-20 mg/kg TMP & 75-100 mg/kg SMZ divided q6h x 14-21d. **Prophylaxis: Adults:** 1 DS tab qd. **Peds:** 150 $mg/m^2/d$ TMP & 750 mg/m^2 SMZ divided bid x 3 consecutive days/wk. **Max:** 320 mg TMP/1600 mg SMZ per d.	■C ❊v **R** CI in pregnancy & nursing.

Septicemia, Bacterial

AMINOGLYCOSIDES

NAME	FORM/STRENGTH	DOSAGE	COMMENTS
Amikacin Sulfate (Amikin)	**Inj:** 50 mg/ml, 250 mg/ml	**IV: Adults, Children & Older Infants:** 7.5 mg/kg q12h or 5 mg/kg IM/IV q8h. **Max:** 1.5 gm/d **Newborns: LD:** 10 mg/kg. **Maint:** 7.5 mg/kg q12h.	■D ❊v **R** [1]
Gentamicin Sulfate (Garamycin)	**Inj:** 40 mg/ml	**IV: Adults:** 3 mg/kg/d given q8h. **Max:** 5 mg/kg/d in 3-4 doses. Reduce to 3 mg/kg/d as soon as clinically indicated. **Peds:** 2-2.5 mg/kg q8h. **Infants/Neonates:** 2.5 mg/kg q8h. **≤1 wk:** 2.5 mg/kg q12h.	■N ❊> **R** [1]
Tobramycin Sulfate (Nebcin)	**Inj:** 10 mg/ml, 40 mg/ml, 1.2 gm	**IV: Adults:** 3 mg/kg/d given q8h. **Max:** 5 mg/kg/d in 3-4 doses. Reduce to 3 mg/kg/d as soon as clinically indicated. **Peds: >1 wk:** 2-2.5 mg/kg q8h or 1.5-1.89 mg/kg q6h. **<1 wk:** Up to 2 mg/kg q12h.	■D ❊> **R** [1]

CEPHALOSPORINS

NAME	FORM/STRENGTH	DOSAGE	COMMENTS
Cefazolin (Ancef, Kefzol)	**Inj:** 500 mg/50 ml, 1 gm/50 ml, 500 mg, 1 gm, 10 gm, 20 gm	**IV: Adults:** 1-1.5 gm q6h. **Peds:** 100 mg/kg/d given as tid-qid.	■B ❊> **R** Safety in neonates not known.
Cefoperazone (Cefobid)	**Inj:** 1 gm, 2 gm, 10 mg	**Adults: IV:** 6-12 gm given as bid-qid.	■B ❊>

Cefotaxime Sodium (Claforan)	**Inj:** 500 mg, 1 gm, 2 gm, 10 gm	**IV: Adults or >50 kg:** 2 gm q4h. **Max:** 12 gm/d. **1 mth-12 yo: <50 kg:** 50-180 mg/kg/d divided into 4-6 doses. **1-4 wks:** 50 mg/kg IV q8h. **0-1 wk:** 50 mg/kg IV q12h.	◙B ❋> **R**
Cefoxitin (Mefoxin)	**Inj:** (Generic) 1 gm, 1 gm/50 ml, 2 gm, 2 gm/50 ml, 10 gm, (Mefoxin) 1 gm/50 ml, 2 gm/ 50 ml	**IV: Adults:** 1 gm q4h or 2 gm q6-8h. **Peds: ≥3 mths:** 80-160 mg/kg/d given as q4-6h. **Max:** 12 gm/d.	◙B ❋> **R**
Ceftazidime (Ceptaz, Fortaz, Tazicef)	**Inj:** 500 mg, 1 gm, 2 gm, 6 gm, 10 gm	**IV: Fortaz/Tazicef: Adults:** 2 gm q8h. **Peds: 1 mth-12 yo:** 30-50 mg/kg q8h, up to 6 gm/d. **0-4 wks:** 30 mg/kg q12h. **Ceptaz: Adults & Peds: ≥12 yo:** 2 gm q8h.	◙B ❋> (Fortaz, Tazicef) ❋v (Ceptaz) **R**
Ceftizoxime (Cefizox)	**Inj:** 500 mg, 1 gm, 2 gm, 10 gm	**IV: Adults:** 3-4 gm q8h. **Peds: ≥6 mths:** 50 mg/kg q6-8h, not to exceed adult dose.	◙B ❋> **R**
Ceftriaxone Sodium (Rocephin)	**Inj:** 1 gm/50 ml, 2 gm/50 ml, 250 mg, 500 mg, 1 gm, 2 gm, 10 gm	**IV: Adults:** 1-2 gm qd (or in equally divided doses bid). **Max:** 4 gm/d. **Peds:** 50-75 mg/kg in divided doses q12h. **Max:** 2 gm/d.	◙B ❋>
Cefuroxime (Kefurox, Zinacef)	**Inj:** 750 mg, 1.5 gm, 7.5 gm	**IV: Adults:** 1.5 gm q6-8h. **Peds: >3 mths:** 100 mg/kg/d given q6-8h. **Max:** 4.5 gm/d.	◙B ❋> **R**
Cephalothin Sodium	**Inj:** 1 gm/50 ml, 2 gm/50 ml	**IV: Adults:** 1-2 gm q4h. **Peds:** 20-30 mg/kg q4h.	◙B ❋> **R**

[1] Potential neurotoxicity, ototoxicity & neuromuscular blockade. Avoid concurrent use with neurotoxic/nephrotoxic agents & diuretics.

NAME	FORM/STRENGTH	DOSAGE	COMMENTS
MONOBACTAMS			
Aztreonam (Azactam)	**Inj:** 500 mg, 1 gm, 2 gm, 1 gm/50 ml, 2 gm/50 ml	**IV: Adults:** 2 gm q6-8h. **Peds:** 30 mg/kg q6-8h.	◙B ❈v **R**
PENICILLINS			
Nafcillin Sodium	**Inj:** 1 gm/50 ml, 1 gm, 2 gm, 10 gm	**Adults: Usual:** 0.5 gm q4-6h (IM) or q4h (IV). **Severe Infection:** 1 gm IM/IV q4h.	◙B ❈>
Oxacillin Sodium	**Inj:** 1 gm/50 ml, 2 gm/50 ml, 1 gm, 2 gm, 10 gm	**Adults:** 1 gm IM/IV q4-6h. **Peds: <40 kg:** 100 mg/kg/d IM/IV divided q4-6h. **Premature & Neonates:** 25 mg/kg/d IM/IV.	◙B ❈>
Piperacillin Sodium	**Inj:** 2 gm, 3 gm, 4 gm	**Adults & Peds: ≥12 yo: IV:** 200-300 mg/kg/d given as q4-6h or 3-4 gm q4-6h.	◙B ❈> **R**
Ticarcillin Disodium/ Clavulanate Potassium (Timentin)	**Inj:** 3 gm-100 mg, 3 gm-100 mg/100 ml, 30 gm-1 gm	**IV: Adults: ≥60 kg:** 300 mg/kg/d ticarcillin given q4h. **<60 kg:** 200-300 mg/kg/d ticarcillin given q4-6h. **Peds: ≥3 mths & <60 kg:** 50 mg/kg/d ticarcillin given q4h. **≥3 mths & ≥60 kg:** 3.1 gm q4h.	◙B ❈> **R**
Ticarcillin (Ticar)	**Inj:** 3 gm, 20 gm	**Adults & Peds:** 200-300 mg/kg/d IV given q4-6h. **0-7 days & <2000 gm:** 75 mg/kg IM/IV q12h. **0-7 days & >2000 gm or >7 days & <2000 gm:** 75 mg/kg IM/IV q8h. **>7 days & >2000 gm:** 100 mg/kg IM/IV q8h.	◙N ❈>
MISCELLANEOUS			
Chloramphenicol (Chloromycetin)	**Inj:** 1 gm	**IV: Adults & Peds:** 50-100 mg/kg/d given q6h. **Infants:** 25 mg/kg/d given q6h.	◙N ❈v **H R** Serious, fatal blood dyscrasias.

Clindamycin (Cleocin)	**Inj:** 150 mg/ml, 300 mg/50 ml, 600 mg/ 50 ml, 900 mg/50 ml	**IV: Adults:** 1200-2700 mg/d given bid-qid. Up to 4800 mg/d. **Peds: 1 mth-16 yo:** 20-40 mg/kg/d given tid-qid. **<1 mth:** 15-20 mg/kg/d given tid-qid.	◉B ❁v Associated with severe, fatal colitis.
Imipenem/Cilastatin Sodium (Primaxin IV)	**Inj:** 250-250 mg, 500-500 mg	**IV: Adults: ≥70 kg: Mild:** 250-500 mg q6h. **Moderate:** 500 mg q6-8h or 1 gm q8h. **Severe:** 500 mg q6h or 1 gm q6-8h. **Max:** 50 mg/kg/d or 4 gm/d, whichever is lower. **Peds: ≥3 mths:** 15-25 mg/kg q6h. **Max:** 4 gm/d. **4 wks-3 mths & ≥1500 gm:** 25 mg/kg q6h. **1-4 wks & ≥1500 gm:** 25 mg/kg q8h. **<1 wk & ≥1500 gm:** 25 mg/kg q12h.	◉C ❁> **R**
Vancomycin	**Inj:** 500 mg, 1 gm, 5 gm, 500 mg/10 ml, 1 gm/20 ml, 5 gm/ 100 ml, 10 gm/100 ml, 500 mg/100 ml, 1 gm/200 ml	**IV: Adults:** 500 mg q6h or 1 gm q12h. **Peds:** 10 mg/kg q6h. **Infants & Neonates:** 15 mg/kg x 1 dose then 10 mg/kg q12h for 1st wk of life, & q8h up to 1 mth of age.	◉C ❁v **R**

Skin/Skin Structure Infection

CARBAPENEM

Ertapenem Sodium (Invanz)	**Inj:** 1 gm	**Adults:**1 gm qd x 7-14d. May give IV up to14d; IM up to 7d.	◉B ❁> **R**
Meropenem (Merrem)	**Inj:** 500 mg, 1 gm	**IV: Adults & Peds: ≥3 mths: >50 kg:** 500 mg q8h. **50 kg:** 10 mg/kg q8h. **Max:** 500 mg q8h.	◉B ❁> **R**

NAME	FORM/STRENGTH	DOSAGE	COMMENTS
CEPHALOSPORINS			
Cefaclor (Ceclor, Ceclor CD)	**Cap:** 250 mg, 500 mg; **Susp:** 125 mg/5 ml, 187 mg/5 ml, 250 mg/5 ml, 375 mg/5 ml; **Tab,ER:** (CD) 375 mg, 500 mg	**Adults: Cap/Susp:** 250 mg q8h. **Tab,ER:** 375 mg q12h. **Peds: ≥1 mth: Cap/Susp:** 20 mg/kg/d given q8h. **Max:**1 gm/d.	B ❀>
Cefadroxil (Duricef)	**Cap:** 500 mg; **Susp:** 250 mg/5 ml, 500 mg/5 ml; **Tab:** 1 gm	**Adults:** 1 gm qd or 500 mg bid. **Peds:** 15 mg/kg q12h (or 30 mg/kg qd for impetigo).	B ❀> **R**
Cefdinir (Omnicef)	**Cap:** 300 mg; **Susp:** 125 mg/5 ml, 250 mg/5 ml	**Adults & Peds: ≥13 yo:** 300 mg cap q12h x 10d. **6 mths-12 yo:** 7 mg/kg susp q12h x 10d.	B ❀> **R**
Cefditoren Pivoxil (Spectracef)	**Tab:** 200 mg	**Adults & Peds: ≥12 yo:** 200 mg bid x 10d.	B ❀> **R**
Cefepime HCl (Maxipime)	**Inj:** 500 mg, 1 gm, 2 gm	**Adults: Moderate-Severe:** 2 gm IV q12h x 10d. **Peds: 2 mths-16 yo: ≤40 kg:** 50 mg/kg IV q12h. **Max:** Do not exceed adult dose.	B ❀> **R**
Cefpodoxime Proxetil (Vantin)	**Susp:** 50 mg/5 ml, 100 mg/5 ml; **Tab:** 100 mg, 200 mg	**Adults & Peds: ≥12 yo:** 400 mg q12h x 7-14d.	B ❀v **R**
Cefprozil (Cefzil)	**Susp:** 125 mg/5 ml, 250 mg/5 ml; **Tab:** 250 mg, 500 mg	**Uncomplicated: Adults & Peds: ≥13 yo:** 250-500 mg q12h or 500 mg q24h x 10d. **2-12 yo:** 20 mg/kg q24h x 10d.	B ❀> **R**

Ceftriaxone Sodium (Rocephin)	**Inj:** 1 gm/50 ml, 2 gm/50 ml, 250 mg, 500 mg, 1 gm, 2 gm, 10 gm	**IM/IV: Adults: Usual:** 1-2 gm qd (or in equally divided doses bid). **Max:** 4 gm/d. **Peds:** 50-75 mg/kg given qd (or in equally divided doses bid). **Max:** 2 gm/d.	◙B ❁>
Cefuroxime Axetil (Ceftin)	**Susp:** 125 mg/5 ml, 250 mg/5 ml; **Tab:** 125 mg, 250 mg, 500 mg	**Adults & Peds: ≥13 yo: Tab:** 250-500 mg bid x 10d. **3 mths-12 yo: Susp:** 15 mg/kg/d bid x 10d for impetigo.	◙B ❁v **R** Tabs & susp not bioequivalent.
Cephalexin (Keflex, Panixine DisperDose)	**Cap:** (Keflex) 250 mg, 333 mg, 500 mg, 750 mg; **Tab, Dispersible:** (Panixine DisperDose) 125 mg, 250 mg.	**Adults:** 500 mg q12h. **Max:** 4 gm/d. **Peds:** 25-50 mg/kg/d given q12h.	◙B ❁>
Cephradine (Velosef)	**Cap:** 250 mg, 500 mg; **Susp:** 250 mg/5 ml	**Adults:** 250 mg q6h or 500 mg q12h. **Peds: >9 mths:** 25-50 mg/kg/d given q6h or q12h (up to adult dose).	◙B ❁> **R**

MACROLIDES

Azithromycin (Zithromax)	**Susp:** 100 mg/5 ml, 200 mg/5 ml, 1 gm/pkt; **Tab:** 250 mg, 500 mg, 600 mg	**Adults: ≥16 yo:** 500 mg qd x 1d, then 250 mg qd on Days 2-5.	◙B ❁>
Clarithromycin (Biaxin)	**Susp:** 125 mg/5 ml, 250 mg/5 ml; **Tab:** 250 mg, 500 mg	**Adults:** 250 mg q12h x 7-14d. **Peds: ≥6 mths:** 7.5 mg/kg q12h x 10d.	◙C ❁> **R**
Dirithromycin (Dynabac)	**Tab,Delay:** 250 mg	**Adults & Peds: ≥12 yo:** 500 mg qd x 5-7d.	◙C ❁>

NAME	FORM/STRENGTH	DOSAGE	COMMENTS
Erythromycin Base	**Tab:** 250 mg	**Adults: Usual:** 250 mg q6h or 500 mg q12h. **Peds: Usual:** 30-50 mg/kg/d in divided doses. **Max:** 4 gm/d.	B >
Erythromycin (Ery-Tab, PCE)	**Tab,Delay:** (Ery-Tab) 250 mg, 333 mg, 500 mg; **Tab,ER:** (PCE) 333 mg, 500 mg	**Adults: Usual:** 250 mg qid, 333 mg q8h, or 500 mg q12h. **Peds: Usual:** 30-50 mg/kg/d in divided doses. **Max:** 4 gm/d.	B >
Erythromycin Ethylsuccinate (E.E.S., EryPed)	**Chewtab:** (EryPed) 200 mg; **Susp:** (EryPed) 100 mg/2.5 ml, 200 mg/5 ml, 400 mg/5 ml, (E.E.S.) 200 mg/5 ml, 400 mg/5 ml; **Tab:** (E.E.S.) 400 mg	**Adults: Usual:** 1600 mg/d given q6h, q8h, or q12h. **Max:** 4 gm/d. **Peds: Usual:** 30-50 mg/kg/d in divided doses q6h, q8h, or q12h. Double dose for more severe infections.	B >
Erythromycin Stearate (Erythrocin)	**Tab:** 250 mg, 500 mg	**Adults: Usual:** 250 mg q6h or 500 mg q12h. **Peds: Usual:** 30-50 mg/kg/d in divided doses. **Max:** 4 gm/d.	B >
MONOBACTAMS			
Loracarbef (Lorabid)	**Cap:** 200 mg, 400 mg; **Susp:** 100 mg/5 ml, 200 mg/5 ml	**Adults & Peds: ≥13 yo:** 200 mg q12h x 7d. **Impetigo: 6 mths-12 yo:** 7.5 mg/kg q12h x 7d.	B > **R**
OXAZOLIDINONE			
Linezolid (Zyvox)	**Inj:** 2 mg/ml; **Susp:** 100 mg/5 ml; **Tab:** 600 mg	**Complicated:** Treat x 10-14d. **Adults & Peds: ≥12 yo:** 600 mg IV/PO q12h. **Birth-11 yo:** 10 mg/kg IV/PO q8h. **Uncomplicated:** Treat x 10-14d. **Adults:** 400 mg PO q12h. **Peds: ≥12 yo:** 600 mg PO q12h. **5-11 yo:** 10 mg/kg PO q12h. **<5 yo:** 10 mg/kg PO q8h.	C >

Amoxicillin (Amoxil, DisperMox,Trimox)	**Cap:** (Amoxil, Trimox) 250 mg, 500 mg; **Chewtab:** (Amoxil) 200 mg, 400 mg; **Susp:** (Amoxil) 50 mg/ml, 125 mg/5 ml, 200 mg/ 5 ml, 250 mg/5 ml, 400 mg/5 ml, (Trimox) 125 mg/5 ml, 250 mg/ 5 ml; **Tab:** (Amoxil) 500 mg, 875 mg; **Tab, Dispersible:** (DisperMox) 200 mg, 400 mg, 600 mg	**Adults & Peds: >40 kg:** 500-875 mg q12h or 250-500 mg q8h, depending on severity. **>3 mths:** 25-45 mg/kg/d divided q12h or 20-40 mg/kg/d divided q8h, depending on severity. **≤3 mths: Usual/Max:** 15 mg/kg q12h.	●B ❋> **R**
Amoxicillin/Clavulanate (Augmentin)	**Chewtab:** 125-31.25 mg, 200-28.5 mg, 250-62.5 mg, 400-57 mg; **Susp:** (per 5 ml)125-31,25 mg, 200-28.5 mg, 250-62.5 mg, 400-57 mg; **Tab:** 250-125 mg, 500-125 mg, 875-125 mg	Dose based on amoxicillin component. **Adults & Peds: ≥40 kg: Tab:** 500-875 mg q12h or 250-500 mg q8h, depending on severity. May use 125 mg/5 ml or 250 mg/5 ml susp in place of 500 mg tab & 200 mg/ 5 ml susp or 400 mg/5 ml susp in place of 875 mg tab. **≥12 wks: Chewtab/Susp:** 25-45 mg/kg/d given q12h or 20-40 mg/kg/d given q8h, depending on severity. **<12 wks: Susp:** 15 mg/kg q12h (use 125 mg/5 ml susp).	●B ❋> **H R** 2- 250 mg tabs are not equivalent to 1- 500 mg tab. Only use 250 mg tab if peds ≥40 kg. Chewtab & tab not interchangeable.
Ampicillin Sodium/ Sulbactam Sodium (Unasyn)	**Inj:** 1-0.5 gm, 2-1 gm, 10-5 gm	**Adults & Peds: ≥1 yo:** 1.5-3 gm IV/IM q6h. **Max:** 4 gm sulbactam/d.	●B ❋> **R**

NAME	FORM/STRENGTH	DOSAGE	COMMENTS
Dicloxacillin Sodium (Dynapen)	**Cap:** 250 mg, 500 mg; **Susp:** 62.5 mg/5 ml	**Adults & Peds: ≥40 kg: Mild-Moderate:** 125 mg q6h. **Severe:** 250 mg q6h. **<40 kg: Mild-Moderate:** 3.125 mg/kg q6h. **Severe:** 6.25 mg/kg q6h.	B >
Penicillin V Potassium (Penicillin VK, Veetids)	**Susp:** 125 mg/5 ml, 250 mg/5 ml; **Tab:** 250 mg, 500 mg	**Adults & Peds: ≥12 yo:** 250-500 mg q6-8h.	B >
Piperacillin/Tazobactam (Zosyn)	**Inj:** 40-5 mg/ml, 60-7.5 mg/ml, 2-0.25 gm, 3-0.375 gm, 4-0.5 gm, 4-0.5 gm/100 ml, 36-4.5 gm	**Adults: IV:** 3.375 gm q6h x 7-10d.	B > **R**

QUINOLONES

NAME	FORM/STRENGTH	DOSAGE	COMMENTS
Ciprofloxacin (Cipro)	**Inj:** 10 mg/ml, 200 mg/100 ml, 400 mg/200 ml; **Susp:** 250 mg/5 ml, 500 mg/5 ml; **Tab:** 250 mg, 500 mg, 750 mg	**Adults: ≥18 yo: Mild-Moderate:** 500 mg PO q12h or 400 mg IV q12h x 7-14d. **Severe/Complicated:** 750 mg PO q12h or 400 mg IV q8h x 7-14d.	C v **R** CI with tizanidine
Levofloxacin (Levaquin)	**Inj:** 5 mg/ml, 25 mg/ml; **Sol:** 25 mg/ml; **Tab:** 250 mg, 500 mg, 750 mg	**Adults: ≥18 yo: Uncomplicated:** 500 mg IV/PO qd x 7-10d. **Complicated:** 750 mg IV/PO qd x 7-14d.	C v **R**
Moxifloxacin HCl (Avelox)	**Inj:** 400 mg/250 ml; **Tab:** 400 mg	**Adults: ≥18 yo: Uncomplicated:** 400 mg IV/PO q24h x 7d. **Complicated:** 400 mg IV/PO q24h x 7-21d.	C v

Ofloxacin (Floxin)	**Tab:** 200 mg, 300 mg, 400 mg	**Adults: ≥18 yo:** 400 mg q12h x 10d.	C v **H R**
STREPTOGRAMIN AGENT			
Dalfopristin/Quinupristin (Synercid)	**Inj:** 350-150 mg; 420-180 mg	**Complicated: Adults & Peds: ≥16 yo:** 7.5 mg/kg IV q12h for at least 7d.	B > **H**
TETRACYCLINES			
Doxycycline Hyclate (Doryx, Vibramycin, Vibra-Tabs)	**Cap:** (Vibramycin) 100 mg; **Cap,Delay:** (Doryx) 75 mg, 100 mg; **Tab:** (Vibra-Tabs) 100 mg	**Adults:** 100 mg q12h on Day 1, then 100 mg qd or 50 mg q12h. **Severe:** 100 mg q12h. **Peds: >8 yo & ≤100 lbs:** 1 mg/lb bid on Day 1, then 1 mg/lb qd or 0.5 mg/lb bid. **Severe:** 2 mg/lb. **>100 lbs:** Adult dose.	D v
Doxycycline Monohydrate (Monodox, Vibramycin)	**Cap:** (Monodox) 50 mg, 100 mg; **Susp:** (Vibramycin) 25 mg/5 ml	**Adults:** 100 mg q12h or 50 mg q6h on Day 1, then 100 mg qd or 50 mg q12h. **Severe:** 100 mg q12h. **Peds: >8 yo & ≤100 lbs:** 1 mg/lb bid on Day 1, then 1 mg/lb qd or 0.5 mg/lb bid. **Severe:** 2 mg/lb. **>100 lbs:** Adult dose.	D v
Minocycline HCl (Dynacin, Minocin)	**Cap:** (Dynacin) 50 mg, 75 mg, 100 mg, (Minocin) 50 mg, 100 mg; **Inj:** (Minocin) 100 mg ; **Tab:** (Dynacin) 50 mg, 75 mg, 100 mg	**Adults:** 200 mg PO/IV, then 100 mg q12h or 50 mg qid. **Peds: >8 yo:** 4 mg/kg PO/IV, then 2 mg/kg q12h.	D v **R**

NAME	FORM/STRENGTH	DOSAGE	COMMENTS
MISCELLANEOUS			
Clindamycin (Cleocin)	**Cap:** 75 mg, 150 mg, 300 mg; **Inj:** 150 mg/ml, 300 mg/50 ml, 600 mg/50 ml, 900 mg/50 ml; **Susp:** 75 mg/5 ml	**IM/IV: Adults:** 600-2700 mg/d in 2-4 doses. **Max:** 600 mg IM single dose. **Peds: 1 mth-16 yo:** 20-40 mg/kg/d in 3-4 doses. **<1 mth:** 15-20 mg/kg/d in 3-4 doses. **PO: Adults:** 150-450 mg q6h. **Peds:** 8-20 mg/kg/d given 3-4 doses.	◉B ❋v (IV) ❋> (PO) Associated with severe, fatal colitis.
Daptomycin (Cubicin)	**Inj:** 250 mg, 500 mg	**Adults: ≥18 yo:** 4 mg/kg IV infusion over 30 min once every 24 h x 7-14d.	◉B ❋> **R**
Tigecycline (Tygacil)	**Inj:** 50 mg/5 ml	**Adults:** 100 mg IV, followed by 50 mg IV q12h x 5-14d.	◉D ❋> **H**

Tuberculosis

Aminosalicylic Acid (Paser)	**Granule:** 4 gm/pkt	**Adults:** 4 gm tid.	◉C ❋>
Ethambutol HCl (Myambutol)	**Tab:** 100 mg, 400 mg	**Adults & Peds: ≥13 yo: Initial:** 15 mg/kg q24h. **Retreatment:** 25 mg/kg q24h x 60d, then decrease to 15 mg/kg q24h.	◉N ❋> **R**
Ethionamide (Trecator)	**Tab:** 250 mg	**Usual: Adults:** 15-20 mg/kg qd or in divided doses. **Max:** 1 gm/d. **Peds: ≥12 yo:** 10-20 mg/kg/d as bid-tid after meals or 15 mg/kg/qd.	◉C ❋>
Isoniazid (Nydrazid)	**Inj:** 100 mg/ml; **Syr:** 50 mg/5 ml; **Tab:** 100 mg, 300 mg	**Active TB: Adults:** 5 mg/kg, up to 300 mg qd, as single dose or15 mg/kg, up to 900 mg/d, 2-3 times/wk. **Peds:** 10-15 mg/kg, up to 300 mg qd, as single dose or 20-40 mg/kg, up to 900 mg/d, 2-3 times/wk. **Prevention: Adults:** 300 mg qd. **Peds:** 10 mg/kg qd, up to 300 mg qd.	◉N ❋> [14]

[14] INH associated with hepatitis. Avoid in acute hepatic diseases.

RECOMMENDED DRUGS FOR THE INITIAL TREATMENT OF TUBERCULOSIS IN CHILDREN* & ADULTS

DOSAGE SCHEDULE**

DRUG	DAILY DOSE (maximum dose)		TWO DOSES PER WEEK (maximum dose)		THREE DOSES PER WEEK (maximum dose)	
	CHILDREN	ADULTS	CHILDREN	ADULTS	CHILDREN	ADULTS
Isoniazid	10-15 mg/kg (300 mg)	5 mg/kg (300 mg)	20-30 mg/kg (900 mg)	15 mg/kg (900 mg)	—	15 mg/kg (900 mg)
Rifampin†	10-20 mg/kg (600 mg)	10 mg/kg (600 mg)	10-20 mg/kg (600 mg)	10 mg/kg (600 mg)	—	10 mg/kg (600 mg)
Pyrazinamide	15-30 mg/kg (2 gm)	18.2-26.8 mg/kg (2 gm)	50 mg/kg (2 gm)	36.4-53.6 mg/kg (4 gm)	—	27.3-44.6 mg/kg (3 gm)
Ethambutol‡	15-20 mg/kg (1 gm)	14.5-21.4 mg/kg (1.6 gm)	50 mg/kg (2.5 gm)	36.4-52.6 mg/kg (4 gm)	—	21.8-35.7 mg/kg (2.4 gm)

* Persons ≤14 yo and ≤40 kg.

Source: *Am J Respir Crit Care Med* 2003; 167: 603-662.

** Based on ideal body weight except adult doses for pyrazinamide and ethambutol (estimated lean body weight).

† Adult dose may need to be adjusted with concomitant use of protease inhibitors or nonnucleoside reverse transcriptase inhibitors.

‡ Caution in children whose vision cannot be monitored (<5 yo). A dose of 15 mg/kg/d can be used in younger children with isoniazid or rifampin resistance.

NAME	FORM/STRENGTH	DOSAGE	COMMENTS
Isoniazid/Pyrazinamide/ Rifampin (Rifater)	**Tab:** 50-300-120 mg	**Adults & Peds: ≥15 yo: Usual: ≤44 kg:** 4 tabs qd, **45-54 kg:** 5 tabs qd. **≥55 kg:** 6 tabs qd. Take 1h before or 2h after a meal. Give pyridoxine to the malnourished, if predisposed to neuropathy, & adolescents.	C v 14
Isoniazid/Rifampin (Rifamate)	**Cap:** 150-300 mg	**Adults: Usual:** 2 caps qd, 1h before or 2h after a meal. Give pyridoxine to the malnourished, if predisposed to neuropathy, & adolescents.	N > 14
Pyrazinamide	**Tab:** 500 mg	**Adults & Peds: Usual:** 15-30 mg/kg qd. **Max:** 3 gm/d. CDC recommends max 2 gm/d w/ daily regimen. **Alternate Regimen:** 50-70 mg/kg BIW. Continue x 2 mths.	C >
Rifampin (Rifadin, Rimactane)	**Cap:** 150 mg, 300 mg; **Inj:** 600 mg	**PO/IV: Adults:** 10 mg/kg qd. **Max:** 600 mg/d. **Peds:** 10-20 mg/kg qd. **Max:** 600 mg/d. Take PO 1h before or 2h after a meal w/ full glass of water. Continue x 2 mths.	C v
Rifapentine (Priftin)	**Tab:** 150 mg	**Adults & Peds: ≥12 yo: Intensive Phase: Initial:** 600 mg BIW w/ interval of not <72h between doses. Continue x 2 mths. **Maint:** 600 mg once wkly x 4 mths. Give pyridoxine to the malnourished, if predisposed to neuropathy, & adolescents.	C v

Upper Respiratory Tract Infection

CEPHALOSPORINS

NAME	FORM/STRENGTH	DOSAGE	COMMENTS
Cefaclor (Ceclor, Ceclor CD)	**Cap:** 250 mg, 500 mg; **Susp:** 125 mg/5 ml, 187 mg/5 ml, 250 mg/	**Adults: Cap/Susp:** 250 mg q8h. **Tab,ER:** 375 mg q12h. **Peds: ≥1 mth: Cap/Susp:** 20 mg/kg/d given q8h. **Max:** 1 gm/d.	B >

	5 ml, 375 mg/5 ml; **Tab,ER:** (CD) 375 mg, 500 mg		
Cefadroxil (Duricef)	**Cap:** 500 mg; **Susp:** 250 mg/5 ml, 500 mg/5 ml; **Tab:** 1 gm	**Adults:** 1 gm qd or 500 mg bid x 10d. **Peds:** 15 mg/kg q12h or 30 mg/kg qd.	◙B ✻> R
Cefdinir (Omnicef)	**Cap:** 300 mg; **Susp:** 125 mg/5 ml; 250 mg/5 ml	**Pharyngitis/Tonsillitis: Adults & Peds: ≥13 yo: Cap:** 300 mg q12h x 5-10d or 600 mg q24h x 10d. **6 mths-12 yo: Susp:** 7 mg/kg q12h x 5-10d or 14 mg/kg q24h x 10d. **Sinusitis: Adults & Peds: ≥13 yo: Cap:** 300 mg q12h or 600 mg q24h x 10d. **6 mths-12 yo: Susp:** 7 mg/kg q12h or 14 mg/kg q24h x 10d.	◙B ✻> R
Cefditoren Pivoxil (Spectracef)	**Tab:** 200 mg	**Pharyngitis/Tonsillitis: Adults & Peds: ≥12 yo:** 200 mg bid x 10d.	◙B ✻> R
Cefixime (Suprax)	**Susp:** 100 mg/5 ml	**Pharyngitis/Tonsillitis: Adults & Peds: >12 yo or >50 kg: Tab/Susp:** 400 mg qd or 200 mg bid. **≤50 kg or >6 mths: Susp:** 8 mg/kg qd or 4 mg/kg bid.	◙B ✻v R
Cefpodoxime Proxetil (Vantin)	**Susp:** 50 mg/5 ml, 100 mg/5 ml; **Tab:** 100 mg, 200 mg	**Pharyngitis/Tonsillitis: Adults & Peds: ≥12 yo:** 100 mg q12h x 5-10d. **2 mths-11 yo:** 5 mg/kg q12h x 5-10d. **Sinusitis: Adults & Peds: ≥12 yo:** 200 mg q12h x 10d. **2 mths-11 yo:** 5 mg/kg q12h x 10d.	◙B ✻v R
Cefprozil (Cefzil)	**Susp:** 125 mg/5 ml, 250 mg/5 ml; **Tab:** 250 mg, 500 mg	**Pharyngitis/Tonsillitis: Adults & Peds: ≥13 yo:** 500 mg q24h x 10d. **2-12 yo:** 7.5 mg/kg q12h x 10d. **Max:** Adult dose. **Sinusitis: Adults & Peds: ≥13 yo:** 250-500 mg q12h x 10d. **6 mths-12 yo:** 7.5-15 mg/kg q12h x 10d. **Max:** Adult dose.	◙B ✻> R

[14] INH associated with hepatitis. Avoid in acute hepatic diseases.

NAME	FORM/STRENGTH	DOSAGE	COMMENTS
Ceftibuten (Cedax)	**Cap:** 400 mg; **Susp:** 90 mg/5 ml	**Pharyngitis/Tonsillitis: Adults & Peds: ≥12 yo:** 400 mg qd x 10d. **≥6 mths:** 9 mg/kg qd x 10d. **Max:** 400 mg/d.	B > **R**
Cefuroxime Axetil (Ceftin)	**Susp:** 125 mg/5 ml, 250 mg/5 ml; **Tab:** 125 mg, 250 mg, 500 mg	**Pharyngitis/Tonsillitis/Sinusitis: Adults & Peds: ≥13 yo: Tab:** 250 mg bid x 10d. **3 mths-12 yo: Pharyngitis/ Tonsillitis: Tab:** 125 mg bid x 10d. **Susp:** 10 mg/kg bid x 10d. **Max:** 500 mg/d. **Sinusitis: Tab:** 250 mg bid x 10d. **Susp:** 15 mg/kg bid x 10d. **Max:** 1 gm/d.	B v **R** Tabs & susp not bioequivalent.
Cephalexin (Keflex, Panixine DisperDose)	**Cap:** (Keflex) 250 mg, 333 mg, 500 mg, 750 mg; **Tab, Dispersible:** (Panixine DisperDose) 125 mg, 250 mg.	**Adults: Usual:** 250 mg q6h. **Streptococcal Pharyngitis:** 500 mg q12h. **Max:** 4 gm/d. **Peds: >1 yo: Usual:** 25-50 mg/kg/d given q12h.	B >
Cephradine (Velosef)	**Cap:** 250 mg, 500 mg; **Susp:** 250 mg/5 ml	**Tonsillitis/Pharyngitis: Adults:** 250 mg q6h or 500 mg q12h. **Peds: >9 mths:** 25-50 mg/kg/d given q6h or q12h (up to adult dose).	B > **R**
KETOLIDES			
Telithromycin (Ketek)	**Tab:** 300 mg, 400 mg	**Sinusitis: Adults:** 800 mg qd x 5d.	C > **H R**
MACROLIDES			
Azithromycin (Zithromax, Zmax)	(Zithromax) **Susp:** 100 mg/ 5 ml, 200 mg/ 5 ml, 1 gm/pkt; **Tab:** 250 mg, 500 mg, 600 mg. (Zmax) **Susp,ER:** 2 gm	**Pharyngitis/Tonsillitis: Zithromax: Adults:** 500 mg qd x 1d, then 250 mg qd on Days 2-5. **Peds: ≥2 yo:** 12 mg/kg qd x 5d. **Acute Bacterial Sinusitis: Zithromax: Adults:** 500 mg qd x 3d. **Peds: ≥6 mths:** 10 mg/kg qd x 3d. **Zmax: Adults:** 2 gm single dose.	B >

Clarithromycin (Biaxin)	**Susp:** 125 mg/5 ml, 250 mg/5 ml; **Tab:** 250 mg, 500 mg; **Tab,ER:** 500 mg	**Adults: Pharyngitis/Tonsillitis: Susp/Tab:** 250 mg q12h x 10d. **Sinusitis: Susp/Tab:** 500 mg q12h x 14d. **Tab,ER:** 1 gm qd x 14d. **Peds: ≥6 mths: Pharyngitis/Tonsillitis/Sinusitis: Susp/Tab:** 7.5 mg/kg q12h x 10d.	●C ❋> **R**
Dirithromycin (Dynabac)	**Tab,Delay:** 250 mg	**Adults & Peds: ≥12 yo:** 500 mg qd x 7-10d.	●C ❋>
Erythromycin Base	**Tab:** 250 mg	**Adults: Usual:** 250 mg q6h or 500 mg q12h. **Peds: Usual:** 30-50 mg/kg/d in divided doses. **Max:** 4 gm/d.	●B ❋>
Erythromycin (Ery-Tab, PCE)	**Tab,Delay:** (Ery-Tab) 250 mg, 333 mg, 500 mg; **Tab,ER:** (PCE) 333 mg, 500 mg	**Adults: Usual:** 250 mg qid, 333 mg q8h, or 500 mg q12h. **Peds: Usual:** 30-50 mg/kg/d in divided doses. **Max:** 4 gm/d.	●B ❋>
Erythromycin Ethylsuccinate (E.E.S., EryPed)	**Chewtab:** (EryPed) 200 mg; **Susp:** (EryPed) 100 mg/2.5 ml, 200 mg/5 ml, 400 mg/5 ml, (E.E.S.) 200 mg/5ml, 400 mg/5 ml; **Tab:** (E.E.S.) 400mg	**Adults: Usual:** 1600 mg/d given q6h, q8h, or q12h. **Max:** 4 gm/d. **Peds: Usual:** 30-50 mg/kg/d in divided doses q6h, q8h, or q12h. Double dose for more severe infections.	●B ❋>
Erythromycin Stearate (Erythrocin)	**Tab:** 250 mg, 500 mg	**Adults: Usual:** 250 mg q6h or 500 mg q12h. **Peds: Usual:** 30-50 mg/kg/d in divided doses. **Max:** 4 gm/d.	●B ❋>
MONOBACTAMS			
Loracarbef (Lorabid)	**Cap:** 200 mg, 400 mg; **Susp:** 100 mg/5 ml, 200 mg/5 ml	**Pharyngitis/Tonsillitis: Adults & Peds: ≥13 yo:** 200 mg q12h x 7d. **6 mths-12 yo:** 7.5 mg/kg q12h x 10d. **Sinusitis: Adults & Peds: ≥13 yo:** 400 mg q12h x 12d. **6 mths-12 yo:** 15mg/kg q12h x 10d.	●B ❋> **R**

PENICILLINS

NAME	FORM/STRENGTH	DOSAGE	COMMENTS
Amoxicillin (Amoxil, DisperMox, Trimox)	**Cap:** (Amoxil, Trimox) 250 mg, 500 mg; **Chewtab:** (Amoxil) 200 mg, 400 mg; **Susp:** (Amoxil) 50 mg/ ml, 125 mg/5 ml, 200 mg/5 ml, 250 mg/5 ml, 400 mg/5 ml, (Trimox) 125 mg/5 ml, 250 mg/ 5 ml; **Tab:** (Amoxil) 500 mg, 875 mg; **Tab, Dispersible:** (DisperMox) 200 mg, 400 mg, 600 mg	**Adults & Peds: >40 kg:** 500-875 mg q12h or 250-500 mg q8h, depending on severity. **>3 mths:** 25-45 mg/kg/d divided q12h or 20-40 mg/kg/d divided q8h, depending on severity. **≤3 mths: Usual/Max:** 15 mg/kg q12h.	◙B ✿> **R**
Amoxicillin/Clavulanate (Augmentin)	**Chewtab:** 125-31.25 mg, 200-28.5 mg, 250-62.5 mg, 400-57 mg; **Susp:** (per 5 ml) 125-31.25 mg, 200-28.5 mg, 250-62.5 mg, 400-57 mg; **Tab:** 250-125 mg, 500-125 mg, 875-125 mg	Dose based on amoxicillin component. **Adults & Peds: ≥40 kg: Tab:** 500-875 mg q12h or 250-500 mg q8h, depending on severity. May use 125 mg/5 ml or 250 mg/5 ml susp in place of 500 mg tab & 200 mg/ 5 ml susp or 400 mg/5 ml susp in place of 875 mg tab. **≥12 wks: Chewtab/Susp:** 25-45 mg/kg/d given q12h or 20-40 mg/kg/d given q8h, depending on severity. **<12 wks: Susp:** 15 mg/kg q12h (use 125 mg/5 ml susp).	◙B ✿> **H R** 2-250 mg tabs are not equivalent to 1- 500 mg tab. Only use 250 mg tab if peds ≥40 kg. Chewtab & tab not interchangeable.
Amoxicillin/Clavulanate (Augmentin XR)	**Tab,ER:** 1000-62.5 mg	**Sinusitis: Adults & Peds: ≥16 yo:** 2 tabs q12h x 10d.	◙ B ✿>

Ampicillin (Principen)	**Cap:** 250 mg, 500 mg; **Susp:** 125 mg/5ml, 250 mg/5ml	**Adults & Peds: >20 kg:** 250 mg qid. **≤20 kg:** 50 mg/kg/d given tid-qid.	◙B ❋>
Ampicillin Sodium	**Inj:** 125 mg, 250 mg, 500 mg, 1 gm, 2 gm, 10 gm	**IM/IV: Adults & Peds: ≥40 kg:** 250-500 mg q6h. **<40 kg:** 25-50 mg/kg/d given q6-8h.	◙B ❋>
Dicloxacillin Sodium (Dynapen)	**Cap:** 250 mg, 500 mg; **Susp:** 62.5 mg/5 ml	**Adults & Peds: ≥40 kg: Mild-Moderate:** 125 mg q6h. **Severe:** 250 mg q6h. **<40 kg: Mild-Moderate:** 3.125 mg/kg q6h. **Severe:** 6.25 mg/kg q6h.	◙B ❋>
Penicillin V Potassium (Penicillin VK, Veetids)	**Susp:** 125 mg/5 ml, 250 mg/5 ml; **Tab:** 250 mg, 500 mg	**Adults & Peds: ≥12 yo: Streptococcal:** 125-250 mg q6-8h x 10d. **Fusospirochetosis:** (Oropharnyx) 250-500 mg q6-8h. **Pneumococcal:** 250-500 mg q6h until afebrile x 2d.	◙B ❋>

QUINOLONES

Ciprofloxacin (Cipro)	**Inj:** 10 mg/ml, 200 mg/100 ml, 400 mg/200 ml; **Susp:** 250 mg/5 ml, 500 mg/5 ml; **Tab:** 250 mg, 500 mg, 750 mg	**Mild/Moderate Acute Sinusitis: Adults: ≥18 yo:** 500 mg PO q12h or 400 mg IV q12h x 10d.	◙C ❋v **R** CI with tizanidine
Levofloxacin (Levaquin)	**Inj:** 5 mg/ml, 25 mg/ml; **Sol:** 25 mg/ml; **Tab:** 250 mg, 500 mg, 750 mg	**Sinusitis: Adults: ≥18 yo:** 500 mg IV/PO qd x 10-14d or 750 mg IV/PO qd x 5d.	◙C ❋v **R**

NAME	FORM/STRENGTH	DOSAGE	COMMENTS
Moxifloxacin HCl (Avelox)	**Inj:** 400 mg/250 ml; **Tab:** 400 mg	**Sinusitis: Adults: ≥18 yo:** 400 mg PO/IV qd x 10d.	C v
TETRACYCLINES			
Demeclocycline (Declomycin)	**Tab:** 150 mg, 500 mg	**Adults:** 150 mg qid or 300 mg bid. **Peds: ≥8 yo:** 3-6 mg/lb/d given bid-qid.	N v
Doxycycline Hyclate (Doryx, Vibramycin, Vibra-Tabs)	**Cap:** (Vibramycin) 100 mg; **Cap,Delay:** (Doryx) 75 mg, 100 mg; **Tab:** (Vibra-Tabs)100 mg	**Adults:** 100 mg q12h on Day 1, then 100 mg qd or 50 mg q12h. **Severe:** 100 mg q12h. **Peds: >8 yo & ≤100 lbs:** 1 mg/lb bid on Day 1, then 1 mg/lb qd or 0.5 mg/lb bid. **Severe:** 2 mg/lb. **>100 lbs:** Adult dose.	D v
Doxycycline Monohydrate (Monodox, Vibramycin)	**Cap:** (Monodox) 50 mg, 100 mg; **Susp:** (Vibramycin) 25 mg/5 ml	**Adults:** 100 mg q12h or 50 mg q6h on Day 1, then 100 mg qd or 50 mg q12h. **Peds: >8 yo & ≤100 lbs:** 1 mg/lb bid on Day 1, then 1 mg/lb qd or 0.5 mg/lb bid. **>100 lbs:** Adult dose.	D v
Minocycline HCl (Dynacin, Minocin)	**Cap:** (Dynacin) 50 mg, 75 mg, 100 mg, (Minocin) 50 mg, 100 mg; **Inj:** (Minocin) 100 mg; **Tab:** (Dynacin) 50 mg, 75 mg, 100 mg	**Adults:** 200 mg PO/IV, then 100 mg q12h or 50 mg qid. **Peds: >8 yo:** 4 mg/kg PO/IV, then 2 mg/kg q12h.	D v **R**
Tetracycline HCl (Sumycin)	**Cap:** 250 mg, 500 mg; **Susp:** 125 mg/5 ml	**Adults:** 250 mg qid or 500 mg bid. **Peds: >8 yo:** 25-50 mg/kg divided bid-qid.	D v **R**

Urinary Tract Infection

CARBAPENEM

Ertapenem Sodium (Invanz)	**Inj:** 1 gm	**Complicated UTI: Adults:** 1 gm qd x 10-14d. May give IV up to 14d; IM up to 7d.	B > **R**

CEPHALOSPORINS

Cefaclor (Ceclor, Ceclor CD)	**Cap:** 250 mg, 500 mg; **Susp:** 125 mg/5 ml, 187 mg/5 ml, 250 mg/5 ml, 375 mg/5 ml	**Adults:** 250 mg q8h. **Peds: ≥1 mth:** 20 mg/kg/d q8h.	B >
Cefadroxil (Duricef)	**Cap:** 500 mg; **Susp:** 250 mg/5 ml, 500 mg/5 ml; **Tab:** 1 gm	**Adults: Uncomplicated Lower UTI:** 1-2 gm/d given qd-bid. **Other UTIs:** 1 gm bid. **Peds:** 15 mg/kg q12h.	B > **R**
Cefepime HCl (Maxipime)	**Inj:** 500 mg, 1 gm, 2 gm	**Adults: Mild-Moderate:** 0.5-1 gm IM/IV q12h x 7-10d. **Severe:** 2 gm IV q12h x 10d. **Peds: 2 mths-16 yo: ≤40 kg:** 50 mg/kg IV q12h. **Max:** Do not exceed adult dose.	B > **R**
Cefixime (Suprax)	**Susp:** 100 mg/5 ml	**Adults & Peds: >12 yo or >50 kg: Tab/Susp:** 400 mg qd or 200 mg bid. **≤50 kg or >6 mths: Susp:** 8 mg/kg qd or 4 mg/kg bid.	B v **R**
Cefpodoxime Proxetil (Vantin)	**Susp:** 50 mg/5 ml, 100 mg/5 ml; **Tab:** 100 mg, 200 mg	**Adults & Peds: ≥12 yo: Uncomplicated UTI:** 100 mg q12h x 7d.	B v **R**

 KEY: PREGNANCY RATING; BREASTFEEDING SAFETY; **H** HEPATIC ADJUSTMENT; **R** RENAL ADJUSTMENT

NAME	FORM/STRENGTH	DOSAGE	COMMENTS
Ceftriaxone Sodium (Rocephin)	**Inj:** 1 gm/50 ml, 2 gm/ 50 ml, 250 mg, 500 mg, 1 gm, 2 gm, 10 gm	**Adults: IM/IV:** 1-2 gm qd (or in equally divided doses bid). **Max:** 4 gm/d.	B >
Cefuroxime Axetil (Ceftin)	**Tab:** 125 mg, 250 mg, 500 mg	**Adults & Peds: ≥13 yo:** 125-250 mg bid x 7-10d.	B v **R**
Cefuroxime (Kefurox, Zinacef)	**Inj:** 750 mg, 1.5 gm, 7.5 gm	**IM/IV: Adults: Uncomplicated UTI:** 750 mg q8h x 5-10d. **Severe/Complicated UTI:** 1.5 gm q8h x 5-10d. **Peds: >3 mths:** 50-100 mg/kg/d given q6-8h. **Max:** 4.5 gm/d.	B > **R**
Cephalexin (Keflex, Panixine DisperDose)	**Cap:** (Keflex) 250 mg, 333 mg, 500 mg, 750 mg; **Tab, Dispersible:** (Panixine DisperDose) 125 mg, 250 mg	**Adults: Usual:** 250 mg q6h. **Uncomplicated Cystitis:** 500 mg q12h x 7-14d. **Max:** 4 gm/d. **Peds: Usual:** 25-50 mg/kg/d in divided doses.	B >
Cephradine (Velosef)	**Cap:** 250 mg, 500 mg; **Susp:** 250 mg/5 ml	**Adults: Uncomplicated:** 500 mg q12h. **Serious (Prostatitis):** 500 mg q6h or 1 gm q12h. **Peds: >9 mths:** 25-50 mg/kg/d given q6h or q12h (up to adult dose).	B > **R**
MONOBACTAMS			
Loracarbef (Lorabid)	**Cap:** 200 mg, 400 mg; **Susp:** 100 mg/5 ml, 200 mg/5 ml	**Adults & Peds: ≥13 yo: Cystitis:** 200 mg qd x 7d. **Pyelonephritis:** 400 mg q12h x 14d.	B > **R**

Amoxicillin (Amoxil, DisperMox, Trimox)	**Cap:** (Amoxil, Trimox) 250 mg, 500 mg; **Chewtab:** (Amoxil) 200 mg, 400 mg; **Susp:** (Amoxil) 50 mg/ ml, 125 mg/5 ml, 200 mg/ 5 ml, 250 mg/5 ml, 400 mg/5 ml, (Trimox) 125 mg/5 ml, 250 mg/ 5 ml; **Tab:** (Amoxil) 500 mg, 875 mg; **Tab, Dispersible:** (DisperMox) 200 mg, 400 mg, 600 mg	**Adults & Peds: >40 kg:** 500-875 mg q12h or 250-500 mg q8h, depending on severity. **>3 mths:** 25-45 mg/kg/d divided q12h or 20-40 mg/kg/d divided q8h, depending on severity. **≤3 mths: Usual/Max:** 15 mg/kg q12h.	B > **R**
Amoxicillin/Clavulanate (Augmentin)	**Chewtab:** 125-31.25 mg, 200-28.5 mg, 250-62.5 mg, 400-57 mg; **Susp:** (per 5 ml) 125-31.25 mg, 200-28.5 mg, 250-62.5 mg, 400-57 mg; **Tab:** 250-125 mg, 500-125 mg, 875-125 mg	Dose based on amoxicillin component. **Adults & Peds: ≥40 kg: Tab:** 500 mg q12h or 250 mg q8h. May use 125 mg/5 ml or 250 mg/5 ml susp in place of 500 mg tab & 200 mg/5 ml or 400 mg/5 ml susp in place of 875 mg tab. **≥12 wks: Chewtab/Susp:** 25 mg/kg/d given q12h or 20 mg/kg/d given q8h. **<12 wks: Susp:** 15 mg/kg q12h (use 125 mg/5 ml susp).	B > **H R** 2- 250 mg tabs are not equivalent to 1- 500 mg tab. Only use 250 mg tab if peds ≥40 kg. Chewtab & tab not interchangeable.
Ampicillin (Principen)	**Cap:** 250 mg, 500 mg; **Susp:** 125 mg/5ml, 250 mg/5ml	**Genitourinary Tract: Adults & Peds: >20 kg:** 500 mg qid. **≤20 kg:** 25 mg/kg qid.	B >

QUINOLONES

NAME	FORM/STRENGTH	DOSAGE	COMMENTS
Ciprofloxacin (Cipro)	**Inj:** 10 mg/ml, 200 mg/100 ml, 400 mg/200 ml; **Susp:** 250 mg/5 ml, 500 mg/5 ml; **Tab:** 250 mg, 500 mg, 750 mg	**Adults: Acute Uncomplicated UTI:** 250 mg PO q12h x 3d. **Mild/Moderate UTI:** 250 mg PO q12h or 200 mg IV q12h x 7-14d. **Severe/Complicated UTI:** 500 mg PO q12h or 400 mg IV q12h x 7-14d. **Chronic Bacterial Prostatitis:** 500 mg PO q12h or 400 mg IV q12h x 28d. **Urethral & Cervical Gonococcal Infections:** 250 mg PO as single dose. **Peds: 1-17 yo: Complicated UTI/Pyelonephritis:** 10-20 mg/kg PO q12h or 6-10 mg/kg IV q8h x 10-21d. **Max:** 750 mg PO or 400 mg IV per dose.	C v **R** CI with tizanidine
Ciprofloxacin (Cipro XR)	**Tab,ER:** 500 mg, 1000 mg	**Adults: ≥18 yrs: Uncomplicated UTI:** 500 mg qd x 3d. **Complicated UTI:** 1000 mg qd x 7-14d. **Acute Uncomplicated Pyelonephritis:** 1000 mg qd x 7-14d.	C v **R** CI with tizanidine
Ciprofloxacin HCl (Proquin XR)	**Tab,ER:** 500 mg	**Adults:** 500 mg qd x 3 days.	C v
Levofloxacin (Levaquin)	**Inj:** 5 mg/ml, 25 mg/ml; **Sol:** 25 mg/ml; **Tab:** 250 mg, 500 mg, 750 mg	**Adults: ≥18 yo: Complicated UTI/Acute Pyelonephritis:** 250 mg IV/PO qd x 10d. **Uncomplicated UTI:** 250 mg IV/PO qd x 3d. **Chronic Bacterial Prostatitis:** 500 mg IV/PO qd x 28d.	C v **R**
Lomefloxacin (Maxaquin)	**Tab:** 400 mg	**Adults: ≥18 yo: Complicated UTI:** 400 mg qd x 14d. **Uncomplicated Cystitis:** 400mg qd x 3d (*E.coli*) or 10d (*K.pneumoniae, P.mirabilis,* or *S.saprophyticus*).	C v **R**

Norfloxacin (Noroxin)	**Tab:** 400 mg	**Adults: ≥18 yo: Uncomplicated UTI:** 400 mg q12h x 3d (*K. pneumoniae, E. coli,* or *P. mirabilis*), or x 7-10d (other organisms). **Complicated UTI:** 400 mg q12h x 10-21d. **Acute/Chronic Prostatitis:** 400 mg q12h x 28d.	C v R
Ofloxacin (Floxin)	**Tab:** 200 mg, 300 mg, 400 mg	**Adults: ≥18 yo: Nongonococcal Cervicitis/Urethritis (*C.trachomatis*) or Mixed Infection of Urethra & Cervix (*C.trachomatis & N.gonorrhoeae*):** 300 mg q12h x 7d. **Acute PID:** 400 mg q12h x 10-14d. **Uncomplicated Cystitis:** 200 mg q12h x 3d (*E.coli* or *K.pneumoniae*) or 7d (other pathogens). **Complicated UTI:** 200 mg q12h x 10d. **Prostatitis (*E.coli*):** 300 mg q12h x 6 wks. **Acute Uncomplicated Urethral & Cervical Gonorrhea:** 400 mg as single dose.	C v H R

SULFONAMIDE

Sulfisoxazole (Gantrisin Pediatric)	**Susp:** 500 mg/5 ml	**Peds: >2 mths: Initial:** 1/2 of 24h dose. **Maint:** 150 mg/kg/d or 4 gm/m²/d in divided doses. **Max:** 6 gm/d.	C v CI in pregnancy & nursing.

SULFONAMIDES AND COMBINATIONS

Sulfamethoxazole/ Trimethoprim (Bactrim, Bactrim DS, Septra, Septra DS, Sulfatrim Pediatric)	**Inj:** 80-16 mg/ml; **Susp:** 200-40 mg/5 ml; **Tab:** (SS) 400-80 mg, (DS) 800-160 mg	**PO: Adults:** 800 mg SMX & 160 mg TMP (1 DS tab, 2 SS tabs, or 20 ml) q12h x 10-14d. **Peds: ≥2 mths:** 4 mg/kg TMP & 20 mg/kg SMX q12h x 10d. **Severe: Adults & Peds: IV:** 8-10 mg/kg/d (based on TMP) given q6-12h up to 14d.	C v R CI in pregnancy & nursing.

NAME	FORM/STRENGTH	DOSAGE	COMMENTS
TETRACYCLINES			
Doxycycline Hyclate (Doryx, Vibramycin, Vibra-Tabs)	**Cap:** (Vibramycin) 100 mg; **Cap,Delay:** (Doryx) 75 mg, 100 mg; **Tab:**(Vibra-Tabs) 100 mg	**Adults:** 100 mg q12h on Day 1, then 100 mg qd or 50 mg q12h. **Peds: >8 yo & ≤100 lbs:** 1 mg/lb bid on Day 1, then 1 mg/lb qd or 0.5 mg/lb bid. **>100 lbs:** Adult dose.	D v
Doxycycline Monohydrate (Monodox, Vibramycin)	**Cap:** (Monodox) 50 mg, 100 mg; **Susp:** (Vibramycin) 25 mg/5 ml	**Adults:** 100 mg q12h or 50 mg q6h on Day 1, then 100 mg qd or 50 mg q12h. **Peds: >8 yo & ≤100 lbs:** 1 mg/lb bid on Day 1, then 1 mg/lb qd or 0.5 mg/lb bid. **>100 lbs:** Adult dose.	D v
Minocycline HCl (Dynacin, Minocin)	**Cap:** (Dynacin) 50 mg, 75 mg, 100 mg, (Minocin) 50 mg, 100 mg; **Inj:** (Minocin) 100 mg; **Tab:** (Dynacin) 50 mg, 75 mg, 100 mg;	**Adults:** 200 mg PO/IV, then 100 mg q12h or 50 mg qid. **Peds: >8 yo:** 4 mg/kg PO/IV, then 2 mg/kg q12h.	D v **R**
Tetracycline HCl (Sumycin)	**Cap:** 250 mg, 500 mg; **Susp:** 125 mg/5 ml	**Adults:** 250 mg qid or 500 mg bid. **Peds: >8 yo:** 25-50 mg/kg divided bid-qid.	D v **R**
MISCELLANEOUS			
Fosfomycin Tromethamine (Monurol)	**Granules:** 3 gm/sachet	**Women: ≥18 yo:** One 3 gm single-dose sachet. Mix w/ 3-4 oz of water.	B v
Nitrofurantoin (Furadantin)	**Susp:** 25 mg/5 ml	**Adults:** 50-100 mg qid x 7d. **Peds: >1 mth:** 5-7 mg/kg/d given as qid x 7d.	B v **R**

Nitrofurantoin, Macrocrystals (Macrobid, Macrodantin)	**Cap:** (Macrobid) 100 mg, (Macrodantin) 25 mg, 50 mg, 100 mg	**Macrobid: Adults & Peds: >12 yo:** 100 mg q12h x 7d. **Macrodantin: Adults:** 50-100 mg qid x 7d. **Peds: ≥1 mth:** 5-7 mg/kg/d given as qid x 7d.	B v **R**
Trimethoprim (Proloprim)	**Tab:** 100 mg, 200 mg	**Adults & Peds: ≥12 yo:** 100 mg bid or 200 mg qd x 10d.	C > **R**

Miscellaneous Anti-Infectives

Iodoquinol (Yodoxin)	**Tab:** 210 mg, 650 mg	**Intestinal Amebiasis: Adults: Usual:** 630-650 mg tid pc x 20d. **Peds: Usual:** 10-13.3 mg/kg tid pc x 20d. **Max:** 1.95 gm/24h.	N >
Tinidazole (Tindamax)	**Tab:** 250 mg, 500 mg	**Giardiasis: Adults:** 2 gm single dose. **>3 yo:** 50 mg/kg single dose. **Max:** 2 gm/d. **Amebiasis: Intestinal: Adults:** 2 gm qd x 3d. **>3 yo:** 50 mg/kg qd x 3d. **Max:** 2 gm/d. **Amebic Liver Abscess: Adults:** 2 gm qd x 3-5d. **>3 yo:** 50 mg/kg qd x 3-5d. **Max:** 2 gm/d. May crush tabs in cherry syrup. Take w/food.	X (1st trimester) C (2nd/3rd trimester) v **R** Avoid unnecessary use.

NAME	FORM/STRENGTH	DOSAGE	COMMENTS

ANTINEOPLASTICS

Antineoplastics

NAME	FORM/STRENGTH	DOSAGE	COMMENTS
Alemtuzumab (Campath)	**Inj:** 30 mg/ml	**B-cell Chronic Lymphocytic Leukemia: Adults: Initial:** 3 mg IV qd. When tolerated, increase to 10 mg/d. **Maint:** When 10 mg tolerated, increase to 30 mg/d TIW up to 12 wks.	C v [63]
Anastrozole (Arimidex)	**Tab:** 1 mg	**Adjuvant/Advanced/Metastatic Breast Cancer: Adults:** 1 mg qd.	D >
Asparaginase (Elspar)	**Inj:** 10,000 IU	**Acute Lymphocytic Leukemia: Adults & Peds:** 1000 IU/kg IV qd x 10d beginning Day 22 of treatment period or 6000 IU/m^2 IM on Days 4, 7, 10, 13, 16, 19, 22, 25, & 28.	C v Be prepared to treat anaphylaxis. [3]
Bevacizumab (Avastin)	**Inj:** 25 mg/ml	**Metastatic Colon/Rectum Carcinoma: Adults:** 5 mg/kg IV infusion over 90 min once q14d until disease progression is detected. If 1st infusion is well tolerated, administer 2nd infusion over 60 min. If 2nd infusion is well tolerated, administer subsequent doses over 30 min.	C v GI perforation. Wound dehiscence. Hemoptysis.
Bicalutamide (Casodex)	**Tab:** 50 mg	**Stage D_2 Metastatic Carcinoma of Prostate: Adults:** 50 mg qd. Intiate w/ LHRH analogue therapy.	X > [3]

Bortezomib (Velcade)	**Inj:** 3.5 mg	**Multiple Myeloma: Adults: Initial:** 1.3 mg/m²/dose IV bolus BIW x 2 wks (days 1, 4, 8, & 11) followed by a 10-day rest period (days 12-21). At least 72 h should elapse between consecutive doses. **Grade 3 Non-Hematological/Grade 4 Hematological Toxicities (excluding neuropathy):** Withhold therapy until symptoms of toxicity resolve. Reinitiate at 25% reduced dose. **Peripheral Neuropathy: Grade 1 w/ pain or Grade 2 (interfering with function but not activities of daily living):** Reduce dose to 1 mg/m². **Grade 2 w/ pain or Grade 3 (interfering with activities of daily living):** Withhold dose until toxicity resolves. Reinitiate at 0.7 mg/m² qwk. **Grade 4 (permanent sensory loss interfering w/ function):** D/C therapy.	◙D ❁v
Busulfan (Myleran)	**Tab:** 2 mg	**CML: Adults & Peds:** 60 mcg/kg/d or 1.8 mg/m²/d.	◙D ❁v Bone marrow hypoplasia. 3
Capecitabine (Xeloda)	**Tab:** 150 mg, 500 mg	**Metastatic Breast Cancer/Colorectal Cancer: Adults ≥18 yo:** 1250 mg/m² bid x 2 wks, then 1 wk rest period. Give as 3 wk cycles. **Dukes' C Colon Cancer: Adjuvant Treatment:** 3 wk cycles for 8 cycles (24 wks). Interrupt and/or reduce dose if toxicity occurs. Readjust according to adverse effects.	◙D ❁v **R** Bleeding & death reported w/coumarin.

3 Give only under supervision of a physician experienced with antineoplastics.
63 Hematologic toxicity & opportunistic infections reported. Gradually increase dose to avoid infusion reactions.

NAME	FORM/STRENGTH	DOSAGE	COMMENTS
Cetuximab (Erbitux)	**Inj:** 2 mg/ml	**Adults:** Pre-medication with H_1 antagonist (eg, diphenhydramine 50 mg IV) is recommended. **Metastatic Colorectal Carcinoma: Initial:** 400 mg/m² IV infusion over 120 min. **Maint:** 250 mg/m² IV infusion over 60 min once wkly. **Squamous Cell Carcinoma of Head & Neck: Combination Therapy: Initial:** 400 mg/m² IV over 120 min 1 wk prior to initiation of a course of radiation treatment. **Maint:** 250 mg/m² over 60 min wkly for duration of radiation therapy. **Recurrent/Metastatic Squamous Cell Carcinoma of Head & Neck: Monotherapy: Initial:** 400 mg/m². **Maint:** 250 mg/m² until disease progression or unacceptable toxicity. Adjust dose based on infusion reactions or dermatologic toxicity. **Max Infusion Rate:** 5 ml/min.	C ✽v Infusion reactions.
Chlorambucil (Leukeran)	**Tab:** 2 mg	**Adults: CLL/Malignant Lymphoma/Hodgkin's Disease: Usual:** 0.1-0.2 mg/kg/d x 3-6 wks. **Lymphocytic Infiltration of Bone Marrow/Hypoplastic Bone Marrow: Max:** 0.1 mg/kg/d.	D ✽v Bone marrow suppression. Infertility. Carcinogenic.
Cinacalcet HCl (Sensipar)	**Tab:** 30 mg, 60 mg, 90 mg	**Hypercalcemia in Parathyroid Carcinoma:** Initial: 30 mg bid. Titrate: Increase q 2-4 wks through sequential doses of 30 mg bid, 60 mg bid, 90 mg bid, & 90 mg tid-qid prn to normalize serum Ca levels.	C ✽v
Cladribine (Leustatin)	**Inj:** 10 mg	**Hairy Cell Leukemia: Adults:** 0.09 mg/kg/d continuous infusion x 7d.	D ✽v Acute nephrotoxicity. [3]
Clofarabine (Clolar)	**Inj:** 1 mg/ml	**Relapsed/Refractory Acute Lymphoblastic Leukemia: Peds: 1-21 yo:** 52 mg/m² IV over 2 h qd x 5d.	D ✽v

Cyclophosphamide (Cytoxan)	**Inj:** 500 mg, 1 gm, 2 gm; **Tab:** 25 mg, 50 mg	**Adults & Peds: Malignant Lymphomas/Leukemias/ Multiple Myeloma/ Mycosis Fungoides/Neuroblastoma/ Ovary Adenocarcinoma/Retinoblastoma/Breast Carcinoma: IV:** 40-50 mg/kg in divided doses over 2-5d, or 10-15 mg/kg q7-10d, or 3-5 mg/kg BIW. **PO:** 1-5 mg/kg/d. **Nonmalignant Disease - Biopsy Proven "minimal changes" Nephrotic Syndrome: Peds:** 2.5-3 mg/kg qd x 60-90d.	D v
Erlotinib (Tarceva)	**Tab:** 25 mg, 100 mg, 150 mg	**Adults: Non-Small Cell Lung Cancer:** 150 mg ≥1 h before or 2 h after food. **Pancreatic Cancer:** 100 mg at least 1 h before or 2 h after food, in combination with gemcitabine. Continue until disease progression or unacceptable toxicity.	D v
Estradiol (Estrace, Gynodiol)	**Tab:** (Estrace) 0.5 mg, 1 mg, 2 mg, (Gynodiol) 0.5 mg, 1 mg, 1.5 mg, 2 mg	**Adults: Advanced Prostate Cancer:** 1-2 mg tid. **Metastatic Breast Cancer:** 10 mg tid for min of 3 mths.	X v [4, 28]
Estramustine (Emcyt)	**Cap:** 140 mg	**Metastatic/Progressive Prostate Carcinoma: Adults:** 14 mg/kg/d given tid-qid.	N >
Estrogens, Conjugated (Premarin)	**Tab:** 0.3 mg, 0.45 mg, 0.625 mg, 0.9 mg, 1.25 mg, 2.5 mg	**Adults: Advanced Prostate Cancer:** 1.25-2.5 mg tid. **Metastatic Breast Cancer:** 10 mg tid for min of 3 mths.	X > [4, 28]

[3] Give only under supervision of a physician experienced with antineoplastics.

[4] Contraindicated in pregnancy. Increased risk of endometrial carcinoma.

[28] Not for prevention of CV disease or dementia. The WHI reported increased risks of MI, stroke, invasive breast cancer, pulmonary emboli, DVT, and probable dementia in postmenopausal women. Prescribe at lowest effective doses for shortest duration.

NAME	FORM/STRENGTH	DOSAGE	COMMENTS
Exemestane (Aromasin)	**Tab:** 25 mg	**Advanced Breast Cancer in Postmenopausal Women/Adjuvant Treatment in Early Breast Cancer: Adults:** 25 mg qd after a meal. Continue in the absence of recurrence until completion of 5 yrs of adjuvant endocrine therapy in early breast cancer treated w/ 2-3 yrs of tamoxifen. Continue until tumor progression is evident in advanced breast cancer. **Concomitant Potent CYP3A4 Inducers:** 50 mg qd after a meal.	◉D ❋>
Fludarabine Phosphate (Fludara)	**Inj:** 50 mg	**B-cell Chronic Lymphocytic Leukemia: Adults:** 25 $mg/m^2/d$ IV over 30 min x 5d, repeat q28d.	◉D ❋v **R** Autoimmune hemolytic anemia. Severe bone marrow suppression.[3]
Flutamide (Eulexin)	**Cap:** 125 mg	**Stage B_2-C Prostatic Carcinoma/Stage D_2 Metastatic Carcinoma: Adults:** 250 mg tid at 8h intervals.	◉D ❋> Hepatic injury.
Fulvestrant (Faslodex)	**Inj:** 50 mg/ml	**Hormone Receptor Positive Metastatic Breast Cancer in Postmenopausal Women: Adults:** 250 mg IM into buttock monthly. Give as either single 5 ml inj or 2 concurrent 2.5 ml inj.	◉D ❋v
Gefitinib (Iressa)	**Tab:** 250 mg	**Adults:** 250 mg/d. **Poorly Tolerated Diarrhea/Skin Adverse Reactions:** Provide brief (up to 14 days) therapy interruption followed by reinstatement of 250 mg/d. **Concomitant Potent CYP3A4 Inducers (eg, rifampicin, phenytoin):** Consider increasing dose to 500 mg/d, in the absence of severe adverse reactions.	◉D ❋v **R**

Gemtuzumab Ozogamicin (Mylotarg)	**Inj:** 5 mg	**CD33 Positive Acute Myeloid Leukemia (1st relapse): Adults: ≥60 yo:** 9 mg/m² IV, repeat after 14d.	D v [3, 64]
Goserelin Acetate (Zoladex)	**Implant:** 3.6 mg	**Adults: Stage B_2-C Prostate Cancer:** 3.6 mg depot SC 8 wks before radiotherapy, then 10.8 mg depot SC 28d later. **Advanced Prostate or Breast Cancer:** 3.6 mg SC in upper abdominal wall q28d.	X v
Goserelin Acetate (Zoladex 3-Month)	**Implant:** 10.8 mg	**Adults: Stage B_2-C Prostate Cancer:** 3.6 mg depot SC 8 wks before radiotherapy, then 10.8 mg depot SC 28d later. **Advanced Prostate Cancer:** 10.8 mg SC q12wks in upper abdominal wall.	X v
Histrelin Acetate (Vantas)	**Implant:** 50 mg	**Advanced Prostate Cancer: Adults:** 50 mg SC into inner aspect of upper arm q12mths. Must remove after 12 mths of therapy.	X v
Hydroxyurea (Hydrea)	**Cap:** 500 mg	**Adults: Solid Tumors: Intermittent:** 80 mg/kg PO as single dose q3d. **Continuous/Resistant CML:** 20-30 mg/kg PO qd. **Head/Neck Carcinoma: Concomitant Therapy w/ Irradiation:** 80 mg/kg PO q3d as single dose.	D v **R**
Imatinib Mesylate (Gleevec)	**Cap:** 100 mg, 400 mg	**Adults: CML: Chronic Phase:** 400 mg/d, may increase to 600 mg qd. **Accelerated Phase/Blast Crisis:** 600 mg/d, may increase to 400 mg bid. **GIST:** 400 mg/d or 600 mg/d. **Peds: ≥3 yrs: CML: Ph+ Chronic Phase: Recurrent After Stem Cell Transplant or Resistant to Interferon-alphaTherapy:** 260 mg/m²/day given qd or split into 2 doses (am & pm). Take w/ food & plenty of water.	D v **H**

[3] Give only under supervision of a physician experienced with antineoplastics.
[64] Severe myelosuppression, hypersensitivity reactions, & hepatotoxicity reported.

NAME	FORM/STRENGTH	DOSAGE	COMMENTS
Interferon alfa-2a (Roferon-A)	**Inj:** 3 MIU, 6 MIU, 9 MIU, 36 MIU	**Adults ≥18 yo: Hairy Cell Leukemia: Induction:** 3 MIU SC qd x 16- 24 wks. **Maint:** 3 MIU SC/IM TIW. **CML: Initial:** 9 MIU SC qd SC/IM.	C v [13]
Interferon alfa-2b (Intron-A)	**Inj:** 10 MIU, 18 MIU, 50 MIU, 10 MIU/ml, 3 MIU/0.2 ml, 5 MIU/ 0.2 ml, 10 MIU/0.2 ml	**Adults: ≥18 yo: Hairy Cell Leukemia:** 2 MIU/m² SC/IM TIW up to 6 mths. **Malignant Melanoma: Induction:** 20 MIU/m² IV x 5d/wk x 4 wks. **Maint:** 10 MIU/m² SC TIW x 48 wks. **Follicular Lymphoma:** 5 MIU SC TIW up to 18 mths. **Condylomata Acuminata:** 1 MIU into lesions TIW x 3 wks. **Kaposi's Sarcoma:** 30 MIU/m² SC/IM TIW.	C v [13]
Leuprolide Acetate (Eligard)	**Inj:** 7.5 mg, 22.5 mg, 30 mg, 45 mg	**Advanced Prostate Cancer: Adults:** 7.5 mg SC monthly, 22.5 mg SC q3mths, 30 mg SC q4mths, or 45 mg SC q6mths. Rotate injection sites.	X >
Leuprolide Acetate (Lupron)	**Inj:** 1 mg/ml	**Advanced Prostate Cancer: Adults:** 1 mg SC qd. Rotate injection sites.	X >
Leuprolide Acetate (Lupron Depot)	**Inj:** (Depot) 7.5 mg, (3 mth) 22.5 mg, (4 mth) 30 mg	**Advanced Prostate Cancer: Adults:** 7.5 mg IM monthly, 22.5 mg IM q3mths, or 30 mg IM q4mths. Give as single dose & rotate injection sites.	X >
Medroxyprogesterone Acetate (Depo-Provera)	**Inj:** 400 mg/ml	**Inoperable, Recurrent, Metastatic Endometrial or Renal Carcinoma: Adults: Initial:** 400-1000 mg IM qwk. **Maint:** 400 mg IM qmth.	N >
Megestrol Acetate (Megace)	**Susp:** 40 mg/ml; **Tab:** 20 mg, 40 mg	**Adults: Advanced Breast Carcinoma:** 40 mg qid. **Advanced Endometrial Carcinoma:** 40-320 mg qd in divided doses. Treat for min of 2 mths **Anorexia/Cachexia/Significant Wt Loss in AIDS: Susp: Initial:** 800 mg/d.	X v

Melphalan (Alkeran)	**Inj:** 50 mg; **Tab:** 2 mg	**Adults: Multiple Myeloma: IV** 16 mg/m² q2wks x 4 doses, then q4wks after recovery from toxicity. **PO:** 6 mg qd x 2-3 wks, then 2 mg qd after WBC & platelets are rising. **Epithelial Ovary Carcinoma:** 0.2 mg/kg/d x 5d. May repeat q4-5wks.	D **R** (Inj) [3, 23]
Mercaptopurine (Purinethol)	**Tab:** 50 mg	**Adults & Peds: ALL: Induction: Initial:** 2.5 mg/kg/d. Calculate to nearest multiple of 25 mg. **Titrate:** May increase to 5 mg/kg/d after 4 wks if needed. **Maint:** 1.5-2.5 mg/kg/d. Dose peds in pm.	D v **H R** [3]
Methotrexate Sodium	**Inj:** 20 mg, 25 mg/ml, 1 gm; **Tab:** 2.5 mg	**Adults: Burkette's Lymphoma: Stages I-II: PO:** 10-25 mg/d x 4-8d for several courses; separate by 7-10d rest period. **Lymphosarcomas: Stage III: PO:** 0.625-2.5 mg/kg/d. **Leukemia: Induction:** 3.3 mg/m² w/ prednisone qd. **Remission Maint:** 15 mg/m² PO/IM twice wkly or 2.5 mg/kg IV q14d. **Mycosis Fungoides:** 5-50 mg qwk. If poor response, give 15-37.5 mg twice wkly. **Osteosarcoma: Initial:** 12 g/m² IV, increase to 15 g/m² if peak levels of 1000 micromolar not reached at end of infusion. **Choriocarcinoma/Trophoblastic Diseases: PO/IM:** 15-30 mg qd x 5d, rest ≥1 wk & repeat 3-5x. **Peds: Meningeal Leukemia: Intrathecal:** Dilute preservative free MTX to 1 mg/ml. Dose q2-5d. **≥3 yo:** 12 mg. **2 yo:** 10 mg. **1 yo:** 8 mg. **<1 yo:** 6 mg.	X v [3, 19]

[3] Give only under supervision of a physician experienced with antineoplastics.
[13] May cause or aggravate neuropsychiatric, autoimmune, ischemic, & infectious disorders; monitor closely.
[19] Monitor for bone marrow, lung, liver & kidney toxicities. Serious toxic reactions.
[23] Chromosomal aberrations. Severe bone marrow suppression.

NAME	FORM/STRENGTH	DOSAGE	COMMENTS
Mitoxantrone (Novantrone)	**Inj:** 2 mg/ml	**Adults: IV: ANLL: Induction:** 12 mg/m² qd on Days 1-3. **Advanced Hormone-Refractory Prostate Cancer Pain:** 12-14 mg/m² q21d.	◙D ❋v Bone marrow suppression. Cardiotoxicity. Secondary AML. [3]
Nelarabine (Arranon)	**Inj:** 5 mg/ml	**T-cell Acute Lymphoblastic Leukemia/T-cell Lymphoblastic Lymphoma: Adults:** 1500 mg/m² IV over 2hrs on Days 1, 3, & 5. Repeat q21d. **Peds:** 650 mg/m²/d IV over 1hr x 5 consecutive days. Repeat q21d.	◙D ❋v [55]
Nilutamide (Nilandron)	**Tab:** 150 mg	**Stage D_2 Prostate Cancer: Adults:** 300 mg qd x 30d, then 150 mg qd. Begin on day of surgical castration.	◙ C ❋> Interstitial pneumonitis.
Oxaliplatin (Eloxatin)	**Inj:** 50 mg, 100 mg	**Metastatic Colon/Rectum Carcinoma: Adults: IV: Day 1:** 85 mg/m² w/ leucovorin (LV) 200 mg/m² over 120 min; followed w/ 5-FU 400 mg/m² bolus, then 5-FU 600 mg/m² as 22h infusion. **Day 2:** LV 200 mg/m² over 120 min; followed by 5-FU 400 mg/m² bolus, then 5-FU 600 mg/m² as 22h infusion. Repeat cycle q2wks. **Adjuvant Therapy:** Recommended cycle q2wks x 6 mths.	◙D ❋v Anaphylactic reactions reported.
Paclitaxel Protein-bound Particles (Abraxane)	**Inj:** 100 mg	**Breast Cancer: Adults: IV:** 260 mg/m² q3wks. Severe neutropenia or severe sensory neuropathy reduce to 220 mg/m²; recurrence reduce to 180 mg/m².	◙D ❋v

Paclitaxel (Taxol)	**Inj:** 6 mg/ml	**Adults: IV: Ovary Carcinoma: Previously Untreated:** 175 mg/m² over 3h or 135 mg/m² over 24h q3wks followed by cisplatin 75 mg/m². **Treated:** 135 or 175 mg/m² over 3h q3wks. **Breast Cancer:** 175 mg/m² over 3h q3wks. **Non-Small Cell Lung Cancer:** 135 mg/m² over 24h q3wks. **Kaposi's Sarcoma:** 135 mg/m² over 3h q3wks or 100 mg/m² over 3h q2wks.	◙D ❁v Anaphylaxis & severe hypersensitivity reactions. [3]
Pemetrexed (Alimta)	**Inj:** 500 mg	**Malignant Pleural Mesothelioma: Adults:** 500 mg/m² IV over 10 min on Day 1 of each 21-day cycle w/ cisplatin 75 mg/m² infused over 2h beginning 30 min after pemetrexed.	◙D ❁v **R**
Procarbazine (Matulane)	**Cap:** 50 mg	**Stage III & IV Hodgkin's Disease: Adults:** 2-4 mg/kg/d x 1st wk then increase to 4-6 mg/kg/d until max response. **Maint:** 1-2 mg/kg/d. **Peds:** 50 mg/m²/d x 1st wk then increase to 100 mg/m²/d until max repsonse. **Maint:** 50 mg/m²/d.	◙D ❁v [3]
Rituximab (Rituxan)	**Inj:** 10 mg/ml	**Adults:** Give as infusion. **Relapsed or Refractory, Low-Grade or Follicular, CD-20 Positive, B-Cell, NHL:** 375 mg/m² IV once wkly x 4 or 8 doses. If develop progressive disease, retreat w/ 375 mg/m² IV once weekly x 4 doses. **Diffuse Large B-Cell NHL:** 375 mg/m² IV given on Day 1 of each cycle of chemotherapy up to 8 infusions.	◙C ❁v [65]

[3] Give only under supervision of a physician experienced with antineoplastics.
[55] Severe neurologic events reported.
[65] Fatal infusion reactions, tumor lysis syndrome & severe mucocutaneous reactions reported.

NAME	FORM/STRENGTH	DOSAGE	COMMENTS
Sorafenib (Nexavar)	**Tab:** 200 mg	**Advanced Renal Cell Carcinoma: Adults:** 400 mg bid w/o food (1 h before or 2 h after eating). Continue until no clinical benefit or unacceptable toxicity. Temporary interruption or reduction to 400 mg qd or qod if serious adverse events suspected.	◉D ✽v
Sunitinib (Sutent)	**Cap:** 12.5 mg, 25 mg, 50 mg	**Adults:** 50 mg qd; 4 weeks on, 2 weeks off. Increase/reduce dose in 12.5 mg increments based on individual safety & tolerability.	◉D ✽v
Tamoxifen Citrate (Nolvadex)	**Tab:** 10 mg, 20 mg	**Adults: Breast Cancer Treatment:** 20 mg qd or qam & qpm. **Ductal Carcinoma in Situ or Reduction of Breast Cancer (High Risk):** 20 mg qd x 5 yrs.	◉D ✽v Uterine malignancies, stroke, & PE reported.
Toremifene (Fareston)	**Tab:** 60 mg	**Metastatic Breast Cancer: Adults:** 60 mg qd.	◉D ✽>
Trastuzumab (Herceptin)	**Inj:** 440 mg	**Metastatic Breast Cancer: Adults: LD:** 4 mg/kg IV over 90 min. **Maint:** 2 mg/kg IV over 30 min qwk.	◉B ✽v Cardiomyopathy. Hypersensitivity, infusion reactions. Pulmonary events.

CARDIOVASCULAR AGENTS

Angina

BETA BLOCKERS

NAME	FORM/STRENGTH	DOSAGE	COMMENTS
Atenolol (Tenormin)	**Inj:** 0.5 mg/ml; **Tab:** 25 mg, 50 mg, 100 mg	**Angina Pectoris: Adults: Initial:** 50 mg qd. **Titrate:** May increase to 100 mg qd after 1 wk. **Max:** 200 mg/d.	◉D ✽> **R**

Metoprolol Succinate (Toprol-XL)	**Tab,ER:** 25 mg, 50 mg, 100 mg, 200 mg	**Angina Pectoris: Adults: Initial:** 100 mg qd. **Titrate:** May increase qwk. **Max:** 400 mg/d.	◉C ❋>
Metoprolol Tartrate (Lopressor)	**Tab:** 50 mg, 100 mg	**Angina Pectoris: Adults: Initial:** 50 mg bid. **Titrate:** May increase qwk. **Maint:** 100-400 mg/d. **Max:** 400 mg/d.	◉C ❋>
Nadolol (Corgard)	**Tab:** 20 mg, 40 mg, 80 mg, 120 mg, 160 mg	**Angina Pectoris: Adults: Initial:** 40 mg qd. **Titrate:** Increase by 40-80 mg q3-7d. **Usual:** 40-80 mg qd. **Max:** 240 mg/d.	◉C ❋v **R** [17]
Propranolol HCl (Inderal, Inderal LA)	**Cap,ER:** 60 mg, 80 mg, 120 mg, 160 mg; **Tab:** 10 mg, 20 mg, 40 mg, 60 mg, 80 mg	**Angina Pectoris: Adults: Inderal LA: Initial:** 80 mg qd. **Titrate:** Increase q3-7d intervals. **Usual:** 160 mg qd. **Max:** 320 mg/d. **Inderal:** 80-320 mg/d given bid-qid.	◉C ❋>
CALCIUM CHANNEL BLOCKER (DIHYDROPYRIDINES)			
Amlodipine Besylate (Norvasc)	**Tab:** 2.5 mg, 5 mg, 10 mg	**Chronic Stable/Vasospastic Angina: Adults:** 5-10 mg qd.	◉C ❋v **H**
Nicardipine (Cardene)	**Cap:** 20 mg, 30 mg	**Chronic Stable Angina: Adults: Initial:** 20 mg tid. **Maint:** 20-40 mg tid.	◉C ❋v **H**
Nifedipine (Procardia, Procardia XL)	(Generic) **Cap:** 10 mg, 20 mg; **Tab,ER:** (XL) 30 mg, 60 mg, 90 mg; (Procardia) **Cap:** 10 mg; **Tab,ER:** (XL) 30 mg, 60 mg, 90 mg	**Vasospastic/Chronic Stable: Adults: Procardia XL: Initial:** 30-60 mg qd. **Titrate:** Increase over 7-14d. **Max:** 120 mg/d. **Procardia: Initial:** 10 mg tid. **Titrate:** Increase over 7-14d. **Usual:** 10-20 mg tid. **Max:** 180 mg/d.	◉C ❋v

[17] Abrupt cessation may induce arrhythmia or MI.

NAME	FORM/STRENGTH	DOSAGE	COMMENTS
CALCIUM CHANNEL BLOCKER (NON-DIHYDROPYRIDINES)			
Bepridil (Vascor)	**Tab:** 200 mg, 300 mg	**Chronic Stable Angina: Adults: Initial:** 200 mg qd. **Titrate:** Adjust after 10d based on response. **Max:** 400 mg qd.	◙ C ❁v
Diltiazem HCl (Cardizem, Cardizem CD, Cardizem LA, Cartia XT, Dilacor XR, Diltia XT, Taztia XT, Tiazac)	**Cap,ER:** (Cardizem CD) 120 mg, 180 mg, 240 mg, 300 mg, 360 mg,(Cartia XT) 120 mg, 180 mg, 240 mg, 300 mg, (Dilacor XR/ Diltia XT) 120 mg, 180 mg, 240 mg, (Taztia XT) 120 mg, 180 mg, 240 mg, 300 mg, 360 mg, (Tiazac) 120 mg, 180 mg, 240 mg, 300 mg, 360 mg, 420 mg; **Tab:** (Cardizem) 30 mg, 60 mg, 90 mg, 120 mg; **Tab,ER:** (Cardizem LA) 120 mg, 180 mg, 240 mg, 300 mg, 360 mg, 420 mg	**Chronic Stable Angina: Adults: Cardizem CD/Cartia XT: Initial:** 120-180 mg qd. **Titrate:** Adjust at 1-2 wk intervals. **Max:** 480 mg/d. **Cardizem: Initial:** 30 mg qid. **Titrate:** Adjust at 1-2d intervals. **Usual:** 180-360 mg/d. **Cardizem LA: Initial:** 180 mg qd. **Titrate:** Adjust at 1-2 wk intervals. **Dilacor XR/Diltia XT: Initial:** 120 mg qd. **Titrate:** Adjust at 1-2 wk intervals. **Max:** 480 mg/d. **Taztia XT/Tiazac: Initial:** 120-180 mg qd. **Titrate:** Adjust at 1-2 wk intervals. **Max:** 540 mg/d.	◙C ❁v
Verapamil (Calan, Covera-HS)	**Tab:** 40 mg, 80 mg, 120 mg; **Tab,ER:**180 mg, 240 mg	**Vasospastic/Unstable/Chronic Stable: Adults: Calan: Usual:** 80-120 mg tid. **Titrate:** Increase by qd or qwk intervals. **Covera-HS: Initial:** 180 mg qhs. **Titrate:** Increase to 240 qhs, then 360 mg qhs, then 480 mg qhs.	◙C ❁v **H** (Calan)

CALCIUM CHANNEL BLOCKER/HMG COA REDUCTASE INHIBITOR

Amlodipine Besylate/Atorvastatin Calcium (Caduet)	**Tab:** 2.5-10 mg, 2.5-20 mg, 2.5-40 mg, 5-10 mg, 5-20 mg, 5-40 mg, 5-80 mg, 10-10 mg, 10-20 mg, 10-40 mg,10-80 mg	Dosing is based on the appropriate combination of recommendations for the monotherapies. **Adults: Amlodipine:** 5-10 mg qd. **Elderly/Hepatic Dysfunction:** 5 mg qd. **Atorvastatin:** See under Antilipidemic Agents for dosing.	◙X ❁v **H**

VASODILATORS

Isosorbide Dinitrate (Dilatrate-SR, Isordil, Isordil Titradose)	**Cap,ER:** (Dilatrate-SR) 40 mg; **Tab,SL:** (Generic) 2.5 mg, 5 mg; **Tab:** (Generic) 5 mg, 10 mg, 20 mg, 30 mg, 40 mg, (Isordil Titradose) 5 mg, 10 mg, 40 mg	**Adults: Prevention: Dilatrate-DR: Usual:** 40 mg bid. Separate doses by 6h. **Max:** 160 mg/d. Take at least 18h nitrate-free interval. **Isordil (Tritradose): Initial:** 5-20 mg bid-tid. **Maint:** 10-40 mg bid-tid. Take at least 14h nitrate-free interval. **Acute Episode/Prevention: Isordil:** 2.5-5 mg SL 15 min before expected episode or to abort acute episode after failure of SL NTG.	◙C ❁>
Isosorbide Mononitrate (Imdur, Ismo, Monoket)	**Tab:** (Monoket) 10 mg, 20 mg, (Ismo) 20 mg; **Tab,ER:** (Imdur) 30 mg, 60 mg, 120 mg	**Prevention/Treatment: Monoket:** 20 mg bid (space 7h apart). **Small Patients: Initial:** 5 mg bid. **Titrate:** Increase to 10 mg by 2nd or 3rd day. **Maint:** 20 mg bid. **Prevention: Ismo:** 20 mg bid, 1st dose on awakening then 7h later. **Imdur: Initial:** 30-60 mg qam. **Titrate:** Increase after several days to 120 mg/d.	◙B (Imdur, Monoket) ◙C (Ismo) ❁>
Nitroglycerin (Minitran, Nitrek, Nitro-Dur)	**Patch:** (mg/h) (Minitran) 0.1, 0.2, 0.4, 0.6; (Nitrek) 0.2, 0.4, 0.6; (Nitro-Dur) 0.1, 0.2, 0.4, 0.6, 0.8	**Prevention: Initial:** 0.2-0.4 mg/h for 12-14h. Remove for 10-12h.	◙C ❁>

NAME	FORM/STRENGTH	DOSAGE	COMMENTS
Nitroglycerin (Nitro-Time)	**Cap,ER:** 2.5 mg, 6.5 mg, 9 mg; **Inj:** 5 mg/ml	**Cap,ER: Initial:** 2.5-6.5 mg tid-qid. **Titrate:** Guide by symptoms and/or side effects. Should have 10-12h nitrate-free period. **Inj: Initial:** 5 mcg/min IV. **Titrate:** Increase by 5 mcg/min q3-5min.	◙C ❋>
Nitroglycerin (Nitro-Bid, Nitrol)	**Oint:** 2% (15 mg/inch)	**Prevention: Initial:** 0.5 inch qam & 6h later. **Titrate:** May increase to 1 inch bid, then to 2 inches bid. Should have 10-12h nitrate-free period.	◙C ❋>
Nitroglycerin (Nitrolingual Spray, Nitroquick, Nitrostat, Nitrotab)	**Spr,SL:** (Nitrolingual) 0.4 mg/spr; **Tab,SL:** 0.3 mg, 0.4 mg, 0.6 mg	**Treatment: Tab:** 1 tab SL q5min, up to 3 tabs/15 min. **Spr:** 1-2 spr SL, up to 3 spr/15 min. **Prophylaxis: Tab/Spr:** Take tab or spr 5-10 min before precipitating activity.	◙C ❋>
MISCELLANEOUS			
Ranolazine (Ranexa)	**Tab,ER:** 500 mg	**Chronic Angina: Adults: Initial:** 500 mg bid. **Max:** 1000 mg bid. Swallow whole; do not crush, break, or chew.	◙C ❋v **H**

Antiarrhythmics

ENDOGENOUS NUCLEOSIDE

NAME	FORM/STRENGTH	DOSAGE	COMMENTS
Adenosine (Adenocard)	**Inj:** 3 mg/ml	**Adults & Peds: ≥50 kg:** 6 mg rapid IV bolus over 1-2 sec. If not converted to NSR within 1-2 min, give 12 mg rapid IV bolus; may give 2nd 12 mg dose if needed. **Max:** 12 mg/dose. **Peds: <50 kg:** 0.05-0.1 mg/kg rapid IV bolus. If not converted to NSR within 1-2 min, give additional bolus doses incrementally increasing amount by 0.05-0.1 mg/kg. Follow each bolus w/ saline flush. Continue process until NSR or a max single dose of 0.3 mg/kg is used.	◙C ❋>

GROUP IA

Disopyramide Phosphate (Norpace, Norpace CR)	**Cap:** 100 mg, 150 mg; **Cap,ER:** 100 mg, 150 mg	**Adults: <50 kg: Cap:** 100 mg q6h. **Cap,ER:** 200 mg q12h. **≥50 kg: Cap:** 150 mg q6h. **Cap,ER:** 300 mg q12h. **Peds: 12-18 yo:** 6-15 mg/kg/d. **4-12 yo:** 10-15 mg/kg/d. **1-4 yo:** 10-20 mg/kg/d. **<1 yo:** 10-30 mg/kg/d.	C v **H R** [5]
Procainamide HCl (Procanbid, Pronestyl, Pronestyl-SR)	(Pronestyl) **Cap:** 250 mg; **Tab:** 250 mg, 375 mg, 500 mg; **Tab,ER:** (SR) 500 mg; (Procanbid) **Tab,ER:** 500 mg,1000 mg	**Adults: Cap/Tab: Initial:** Up to 50 mg/kg/d in divided doses q3h. May give q3h, q4h, or q6h; adjust by patient response. **Tab,ER: Initial:** Up to 50 mg/kg/d given q6h. Adjust by patient response. **Procanbid: Initial:** Up to 50 mg/kg/d given q12h. Adjust by patient response.	C v **H R** May cause positive ANA titer. [5]
Quinidine Sulfate (Quinidex Extentabs)	**Tab,ER:** 300 mg	**Adults: A-Fib/Flutter Conversion: Initial:** 300 mg q8-12h. **Titrate:** Increase cautiously if no result & levels within therapeutic range. **A-Fib/Flutter Relapse Reduction:** 300 mg q8-12h. **Titrate:** Increase cautiously if needed. **Ventricular Arrhythmia:** Dosing regimens not adequately studied. Monitor ECG for QTc prolongation.	C v

GROUP IB

Lidocaine HCl (Xylocaine)	**Inj:** 0.5%, 1%, 2%	**Adults: Initial:** 50-100 mg IV given 25-50 mg/min, may repeat after 5 min. **Max:** 200-300 mg/h. Following bolus, initiate w/ 1-4 mg min continuous infusion. **Maint:** Adjust according to cardiac rhythm & toxicity. **Peds:** 1 mg/kg bolus, then 30 mcg/kg/min.	B >
Mexiletine HCl	**Cap:** 150 mg, 200 mg, 250 mg	**Adults: Initial:** 200 mg q8h. **Titrate:** Increase by 50-100 mg q2-3d. **Max:** 1200 mg/d.	C v **H** [5]

[5] Proarrhythmic properties/drug should only be used in life-threatening arrhythmias.

NAME	FORM/STRENGTH	DOSAGE	COMMENTS
GROUP IC			
Flecainide Acetate (Tambocor)	**Tab:** 50 mg, 100 mg, 150 mg	**Adults: PSVT/PAF: Initial:** 50 mg q12h. **Titrate:** Increase by 50 mg bid q4d. **Max:** 300 mg/d. **Sustained VT: Initial:** 100 mg q12h. **Titrate:** Increase by 50 mg bid q4d. **Max:** 400 mg/d. **Peds: <6 mths: Initial:** 50 mg/m^2/d given bid-tid. **>6 mths:** 100 mg/m^2/d given bid-tid. **Max:** 200 mg/m^2/d.	●C ✽> **R**
Propafenone HCl (Rythmol, Rythmol SR)	**Cap,ER:** (SR) 225 mg, 325 mg, 425 mg; **Tab:** 150 mg, 225 mg, 300 mg	**Adults: Tab: Initial:** 150 mg q8h, may increase q3-4d to 225 mg q8h, then to 300 mg q8h. **Max:** 900 mg/d. **Cap,ER: Initial:** 225 mg q12h, may increase at min 5d intervals to 325 mg q12h, then to 425 mg q12h if needed.	●C ✽v (Rythmol) ✽> (Rythmol SR) **H** 5
GROUP II			
Acebutolol HCl (Sectral)	**Cap:** 200 mg, 400 mg	**Ventricular Arrhythmia: Adults: Initial:** 200 mg bid. **Maint:** Increase gradually to 600-1200 mg/d.	●B ✽v **R**
Esmolol HCl (Brevibloc)	**Inj:** 10 mg/ml, 20 mg/ml, 250 mg/ml	**Adults: SVT: Initial:** 500 mcg/kg/min x 1 min, then 50 mcg/kg/min x 4 min. **Maint:** 50-200 (avg 100) mcg/kg/min. **Intra-/Post-op Tachycardia: Initial: Rapid:** 80 mg IVP, then 150 mcg/kg/min infusion. **Gradual:** 500 mcg/kg/min x 1 min, then 50 mcg/kg/min x 4 min. If inadequate response within 5 min, repeat LD & give maint 100 mcg/kg/min.	●C ✽>
Propranolol HCl (Inderal)	**Inj:** 1 mg/ml; **Tab:** 10 mg, 20 mg, 40 mg, 60 mg, 80 mg	**Adults: PO:** 10-30 mg tid-qid, given ac & qhs. **IV:** 1-3 mg IV at 1 mg/min.	●C ✽>

Amiodarone HCl (Cordarone, Pacerone)	(Cordarone) **Inj:** 50 mg/ml; **Tab:** 200 mg; (Pacerone) **Tab:** 100 mg, 200 mg, 300 mg, 400 mg	**Adults: PO: LD:** 800-1600 mg/d PO x 1-3 wks until response. Reduce to 600-800 mg/d x 1 mth. **Maint:** 400 mg/d. **IV: LD:** 150 mg over 1st 10 min (15 mg/min), then 360 mg over next 6h (1 mg/min), then 540 mg over remaining 18h (0.5 mg/min). **Maint:** 0.5 mg/min x 2-3 wks.	◙D ❖v
Bretylium Tosylate	**Inj:** 50 mg/ml	**Adults: Life-Threatening Ventricular Arrhythmias: Initial:** 5 mg/kg IV, increase to 10 mg/kg if needed. **Maint:** 5-10 mg/kg q6h. **Other Ventricular Arrhythmias: Initial:** 5-10 mg/kg IM/IV repeat at 1-2h if needed. **Maint:** 5-10 mg/kg IV q6h or 5-10 mg/kg IM q6-8h.	◙C ❖>
Dofetilide (Tikosyn)	**Cap:** 0.125 mg, 0.25 mg, 0.5 mg	**A-Fib/Flutter: Adults: ≥18 yo: Usual:** 500 mcg bid, modify using algorithm based on ECG, HR & CrCl. Re-evaluate q3mths based on QTc & renal function.	◙C ❖v **R** Should be inpatient at least 3d when initiate. Monitor ECG.
Sotalol HCl (Betapace, Betapace AF)	**Tab:** (Betapace) 80 mg, 120 mg, 160 mg, 240 mg; **Cap:** (Betapace AF) 80 mg, 120 mg, 160 mg	**Adults: Life-Threatening Ventricular Arrhythmia: Betapace: Initial:** 80 mg bid. **Titrate:** Increase q3d prn to 120-160 mg bid. **Usual:** 160-320 mg/d given bid-tid. **Adults: NSR Maint in A-Fib/Flutter: Betapace AF:** Dose according to CrCl, refer to PI. **Peds: Betapace/Betapace AF: ≥2 yo: Initial:** 30 mg/m² tid. **Titrate:** Wait ≥36h between dose increases. Guide dose by response, HR & QT_C. **Max:** 60 mg/m². **<2 yo:** See dosing chart in PI. Reduce dose or d/c if QT_C >550 msec.	◙B ❖v **R** Should be inpatient at least 3d when initiate. Monitor ECG &CrCl. [5]

[5] Proarrhythmic properties/drug should only be used in life-threatening arrhythmias.

NAME	FORM/STRENGTH	DOSAGE	COMMENTS
GROUP IV			
Verapamil HCl (Calan)	**Tab:** 40 mg, 80 mg, 120 mg	**Adults: A-Fib (Digitalized): Usual:** 240-320 mg/d given tid-qid. **PSVT Prophylaxis (Non-Digitalized):** 240-480 mg/d given tid-qid. **Max:** 480 mg/d.	◙C ✽v
MISCELLANEOUS			
Digoxin (Digitek, Lanoxicaps, Lanoxin, Lanoxin Pediatric)	**Cap:** (Lanoxicaps) 0.05 mg, 0.1 mg, 0.2 mg; **Inj:** (Lanoxin Pediatric) 0.1 mg/ml, (Lanoxin) 0.25 mg/ml; **Sol:** (Lanoxin Pediatric) 0.05 mg/ml; **Tab:** (Digitek, Lanoxin) 0.125 mg, 0.25 mg	**A-Fib: Adults:** Titrate to minimum effective dose for desired response.	◙C ✽> **R**
Ibutilide Fumarate (Corvert)	**Inj:** 0.1 mg/ml	**A-Fib/Flutter: Adults: ≥18 yo: 1st Infusion: ≥60 kg:** 1 mg over 10 min. **<60 kg:** 0.01 mg/kg over 10 min. **2nd Infusion:** Repeat equal strength infusion 10 min after 1st dose if arrhythmia still present.	◙C ✽v [5]

Antilipidemic Agents

NAME	FORM/STRENGTH	DOSAGE	COMMENTS
BILE ACID SEQUESTRANTS			
Cholestyramine (Questran, Questran Light, Prevalite)	**Pow:** 4 gm/pkt or scoopful	**Adults: Initial:** 1 pkt or scoopful qd or bid. **Maint:** 2-4 pkts or scoopfuls/d divided into 2 doses. **Max:** 6 pkts or scoopfuls/d. **Peds: Usual:** 240 mg/kg/d of anhydrous cholestyramine resin in 2-3 divided doses. **Max:** 8 g/d.	◙C ✽> May decrease vitamin content in breast milk.

Colesevelam (WelChol)	**Tab:** 625 mg	**Adults: Initial:** 3 tabs bid or 6 tabs qd w/ meal. May increase to 7 tabs/d.	B >
Colestipol Hydrochloride (Colestid)	**Granules:** 5 gm/pkt or scoopful; **Tab:** 1 gm	**Adults: Initial:** 2 gm (tabs) or 5 gm (1 pkt or scoopful) qd-bid. **Titrate:** Increase by 2 gm qd or bid at 1-2 mth intervals. **Usual:** 2-16 gm/d (tab) or 1-6 pkts or scoopfuls qd or in divided doses.	N >
CALCIUM CHANNEL BLOCKER/HMG COA REDUCTASE INHIBITOR			
Amlodipine Besylate/Atorvastatin Calcium (Caduet)	**Tab:** 2.5-10 mg, 2.5-20 mg, 2.5-40 mg, 5-10 mg, 5-20 mg, 5-40 mg, 5-80 mg, 10-10 mg, 10-20 mg, 10-40 mg, 10-80 mg	Dosing is based on the appropriate combination of recommendations for the monotherapies. **Amlodipine:** See under Angina & Hypertension for dosing. **Atorvastatin: Adults: Hypercholesterolemia/Mixed Dyslipidemia: Initial:** 10-20 mg qd (or 40 mg qd for LDL-C reduction >45%). **Titrate:** Adjust dose at 2-4 wk intervals. **Usual:** 10-80 mg qd. **Homozygous Familial Hypercholesterolemia:** 10-80 mg qd. **Peds: 10-17 yo (postmenarchal): Heterozygous Familial Hypercholesterolemia: Initial:** 10 mg/d. **Titrate:** Adjust dose at ≥4 wks intervals. **Max:** 20 mg/d.	X v H

[5] Proarrhythmic properties/drug should only be used in life-threatening arrhythmias.

NAME	FORM/STRENGTH	DOSAGE	COMMENTS

CHLOESTEROL ABSORPTION INHIBITOR/HMG COA REDUCTASE INHIBITOR

NAME	FORM/STRENGTH	DOSAGE	COMMENTS
Ezetimibe/Simvastatin (Vytorin)	**Tab:** 10/10 mg, 10/20 mg, 10/40 mg, 10/80 mg	**Adults:** Take once daily in the evening. **Initial:** 10/20 mg qd. **Less aggressive LDL-C reductions: Initial:** 10/10 mg qd. **LDL-C reduction >55%: Initial:** 10/40 mg qd. **Titrate:** Adjust at ≥2 wks. **Homozygous Familial Hypercholesterolemia:** 10/40 mg or 10/80 mg qd. **Concomitant Bile Acid Sequestrant:** Take either ≥2 hours before or ≥4 hours after bile acid sequestrant. **Concomitant Cyclosporine:** Avoid unless tolerant of ≥5 mg of simvastatin. **Max:** 10/10 mg/d. **Concomitant Amiodarone/Verapamil: Max:** 10/20 mg/d.	X v R

CHOLESTEROL ABSORPTION INHIBITOR

NAME	FORM/STRENGTH	DOSAGE	COMMENTS
Ezetimibe (Zetia)	**Tab:** 10 mg	**Adults:** 10 mg qd. May give w/ HMG-CoA reductase inhibitor (primary hypercholesterolemia) or fenofibrate (mixed hyperlipidemia) for incremental effect. Give either ≥2h before or ≥4h after bile acid sequestrant.	C v

FIBRIC ACIDS

NAME	FORM/STRENGTH	DOSAGE	COMMENTS
Clofibrate	**Cap:** 500 mg	**Adults:** 2 gm/d in divided doses.	C v H R
Fenofibrate (Antara, Lofibra, Tricor, Triglide)	**Cap:** (Antara) 43 mg, 87 mg, 130 mg. (Lofibra) 67 mg, 134 mg, 200 mg. **Tab:** (Tricor) 48 mg, 145 mg. (Triglide) 50 mg, 160 mg.	**Adults: Hypercholesterolemia/Mixed Dyslipidemia: Initial:** (Antara) 130 mg/d. (Lofibra) 200 mg/d. (Tricor) 145 mg/d. (Triglide) 160 mg/d. **Hypertriglyceridemia: Initial:** (Antara) 43-130 mg/d. (Lofibra) 67-200 mg/d. (Tricor) 48-145 mg/d. (Triglide) 50-160 mg/d. **Max:** (Antara) 130 mg/d. (Lofibra) 200 mg/d. (Tricor) 145 mg/d. (Triglide) 160 mg/d.	C v H R

Gemfibrozil (Lopid)	**Tab:** 600 mg	**Adults:** 600 mg bid 30 min ac.	C v **H R**

HMG COA REDUCTASE INHIBITOR/NICOTINIC ACID

Lovastatin/Niacin (Advicor)	**Tab:** 20-500 mg, 20-750 mg, 20-1000mg	**Adults:** ≥**18 yo: Initial:** 20-500 mg qhs. **Titrate:** Increase by ≤500 mg of niacin q4wks. **Max:** 40-2000 mg. Adjust w/ cyclosporine or fibrates. May pretreat w/ ASA/NSAID to reduce flushing.	X v **H**

HMG COA REDUCTASE INHIBITORS

Atorvastatin Calcium (Lipitor)	**Tab:** 10 mg, 20 mg, 40 mg, 80 mg	**Adults: Hypercholesterolemia/Mixed Dyslipidemia: Initial:** 10-20 mg qd (or 40 mg qd for LDL-C reduction >45%). **Titrate:** Adjust at 2-4 wk intervals. **Usual:** 10-80 mg qd. **Homozygous Familial Hypercholesterolemia:** 10-80 mg qd. **Peds: 10-17 yo (postmenarchal): Heterozygous Familial Hypercholesterolemia: Initial:** 10 mg/d. **Titrate:** Adjust at ≥4 wk intervals. **Max:** 20 mg/d.	X v
Fluvastatin Sodium (Lescol, Lescol XL)	**Cap:** (Lescol) 20 mg, 40 mg; **Tab,ER:** (Lescol XL) 80 mg	**Adults:** ≥**18 yrs: Initial:** (LDL-C reduction ≥25%) 40 mg cap qpm or 80 mg XL tab at anytime of day (or 40 mg cap bid). (LDL-C reduction <25%) 20 mg cap qpm. **Usual:** 20-80 mg/day. Take 2h after bile-acid resins qhs. **Peds: 10-16 yo (≥1 yr post-menarche): Heterozygous Familial Hypercholesterolemia:** Individualize dose: **Initial:** 20 mg cap. **Titrate:** Adjust dose at 6 wk intervals. **Max:** 40 mg cap bid or 80 mg XL tab qd.	X v **H**

NAME	FORM/STRENGTH	DOSAGE	COMMENTS
Lovastatin (Altoprev)	**Tab,ER:** 10 mg, 20 mg, 40 mg, 60 mg	**Adults: Initial:** 20, 40, or 60 mg qhs. Use 10 mg/d if patient requires smaller reductions. May adjust q4wks or more. Adjust w/ cyclosporine, fibrates, niacin, amiodarone, verapamil.	◙X ❁v **H R**
Lovastatin (Mevacor)	**Tab:** 20 mg, 40 mg	**Adults: Initial:** 20 mg qd w/ pm meal (10 mg/d if need LDL-C reduction <20%). **Usual:** 10-80 mg/d as qd-bid. **Peds: 10-17 yo: Heterozygous Familial Hypercholesterolemia: Initial:** 20 mg qd (10 mg qd if need LDL-C reduction <20%). **Titrate:** May adjust q4wks. **Max:** 40 mg/d. Adjust w/ cyclosporine, fibrates, niacin, verapamil, or amiodarone.	◙X ❁v **H R**
Pravastatin Sodium (Pravachol)	**Tab:** 10 mg, 20 mg, 40 mg, 80 mg	**Adults: ≥18 yo: Initial:** 40 mg qd. **Titrate:** Increase to 80 mg qd. **Heterozygous Familial Hypercholesterolemia: Peds: 14-18 yo:** 40 mg qd. **8-13 yo:** 20 mg qd. Adjust w/ cyclosporine. Take at least 1h before or 4h after the resin.	◙X ❁v **H R**
Rosuvastatin (Crestor)	**Tab:** 5 mg, 10 mg, 20 mg, 40 mg	**Adults: Hypercholesterolemia/Mixed Dyslipidemia: Initial:** 10 mg qd (or 5 mg qd for less aggressive LDL-C reductions; 20 mg qd w/ LDL-C >190 mg/dL). **Titrate:** Adjust dose if needed at 2-4 wk intervals. **Range:** 5-40 mg qd. **Homozygous Familial Hypercholesterolemia:** 20 mg qd. Max: 40 mg qd. Adjust w/ cyclosporine, gemfibrozil.	◙X ❁v **H R**

Simvastatin (Zocor)	**Tab:** 5 mg, 10 mg, 20 mg, 40 mg, 80 mg	**Adults: Initial:** 20-40 mg qpm, 40 mg if at high risk for CHD events. **Usual:** 5-80 mg/d. **Homozygous Familial Hypercholesterolemia:** 40 mg qpm or 80 mg/d given as 20 mg bid plus 40 mg qpm. Adjust w/ cyclosporine, fibrates, amiodarone, verapamil, or niacin. **10-17 yo (at least 1-yr postmenarchal): Heterozygous Familial Hypercholesterolemia: Initial:** 10 mg qpm. **Usual:** 10-40 mg/d. **Titrate:** Adjust at ≥4 wk intervals. **Max:** 40 mg/d.	◙X ❁v **H R**

NICOTINIC ACID

Niacin (Niaspan)	**Tab,ER:** 500 mg, 750 mg, 1000 mg	**Adults: Initial:** 500 mg qhs. **Titrate:** Increase by 500 mg q4wks. **Maint:** 1-2 gm qhs. May pretreat w/ ASA/NSAID to reduce flushing.	◙C ❁v **H**

SALICYLATE/HMG-COA REDUCTASE INHIBITOR

Aspirin/Pravastatin Sodium (Pravigard PAC)	**Tab:** 81-20 mg, 325-20 mg, 81-40 mg, 325-40 mg, 81-80 mg, 325-80 mg	**Adults: Usual:** 81-40 mg or 325-40 mg qd. May increase to 81-80 mg or 325-80 mg qd.	◙X ❁v **H**

MISCELLANEOUS

Omega-3-acid ethyl esters (Omacor)	**Cap:** 1 gm	**Adults:** 4 gm qd. Given as a single 4-gm dose or as two 2-gm doses.	◙C ❁>

NAME	FORM/STRENGTH	DOSAGE	COMMENTS

Coagulation Modifiers

DIRECT THROMBIN INHIBITORS

NAME	FORM/STRENGTH	DOSAGE	COMMENTS
Argatroban	**Inj:** 100 mg/ml	**Adults: ≥18 yo: Thrombosis in HIT:** D/C heparin & obtain baseline aPTT. **Initial:** 2 mcg/kg/min IV. Check aPTT after 2h. **Titrate:** Increase until aPTT is 1.5-3 x initial baseline. **Max:** 10 mcg/kg/min. **HIT w/ PCI: Initial:** 350 mcg/kg bolus w/ 25 mcg/kg/min IV. Adjust based on ACT. Continue infusion dose once therapeutic ACT (300-400 sec) achieved.	B v **H**
Bivalirudin (Angiomax)	**Inj:** 250 mg	**Adults:** 0.75 mg/kg IV bolus, then 1.75 mg/kg/h for duration of PCI procedure. Additional bolus of 0.3 mg/kg can be given if needed based on ACT. Continuation of infusion drip for up to 4 h post-procedure is optional. After 4 h, if needed, an additional 0.2 mg/kg/h IV for up to 20 h may be initiated.	B > **R**

GLYCOPROTEIN IIB/IIIA INHIBITORS

NAME	FORM/STRENGTH	DOSAGE	COMMENTS
Abciximab (ReoPro)	**Inj:** 2 mg/ml	**Adults: PCI:** 0.25 mg/kg IV bolus given 10-60 min before PCI, then 0.125 mcg/kg/min IV infusion (Max: 10 mcg/min) x 12h. **Unstable Angina (PCI within 24h):** 0.25 mg/kg IV bolus, then 10 mcg/min infusion x 18-24h, concluding 1h after PCI.	C >
Eptifibatide (Integrilin)	**Inj:** 2 mg/ml, 0.75 mg/ml	**Adults: Acute Coronary Syndrome:** 180 mcg/kg IV bolus, then 2 mcg/kg/min IV infusion up to 72h. **PCI:** 180 mcg/kg IV bolus before PCI, then 2 mcg/kg/min IV infusion x 18-24h post-PCI. Give 2nd 180 mcg/kg IV bolus 10 min after 1st bolus.	B > **R**

Tirofiban HCl (Aggrastat)	**Inj:** 0.05 mg/ml, 0.25 mg/ml	**Acute Coronary Syndrome: Adults: ≥18 yo: Initial:** 0.4 mcg/kg/min IV x 30 min. **Maint:** 0.1 mcg/kg/min IV. Continue through angiography & 12-24h after angioplasty/atherectomy.	◙B ❋v **R** Use with ASA & heparin unless CI.
GLYCOSAMINOGLYCAN			
Heparin Sodium	**Inj:** 1000 U/ml, 2500 U/ml, 5000 U/ml, 7500 U/ml, 10,000 U/ml	**Adults: Based on 68 kg: LD:** 5000 U IV, then 10,000-20,000 U SC. **Maint:** 8000-10,000 U q8h or 15,000-20,000 U q12h. **Intermittent IV Injection: LD:** 10,000 U. **Maint:** 5000-10,000 U q4-6h. **IV Infusion: LD:** 5,000 U. **Maint:** 20,000-40,000 U/d. **Peds: Initial:** 50 U/kg IV. **Maint:** 100 U/kg IV q4h or 20,000 U/m²/d continuous IV.	◙C ❋ ∧
LOW MOLECULAR WEIGHT HEPARINS			
Dalteparin Sodium (Fragmin)	**Inj:** 2500 IU/0.2 ml, 5000 IU/0.2 ml, 7500 IU/0.3 ml, 10,000 IU/ml, 25,000 IU/ml	**Adults: SC: Unstable Angina/Non-Q-Wave MI:** 120 U/kg, up to 10,000 IU q12h w/ 75-165 mg/d ASA x 5-8d. **Hip Replacement Surgery: Initial:** 2500 IU 2h pre-op, then 2500 IU 4-8h post-op. **Maint:** 5000 IU qd x 5-10d post-op (up to 14d) (refer to full PI for alternate dosing). **Abdominal Surgery:** 2500 IU 1-2h pre-op, then qd x 5-10d post-op (refer to full PI for high risk dosing). **Severely Restricted Mobility During Acute Illness:** 5000 IU qd x 12-14d.	◙B ❋> [6]
Danaparoid Sodium (Orgaran)	**Inj:** 750 U/0.6 ml	**DVT/PE Prevention w/ Hip Replacement Surgery: Adults:** 750 U SC bid; 1-4h pre-op, then not before 2h post-op. Continue x 7-10d (up to 14d).	◙B ❋> [6]

[6] Risk of paralysis by spinal/epidural hematoma with neuraxial anesthesia/lumbar puncture. Increased risk with concomitant anticoagulation, NSAIDS, or traumatic/repeated lumbar puncture.

NAME	FORM/STRENGTH	DOSAGE	COMMENTS
Enoxaparin (Lovenox)	**Inj:** 30 mg/0.3 ml, 40 mg/0.4 ml, 60 mg/0.6 ml, 80 mg/0.8 ml, 100 mg/ml, 120 mg/0.8 ml, 150 mg/ml, 300 mg/3 ml	**Adults: SC: Hip/Knee Replacement Surgery:** 30 mg q12h 12-24h post-op x 7-10d (up to 14d). Hip (alternative dosing): 40 mg qd 12h pre-op, then 40 mg qd x 3 wks. **Abdominal Surgery:** 40 mg qd, 2h pre-op x 7-10d (up to 14d). **DVT Outpatient Treatment:** 1 mg/kg q12h w/ warfarin (goal INR 2-3) x 7d (up to 17d). **DVT/PE Inpatient Treatment:** 1 mg/kg q12h or 1.5 mg/kg qd w/ warfarin (goal INR 2-3) x 7d (up to 17d). **Unstable Angina/Non-Q-Wave MI:** 1 mg/kg q12h with 100-325 mg/d ASA x 2-8d (up to 12.5d). **Acute Illness:** 40 mg qd x 6-11d (up to 14d).	●B ❄> **R** 6
Tinzaparin (Innohep)	**Inj:** 20,000 IU/ml	**DVT/PE Treatment: Adults:** 175 IU/kg SC qd for at least 6d & until anticoagulated w/ warfarin.	●B ❄> 6
PHOSPHODIESTERASE/PLATELET AGGREGATION-ADHESION INHIBITORS			
Anagrelide HCl (Agrylin)	**Cap:** 0.5 mg, 1 mg	**Thrombocythemia: Initial: Adults:** 0.5 mg qid or 1 mg bid x 1 wk. **Peds:** 0.5 mg qd. **Titrate:** May increase by 0.5 mg/d qwk. Adjust based on platelet count. **Max:** 10 mg/d or 2.5 mg/dose.	●C ❄v **H R**
Aspirin (Bayer Aspirin, Ecotrin)	**Chewtab:** 81 mg; **Tab:** 81 mg, 325 mg; **Tab,Delay:** 81 mg, 325 mg, 500 mg	**Adults: Stroke/TIA:** 50-325 mg qd. **Suspected AMI: Initial:** 160-162.5 mg qd as soon as suspect MI. **Maint:** 160-162.5 mg x 30d post-infarct. **Prevention or Recurrent MI:** 75-325 mg qd.	●N ❄> **H R** Avoid use during 3rd trimester.
Cilostazol (Pletal)	**Tab:** 50 mg, 100 mg	**Intermittent Claudication: Adults:** 100 mg bid, 1/2h before or 2h after breakfast & dinner. Dose 50 mg bid w/ certain drugs.	●C ❄v CI in CHF.

Clopidogrel Bisulfate (Plavix)	**Tab:** 75 mg	**Adults: MI/Stroke/Peripheral Arterial Disease:** 75 mg qd. **Acute Coronary Syndrome: LD:** 300 mg. **Maint:** 75 mg qd. Take w/ 75-325 mg ASA qd.	B v
Dipyridamole (Persantine)	**Tab:** 25 mg, 50 mg, 75 mg	**Prophylaxis to Thromboembolism after Cardiac Valve Replacement: Adults:** 75-100 mg qid as an adjunct to warfarin.	B >
Dipyridamole/ASA (Aggrenox)	**Cap,ER:** 200-25 mg	**Risk Reduction of Stroke: Adults:** 1 cap qam & qpm.	B (Dipyridamole) D (ASA) > **H R**
Ticlopidine HCl (Ticlid)	**Tab:** 250 mg	**Adults: Stroke:** 250 mg bid. **Coronary Artery Stenting:** 250 mg bid w/ ASA up to 30d after stent implant. Take w/ food.	B v **H R** [15]
SPECIFIC FACTOR XA INHIBITOR			
Fondaparinux Sodium (Arixtra)	**Inj:** 2.5 mg/0.5 ml, 5 mg/0.4 ml, 7.5 mg/0.6 ml, 10 mg/0.8 ml	**Adults: SC: DVT Prophylaxis for Hip Fracture or Replacement Surgery/Knee Replacement Surgery/Abdominal Surgery:** 2.5 mg qd, starting 6-8h post-op x 5-9d (Hip/Knees: up to 11d; Abdominal: up to 10d). **Hip Fracture Surgery:** Extended prophylaxis up to 24 additional days. **DVT/PE Treatment: <50 kg:** 5 mg qd. **50-100 kg:** 7.5 mg qd. **>100 kg:** 10 mg qd. Add concomitant warfarin ASAP (usually within 72 h) & continue x 5-9d (up to 26d) until INR=2-3.	B > **R** [6]

[6] Risk of paralysis by spinal/epidural hematoma with neuraxial anesthesia/lumbar puncture. Increased risk with concomitant anticoagulation, NSAIDS, or traumatic/repeated lumbar puncture.

[15] Neutropenia. Agranulocytosis. TTP. Aplastic anemia.

NAME	FORM/STRENGTH	DOSAGE	COMMENTS
THROMBOLYTICS			
Alteplase (Activase)	**Inj:** 50 mg, 100 mg	**Adults: Acute MI: Accelerated Infusion: >67 kg:** 15 mg IV bolus, then 50 mg over 30 min, then 35 mg infused over the next 60 min. **≤67 kg:** 15 mg IV bolus, then 0.75 mg/kg over next 30 min up to 50 mg, & then 0.50 mg/kg over the next 60 min up to 35 mg. **3h-Infusion:** 60 mg infused over 1st hr (of which 6-10 mg IV bolus), then 20 mg over the 2nd hr, & 20 mg over the 3rd hr. **<65kg:** 1.25 mg/kg over 3h. **Acute Ischemic Stroke:** 0.9 mg/kg up to 90 mg over 60 min (10% of total dose given as initial bolus over 1 min). **PE:** 100 mg IV over 2h.	C ✽>
Alteplase (Cathflo Activase)	**Inj:** 2 mg	**Obstructed Catheters: Adults & Peds: ≥30 kg:** 2 mg in 2 ml. **<30 kg:** 110% of catheter internal lumen volume, not to exceed 2 mg in 2 ml. Repeat if function not restored after 120 min. **Max:** 2 mg/dose. Reconstitute to 1 mg/ml.	C ✽>
Reteplase (Retavase)	**Inj:** 10.4 U	**Acute MI: Adults:** 10 U IV over 2 min, repeat in 30 min.	C ✽>
Streptokinase (Streptase)	**Inj:** 250,000 IU, 750,000 IU, 1.5 MIU	**Adults: Acute MI:** 1.5 MIU IV within 60 min. **PE/DVT:** 250,000 IU over 30 min, then 100,000 IU/h x 24h (72h if DVT). **Thrombosis/Embolism:** 250,000 IU over 30 min, then 100,000 IU/h x 24-72h.	C ✽>
Tenecteplase (TNKase)	**Inj:** 50 mg	**Adults: Acute MI: <60 kg:** 30 mg. **60 to <70 kg:** 35 mg. **70 to <80 kg:** 40 mg. **80 to <90 kg:** 45 mg. **≥90 kg:** 50 mg. Give IV over 5 sec. **Max:** 50 mg/dose.	C ✽>

Urokinase (Abbokinase)	**Inj:** 250,000 IU	**PE: Adults: LD:** 4400 IU/kg IV at 90 ml/h over 10 min. **Maint:** 4400 IU/kg/h IV at 15 ml/h for 12h. Flush line after each cycle.	B >
Urokinase (Abbokinase Open-Cath)	**Inj:** 5000 IU, 9000 IU	**Obstructed Catheters: Adults:** Amount of drug should equal the internal volume of the catheter, may repeat in resistant cases. Specialized administration.	B >

VITAMIN K-DEPENDENT COAGULATION FACTOR INHIBITOR

Warfarin Sodium (Coumadin)	**Inj:** 5 mg; **Tab:** 1 mg, 2 mg, 2.5 mg, 3 mg, 4 mg, 5 mg, 6 mg, 7.5 mg, 10 mg	**Adults: ≥18 yo:** Adjust dose based on PT/INR. Give IV as alternate to PO. **Initial:** 2-5 mg qd. **Maint:** 2-10 mg qd. **Venous Thromboembolism (including PE):** INR of 2-3. **A-Fib:** INR of 2-3. **Post-MI:** Initiate 2-4 wks post-infarct & maintain INR of 2.5-3.5. **Mechanical/Bioprosthetic Heart Valve:** INR of 2-3 x 12 wks after valve insertion, then INR of 2.5-3.5 long term.	X > **H**

CV Risk Reduction

ACE INHIBITORS

Perindopril Erbumine (Aceon)	**Tab:** 2 mg, 4 mg, 8 mg	**Risk Reduction of CV Mortality/MI in Stable CAD: Adults: Initial:** 4 mg qd for 2 wks. **Maint:** 8 mg qd. **Elderly (>70 yrs): Initial:** 2 mg qd for 1 wk. **Titrate:** 4 mg qd for 1 wk. **Maint:** 8 mg qd.	C (1st trimester) D (2nd/3rd trimester) v **R** [7]

[7] ACE Inhibitors can cause injury & death to developing fetus in 2nd & 3rd trimesters.

NAME	FORM/STRENGTH	DOSAGE	COMMENTS
Ramipril (Altace)	**Cap:** 1.25 mg, 2.5 mg, 5 mg, 10 mg	**Risk Reduction of MI, Stroke, Death (≥55 yrs): Adults: Initial:** 2.5 mg qd for 1 wk. Increase to 5 mg qd for the next 3 wks. **Maint:** 10 mg qd. Reduce/discontinue diuretic if possible. **Volume Depletion/Renal Artery Stenosis: Initial:** 1.25 mg qd.	C (1st trimester) D (2nd/3rd trimester) v **R** [7]

ANGIOTENSIN II RECEPTOR ANTAGONISTS

NAME	FORM/STRENGTH	DOSAGE	COMMENTS
Valsartan (Diovan)	**Tab:** 40 mg, 80 mg, 160 mg, 320 mg	**Reduction of CV Mortality Post-MI: Adults: Initial:** 20 mg bid. **Titrate:** Increase to 40 mg bid within 7d, then titrate up to 160 mg bid.	C (1st trimester) D (2nd/3rd trimester) v **R** [9]

Heart Failure

ACE INHIBITORS

NAME	FORM/STRENGTH	DOSAGE	COMMENTS
Captopril (Capoten)	**Tab:** 12.5 mg, 25 mg, 50 mg, 100 mg	**Adults: CHF: Initial:** 25 mg tid. **Usual:** 50-100 mg tid. **Max:** 450 mg/d. **Left Ventricular Dysfunction Following MI: Initial:** 6.25 mg single dose, then 12.5 mg tid. **Titrate:** Increase to 25 mg tid over next several days, then to 50 mg tid over next several wks. **Usual:** 50 mg tid.	C (1st trimester) D (2nd/3rd trimester) v **R** [7]
Enalapril Maleate (Vasotec)	**Tab:** 1.25 mg, 2.5 mg, 5 mg, 10 mg, 20 mg	**Adults: Initial:** 2.5 mg qd. **Titrate:** Increase over few days or wks. **Usual:** 2.5-20 mg given bid. **Max:** 40 mg/d.	C (1st trimester) D (2nd/3rd trimester) v **R** [7]
Fosinopril Sodium (Monopril)	**Tab:** 10 mg, 20 mg, 40 mg	**Adults: Initial:** 10 mg qd. **Titrate:** Increase over several wk period. **Usual:** 20-40 mg qd. **Max:** 40mg/d.	C (1st trimester) D (2nd/3rd trimester) v **R** [7]

Lisinopril (Prinivil, Zestril)	**Tab:** 2.5 mg, 5 mg, 10 mg, 20 mg, 30 mg, 40 mg	**Adults: CHF: Initial:** 5 mg qd. **Titrate:** (Zestril) ≤10 mg q2wks. **Usual:** (Prinivil) 5-20 mg qd. (Zestril) 5-40 mg qd. **Max:** (Prinivil) 20 mg/d. (Zestril) 40 mg/d. **AMI: Initial:** 5 mg within 24 h, then 5 mg after 24 h, then 10 mg after 48 h, then 10 mg qd. Use 2.5 mg during 1st 3 days w/ low systolic BP. **Maint:** 10 mg qd for 6 wks, 2.5-5 mg w/ hypotension. D/C w/ prolonged hypotension.	C (1st trimester) D (2nd/3rd trimester) ❊v **R** [7]
Quinapril HCl (Accupril)	**Tab:** 5 mg, 10 mg, 20 mg, 40 mg	**Adults: Initial:** 5 mg bid. **Titrate:** Increase at wkly intervals. **Usual:** 10-20 mg bid. **Max:** 40 mg/d.	C (1st trimester) D (2nd/3rd trimester) ❊v **R** [7]
Ramipril (Altace)	**Cap:** 1.25 mg, 2.5 mg, 5 mg, 10 mg	**Adults: Post-MI CHF: Initial: 2.5 mg bid, 1.25 mg bid if hypotensive.** Titrate: Increase to 5 mg bid. **CrCl <40ml/min: Initial:** 1.25 mg qd. **Titrate:** May increase to 1.25 mg bid. **Max:** 2.5 mg bid. Reduce/discontinue diuretic if possible. **Volume Depletion/Renal Artery Stenosis: Initial:** 1.25 mg qd.	C (1st trimester) D (2nd/3rd trimester) ❊v **R** [7]
Trandolapril (Mavik)	**Tab:** 1 mg, 2 mg, 4 mg	**Post-MI CHF: Adults: Initial:** 1 mg qd. **Usual:** 4 mg qd. **Max:** 4 mg/d.	C (1st trimester) D (2nd/3rd trimester) ❊v **R** [7]
ALDOSTERONE BLOCKER			
Eplerenone (Inspra)	**Tab:** 25 mg, 50 mg	**CHF Post-MI: Adults: Initial:** 25 mg qd. **Titrate:** To 50 mg qd within 4 wks. **Maint:** 50 mg qd. **Adjust dose based on K+ level:** See labeling.	B ❊v **R**

[7] ACE Inhibitors can cause injury & death to developing fetus in 2nd & 3rd trimesters.

[9] Drugs acting directly on the renin-angiotensin system can cause fetal/neonatal morbidity & death, primarily during 3rd trimester.

NAME	FORM/STRENGTH	DOSAGE	COMMENTS
ALPHA/BETA BLOCKERS			
Carvedilol (Coreg)	**Tab:** 3.125 mg, 6.25 mg,12.5 mg, 25 mg	**Mild-Severe HF: Adults: Initial:** 3.125 mg bid x 2 wks. **Titrate:** Double dose q2wks. **Max:** 50 mg bid if >85 kg. Reduce dose if HR <55 beats/min. Take w/ food.	◙C ❋v
ANGIOTENSIN II RECEPTOR ANTAGONISTS			
Candesartan Cilexetil (Atacand)	**Tab:** 4 mg, 8 mg, 16 mg, 32 mg	**Adults: Initial:** 4 mg qd. **Titrate:** Double dose at 2 wk intervals. **Target:** 32 mg qd.	◙C (1st trimester) ◙D (2nd/3rd trimester) ❋v **R** [9]
Valsartan (Diovan)	**Tab:** 40 mg, 80 mg, 160 mg, 320 mg	**Adults: CHF: Initial:** 40 mg bid. **Titrate:** Increase to 80 mg or 160 mg bid (use highest dose tolerated). **Max:** 320 mg/d in divided doses.	◙C (1st trimester) ◙D (2nd/3rd trimester) ❋v **R** [9]
BETA BLOCKERS			
Metoprolol Succinate (Toprol-XL)	**Tab,ER:** 25 mg, 50 mg, 100 mg, 200 mg	**Adults: Initial: Class II HF:** 25 mg qd x 2 wks. **Severe HF:** 12.5 mg qd x 2 wks. **Titrate:** Double dose q2wks as tolerated. **Max:** 200 mg/d.	◙C ❋>
DIURETICS (INDOLINE)			
Indapamide (Lozol)	(Lozol) **Tab:** 1.25 mg; (Generic) **Tab:** 1.25 mg, 2.5 mg	**Adults: Initial:** 2.5 mg qam. **Titrate:** After 1 wk, may increase to 5 mg qd. **Max:** 5 mg qd.	◙B ❋v
DIURETICS (LOOP)			
Bumetanide (Bumex)	(Bumex) **Tab:** 0.5 mg, 1 mg, 2 mg; (Generic) **Inj:** 0.25 mg/ml; **Tab:** 0.5 mg, 1 mg, 2 mg	**Adults: ≥18 yo: PO: Usual:** 0.5-2 mg qd. **Maint:** Give qod or q3-4d. **Max:** 10 mg/d. **IV/IM: Initial:** 0.5-1 mg, may repeat q2-3h x 2-3 doses. **Max:** 10 mg/d.	◙C ❋v [8]

Furosemide (Lasix)	(Generic) **Inj:** 10 mg/ml; **Sol:** 10 mg/ml, 40 mg/5 ml; **Tab:** 20 mg, 40 mg, 80 mg; (Lasix) **Tab:** 20 mg, 40 mg, 80 mg	**Adults: PO: Usual:** 20-80 mg as single dose, may repeat or increase by 20-40 mg after 6-8h. **Max:** 600 mg/d. **IV/IM:** 20-40 mg. May repeat or increase by 20 mg after 2h. **Peds: PO: Usual:** 2 mg/kg as single dose, may increase by 1-2 mg/kg after 6-8h. **Max:** 6 mg/kg. **IV/IM:** 1 mg/kg single dose. May increase by 1 mg/kg after 2h. **Max:** 6 mg/kg.	C > [8]
Torsemide (Demadex)	**Inj:** 10 mg/ml; **Tab:** 5 mg, 10 mg, 20 mg, 100 mg	**Adults: PO/IV: Initial:** 10-20 mg qd. **Titrate:** Double dose until desired diuretic response. **Max:** 200 mg/d.	B >
DIURETICS (POTASSIUM SPARING)			
Amiloride HCl (Midamor)	**Tab:** 5 mg	**Adults: Initial:** 5 mg qd. **Titrate:** Increase to 10 mg/d. If hyperkalemia persists, may increase to 15 mg/d then to 20 mg/d. **Maint:** May give on an intermittent basis.	B v
Spironolactone (Aldactone)	**Tab:** 25 mg, 50 mg, 100 mg	**Adults: Initial:** 100 mg/d in single or divided doses. **Usual:** 25-200 mg/d.	C v [16]
Triamterene (Dyrenium)	**Cap:** 50 mg, 100 mg	**Adults: Initial:** 100 mg bid. **Max:** 300 mg/d.	C v
DIURETICS (POTASSIUM SPARING/THIAZIDE)			
Amiloride/HCTZ (Moduretic)	**Tab:** 5-50 mg	**Adults: Initial:** 1 tab qd. **Maint:** May be given on intermittent basis. **Max:** 2 tabs qd.	B v

[8] Excess amounts may lead to water & electrolyte depletion.
[9] Drugs acting directly on the renin-angiotensin system can cause fetal/neonatal morbidity & death, primarily during 3rd trimester.
[16] Tumorigenic in chronic toxicity studies. Avoid unnecessary use.

NAME	FORM/STRENGTH	DOSAGE	COMMENTS
Spironolactone/HCTZ (Aldactazide)	**Tab:** 25-25 mg, 50-50 mg	**Adults: Usual:** 100 mg/d per component qd or in divided doses. **Maint:** 25-200 mg/d per component.	◙C ❋v Not for initial therapy. 16
Triamterene/HCTZ (Dyazide, Maxzide)	**Cap:** (Dyazide) 37.5-25 mg; **Tab:** (Maxzide) 37.5-25 mg, 75-50 mg	**Adults: Usual:** (37.5-25 mg cap/tab) 1-2 caps or tabs qd. (75-50 mg tab) 1 tab qd.	◙C ❋v
DIURETICS (QUINAZOLINE)			
Metolazone (Zaroxolyn)	**Tab:** 2.5 mg, 5 mg, 10 mg	**Adults:** 5-20 mg qd.	◙B ❋v Rapid and slow formulations are not equivalent.
DIURETICS (THIAZIDE)			
Chlorothiazide (Diuril)	**Inj:** 0.5 gm; **Susp:** 250 mg/5 ml; **Tab:** 250 mg, 500 mg	**Adults: PO/IV:** 0.5-1 gm qd-bid. May give qod or 3-5d per wk. **Peds: PO: Usual:** 10-20 mg/kg/d given qd-bid. **Max: 2-12 yo:** 1 gm/d. **≤2 yo:** 375 mg/d. **<6 mths:** 15 mg/kg bid.	◙C ❋v
Hydrochlorothiazide	**Cap:** 12.5 mg; **Tab:** 25 mg, 50 mg, 100 mg	**Adults: Usual:** 25-100 mg qd. May give qod or 3-5d per wk. **Peds:** 1-2 mg/kg/d given qd-bid. **Max: 2-12 yo:** 100 mg/d. **≤2 yo:** 37.5 mg/d. **<6 mths:** 1.5 mg/kg bid.	◙B ❋v

INOTROPIC AGENTS

Digoxin (Digitek, Lanoxicaps, Lanoxin, Lanoxin Pediatric)	**Cap:** (Lanoxicaps) 0.05 mg, 0.1 mg, 0.2 mg; **Inj:** (Lanoxin Pediatric) 0.1 mg/mL, (Lanoxin) 0.25 mg/mL; **Sol:** (Lanoxin Pediatric) 0.05 mg/mL; **Tab:** (Digitek, Lanoxin) 0.125 mg, 0.25 mg	**HF: Adults: Rapid Digitalization: LD:** (Cap/Inj) 0.4-0.6 mg PO/IV or (Tab) 0.5-0.75 mg PO. May give additional (Cap/Inj) 0.1-0.3 mg or (Tab) 0.125-0.375 mg at 6-8h intervals until clinical effect. **Maint:** (Tab) 0.125-0.5 mg qd. **Peds: Sol/Ped Inj: Digitalizing Dose: Premature Infants:** 20-30 mcg/kg PO or 15-25 mcg/kg IV. **Full-Term Infants:** 25-35 mcg/kg PO or 20-30 mcg/kg IV. **1-24 mths:** 35-60 mcg/kg PO or 30-50 mcg/kg IV. **2-5 yo:** 30-40 mcg/kg PO or 25-35 mcg/kg IV. **5-10 yo:** 20-35 mcg/kg PO or 15-30 mcg/kg IV. **>10 yo:** 10-15 mcg/kg PO or 8-12 mcg/kg IV. **Maint: Premature Infants:** 20-30% of digitalizing dose. **Full-Term Infants to >10 yo:** 25-35% of digitalizing dose. **Cap: Digitalizing Dose: 2-5 yo:** 25-35 mcg/kg. 5-10 yo: 15-30 mcg/kg. **>10 yo:** 8-12 mcg/kg. **Maint: ≥2 yo:** 25-35% of digitalizing dose. **Tab: Maint: 2-5 yo:** 10-15 mcg/kg. **5-10 yo:** 7-10 mcg/kg. **>10 yo:** 3-5 mcg/kg.	C > R

MISCELLANEOUS

Isosorbide Dinitrate/ Hydralazine HCl (BiDil)	**Tab:** 20-37.5 mg	**Adults: Initial:** 1 tab bid. **Max:** 2 tabs tid.	C >

[16] Tumorigenic in chronic toxicity studies. Avoid unnecessary use.

Hypertension

ACE INHIBITORS

NAME	FORM/STRENGTH	DOSAGE	COMMENTS
Benazepril HCl (Lotensin)	**Tab:** 5 mg, 10 mg, 20 mg, 40 mg	**Adults: Initial:** 10 mg qd; 5 mg qd if on diuretic. **Maint:** 20-40 mg/d as qd-bid. **Max:** 80 mg/d. **Peds: ≥6 yo: Initial:** 0.2 mg/kg qd. **Max:** 0.6 mg/kg.	◙C (1st trimester) ◙D (2nd/3rd trimester) ❋> **R**[7]
Captopril (Capoten)	**Tab:** 12.5 mg, 25 mg, 50 mg, 100 mg	**Adults: Initial:** 25 mg bid-tid. **Titrate:** Increase to 50 mg bid-tid after 1-2 wks. **Usual:** 25-150 mg bid-tid. **Max:** 450 mg/d.	◙C (1st trimester) ◙D (2nd/3rd trimester) ❋v **R**[7]
Enalapril Maleate (Vasotec)	**Tab:** 1.25 mg, 2.5 mg, 5 mg, 10 mg, 20 mg	**Adults: Initial:** 5 mg qd, 2.5 mg if on diuretic. **Usual:** 10-40 mg/d as qd-bid. **Peds: 1 mth-16 yo: Initial:** 0.08 mg/kg (up to 5 mg) qd. **Max:** 0.58 mg/kg/dose (or 40 mg/dose).	◙C (1st trimester) ◙D (2nd/3rd trimester) ❋v **R**[7]
Enalaprilat (Vasotec IV)	**Inj:** 1.25 mg/ml	**Adults: Usual:** 1.25 mg over 5 min q6h. **Max:** 20 mg/d. **Concomitant Diuretic: Initial:** 0.625 mg over 5 min, may repeat after 1h. **Maint:** 1.25 mg q6h. **PO/IV Conversion:** 5 mg/d PO or 1.25 mg IV q6h & 2.5 mg/d PO or 0.625 mg q6h IV.	◙C (1st trimester) ◙D (2nd/3rd trimester) ❋v **R**[7]
Fosinopril Sodium (Monopril)	**Tab:** 10 mg, 20 mg, 40 mg	**Adults: Initial:** 10 mg qd. **Usual:** 20-40 mg qd. **Max:** 80 mg/d. **Peds: >50 kg:** 5-10 mg qd.	◙C (1st trimester) ◙D (2nd/3rd trimester) ❋v[7]
Lisinopril (Prinivil, Zestril)	**Tab:** 2.5 mg, 5 mg, 10 mg, 20 mg, 30 mg, 40 mg	**Adults: Initial:** 10 mg qd, 5 mg qd if on diuretic. **Usual:** 20-40 mg qd. **Max:** 80 mg/d.	◙C (1st trimester) ◙D (2nd/3rd trimester) ❋v **R**[7]

Moexipril HCl (Univasc)	**Tab:** 7.5 mg, 15 mg	**Adults: Initial:** 7.5 mg qd, 3.75 mg if on diuretic. **Usual:** 7.5-30 mg/d as qd-bid. **Max:** 60 mg/d.	C (1st trimester) D (2nd/3rd trimester) v **R** [7]
Perindopril Erbumine (Aceon)	**Tab:** 2 mg, 4 mg, 8 mg	**Adults: Initial:** 4 mg qd, 2-4 mg/d if on diuretic. **Usual:** 4-8 mg/d as qd-bid. **Max:** 16 mg qd.	C (1st trimester) D (2nd/3rd trimester) v **R** [7]
Quinapril HCl (Accupril)	**Tab:** 5 mg, 10 mg, 20 mg, 40 mg	**Adults: Initial:** 10-20 mg qd; 5 mg qd if on diuretic. **Usual:** 20-80 mg/d given qd-bid.	C (1st trimester) D (2nd/3rd trimester) v **R** [7]
Ramipril (Altace)	**Tab:** 1.25 mg, 2.5 mg, 5 mg, 10 mg	**Adults: Initial:** 2.5 mg bid, 1.25 mg bid if on a diuretic. **Usual:** 2.5-20 mg/d given qd-bid.	C (1st trimester) D (2nd/3rd trimester) **H R** [7]
Trandolapril (Mavik)	**Tab:** 1 mg, 2 mg, 4 mg	**Post-MI CHF/Left-Ventricular Dysfunction: Adults: Initial**: 1 mg qd in non-black patients; 2 mg qd in black patients; 0.5 mg if on diuretic. **Titrate:** Adjust at 1 wk intervals. **Usual:** 2-4 mg qd. **Max:** 8 mg/d.	C (1st trimester) D (2nd/3rd trimester) v **H R** [7]

ACE INHIBITORS/CALCIUM CHANNEL BLOCKERS

Amlodipine/Benazepril (Lotrel)	**Cap:** 2.5-10 mg, 5-10 mg, 5-20 mg, 5-40 mg, 10-20 mg, 10-40 mg	**Adults: Usual:** If not controlled on monotherapy, or unacceptable edema w/ amlodipine, then 2.5-10 mg amlodipine & 10-80 mg benazepril per day.	C (1st trimester) D (2nd/3rd tri-mester) v **H R** [7, 24]

[7] ACE Inhibitors can cause injury & death to developing fetus in 2nd & 3rd trimesters.
[24] Avoid if CrCl <30 ml/min.

JOINT NATIONAL COMMITTEE (JNC) VII ALGORITHM FOR HYPERTENSION

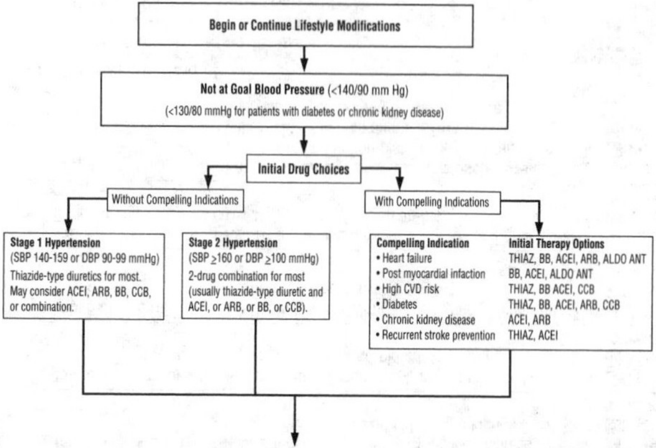

Begin or Continue Lifestyle Modifications
Not at Goal Blood Pressure (<140/90 mm Hg)
(<130/80 mmHg for patients with diabetes or chronic kidney disease)
Initial Drug Choices
Without Compelling Indications
With Compelling Indications
Stage 1 Hypertension
(SBP 140-159 or DBP 90-99 mmHg)
Thiazide-type diuretics for most. May consider ACEI, ARB, BB, CCB, or combination.
Stage 2 Hypertension
(SBP ≥160 or DBP ≥100 mmHg)
2-drug combination for most (usually thiazide-type diuretic and ACEI, or ARB, or BB, or CCB).
Compelling Indication
Initial Therapy Options
• Heart failure — THIAZ, BB, ACEI, ARB, ALDO ANT
• Post myocardial infaction — BB, ACEI, ALDO ANT
• High CVD risk — THIAZ, BB ACEI, CCB
• Diabetes — THIAZ, BB, ACEI, ARB, CCB
• Chronic kidney disease — ACEI, ARB
• Recurrent stroke prevention — THIAZ, ACEI

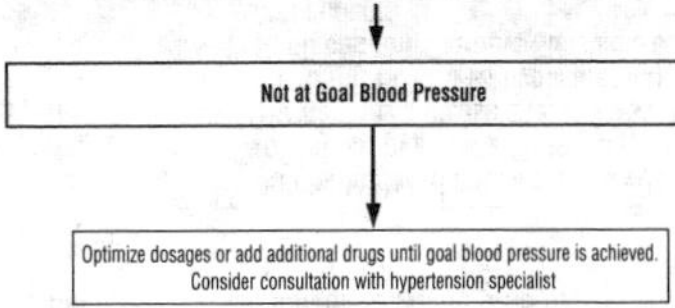
Not at Goal Blood Pressure
Optimize dosages or add additional drugs until goal blood pressure is achieved.
Consider consultation with hypertension specialist

Key:
THIAZ = thiazide diuretic
ACEI = angiotensin converting enzyme inhibitor
ARB = angiotension receptor blocker
BB = beta blocker
CCB = calcium channel blocker
ALDO ANT = aldosterone antagonist

NAME	FORM/STRENGTH	DOSAGE	COMMENTS
Trandolapril/Verapamil HCl (Tarka)	**Tab:** 2-180 mg, 1-240 mg, 2-240 mg, 4-240 mg	**Replacement Therapy: Adults:** 1 tab qd w/ food.	◙C (1st trimester) ◙D (2nd/3rd trimester) ❁v **H R** [7]

[7] ACE Inhibitors can cause injury & death to developing fetus in 2nd & 3rd trimesters.

ACE INHIBITORS/THIAZIDES

NAME	FORM/STRENGTH	DOSAGE	COMMENTS
Benazepril/HCTZ (Lotensin HCT)	**Tab:** 5-6.25 mg, 10-12.5 mg, 20-12.5 mg, 20-25 mg	**Adults: Initial (if not controlled on benazepril monotherapy):** 10-12.5 mg tab or 20-12.5 mg tab. **Titrate:** May increase after 2-3 wks. **Initial (if controlled on 25 mg HCTZ/d w/ hypokalemia):** 5-6.25 mg tab. **Replacement Therapy:** Substitute combination for titrated components.	C (1st trimester) D (2nd/3rd trimester) **R** [7, 24]
Captopril/HCTZ (Capozide)	**Tab:** 25-15 mg, 25-25 mg, 50-15 mg, 50-25 mg	**Adults: Initial:** 25-15 mg tab qd. **Titrate:** Adjust dose at 6-wk intervals. **Max:** 150 mg captopril/50 mg HCTZ per day. **Replacement Therapy:** Substitute combination for titrated components.	C (1st trimester) D (2nd/3rd trimester) v **R** [7]
Enalapril/HCTZ (Vaseretic)	**Tab:** 5-12.5 mg, 10-25 mg	**Adults: Initial (if not controlled on enalapril/HCTZ monotherapy):** 5-12.5 mg tab or 10-25 mg tab qd. **Titrate:** May increase after 2-3 wks. **Max:** 20 mg enalapril/50 mg HCTZ per day. **Replacement Therapy:** Substitute combination for titrated components.	C (1st trimester) D (2nd/3rd trimester) v **R** [7, 24]
Fosinopril Sodium/HCTZ (Monopril HCT)	**Tab:** 10-12.5 mg, 20-12.5 mg	**Adults: Initial (if not controlled w/ fosinopril or HCTZ monotherapy):** 10-12.5 mg tab or 20-12.5 mg tab qd.	C (1st trimester) D (2nd/3rd trimester) v **R** [7, 24]
Lisinopril/HCTZ (Prinzide, Zestoretic)	**Tab:** 10-12.5 mg, 20-12.5 mg, 20-25 mg	**Adults: Initial (if not controlled w/ lisinopril/HCTZ monotherapy):** 10-12.5 mg tab or 20-12.5 mg tab daily. **Titrate:** May increase after 2-3 wks. **Initial (if controlled on 25 mg HCTZ/d w/ hypokalemia):** 10-12.5 mg tab. **Replacement Therapy:** Substitute combination for titrated components.	C (1st trimester) D (2nd/3rd trimester) v **R** [7, 24]

Moexipril/HCTZ (Uniretic)	**Tab:** 7.5-12.5 mg, 15-12.5 mg, 15-25 mg	**Adults: Initial (if not controlled on moexipril/HCTZ monotherapy):** Switch to 7.5-12.5 mg tab, 15-12.5 mg tab, or 15-25 mg tab qd. **Titrate:** May increase after 2-3 wks. **Initial (if controlled on 25 mg HCTZ/d w/ hypokalemia):** 3.75-6.25 mg (1/2 of 7.5-12.5 mg tab). **Replacement Therapy:** Substitute combination for titrated components.	◙C (1st trimester) ◙D (2nd/3rd trimester) ❁v Avoid if CrCl ≤40 ml/min. [7]
Quinapril/HCTZ (Accuretic)	**Tab:** 10-12.5 mg, 20-12.5 mg, 20-25 mg	**Adults: Initial (if not controlled on quinapril monotherapy):** 10-12.5 mg or 20-12.5 mg tab qd. **Titrate:** May increase after 2-3 wks. **Initial (if controlled on 25 mg HCTZ/d w/ hypokalemia):** 10-12.5 mg or 20-12.5 mg tab qd.	◙C (1st trimester) ◙D (2nd/3rd trimester) ❁v [7, 24]
ALDOSTERONE BLOCKER			
Eplerenone (Inspra)	**Tab:** 25 mg, 50 mg	**Adults: Initial:** 50 mg qd. May increase to 50 mg bid if inadequate effect. **With Weak CYP450 3A4 Inhibitors: Initial:** 25 mg qd.	◙B ❁v **R**
ALPHA ADRENERGIC BLOCKERS			
Clonidine HCl (Catapres, Catapres-TTS)	**Tab:** 0.1 mg, 0.2 mg, 0.3 mg; **Patch:** (TTS) 0.1 mg/24 h, 0.2 mg/24 h, 0.3 mg/24 h	**Adults: Patch: Initial:** 0.1 mg/24h patch wkly. **Titrate:** May increase after 1-2 wks. **Max:** 0.6 mg/24h. **Tab: Initial:** 0.1 mg bid. **Titrate:** May increase by 0.1 mg wkly. **Usual:** 0.2-0.6 mg/d. **Max:** 2.4 mg/d.	◙C ❁> **R**
Doxazosin Mesylate (Cardura)	**Tab:** 1 mg, 2 mg, 4 mg, 8 mg	**Adults: Initial:** 1 mg qd. **Titrate:** May double the dose q1-2wks. **Max:** 8 mg/d.	◙C ❁>

[7] ACE Inhibitors can cause injury & death to developing fetus in 2nd & 3rd trimesters.
[24] Avoid if CrCl <30 ml/min.

NAME	FORM/STRENGTH	DOSAGE	COMMENTS
Guanfacine HCl (Tenex)	**Tab:** 1 mg, 2 mg	**Adults: Initial:** 1 mg qhs, may increase to 2 mg qhs after 3-4 wks. **Max:** 3 mg/d.	◙B ❋>
Methyldopa (Aldomet)	**Tab:** 125 mg, 250 mg, 500 mg	**Adults: Initial:** 250 mg bid-tid x 48h. **Titrate:** Adjust to desired response q2d. **Maint:** 500 mg-2 gm/d given bid-qid. **Max:** 3 gm/d. **Peds: Initial:** 10 mg/kg/d given bid-qid. **Max:** 65 mg/kg/d or 3 gm/d.	◙B ❋> **R**
Methyldopate HCl	**Inj:** 50 mg/ml	**Usual:** 250-500 mg infused over 30-60 min q6h. **Max:** 1 gm q6h. **Peds:** 20-40 mg/kg/d IV given q6h. **Max:** 65 mg/kg/d or 3 g/d.	◙C ❋> **R**
Prazosin HCl (Minipress)	**Tab:** 1 mg, 2 mg, 5 mg	**Adults: Initial:** 1 mg bid-tid. **Usual:** 6-15 mg/d in divided doses. **Max:** 40 mg/d.	◙C ❋> Syncope w/ 1st dose.
Reserpine	**Tab:** 0.1 mg, 0.25 mg	**Adults: Initial:** 0.5 mg qd x 1-2 wks. **Maint:** 0.1-0.25 mg qd.	◙C ❋v
Terazosin HCl (Hytrin)	**Cap:** 1 mg, 2 mg, 5 mg, 10 mg	**Adults: Initial:** 1 mg qhs. **Titrate:** Increase stepwise as needed. **Usual:** 10 mg qd. May increase to 20 mg/day after 4-6 wks. **Max:** 20 mg/d. If d/c for several days, restart at initial dose.	◙C ❋> Syncope w/ 1st dose.

ALPHA ADRENERGIC BLOCKERS/THIAZIDES

NAME	FORM/STRENGTH	DOSAGE	COMMENTS
Methyldopa/HCTZ	**Tab:** 250-15 mg, 250-25 mg, 500-30 mg	**Adults: Initial:** 250-15 mg tab bid-tid, 250-25 mg tab bid, or 500-30 mg qd. **Max:** 50 mg HCTZ/d or 3 gm methyldopa/d.	◙C ❋v Not for initial therapy.

ALPHA/BETA BLOCKERS

Carvedilol (Coreg)	**Tab:** 3.125 mg, 6.25 mg, 12.5 mg, 25 mg	**Adults: Initial:** 6.25 mg bid x 7-14d. **Titrate:** Double dose q7-14d as tolerated. **Max:** 50 mg/d. Take w/ food.	C v
Labetalol HCl (Normodyne)	**Inj:** 5 mg/ml; **Tab:** 100 mg, 200 mg, 300 mg	**Adults: PO: Initial:** 100 mg bid. **Titrate:** Increase by 100 mg bid q2-3d. **Maint:** 200-400 mg bid. **Max:** 2400 mg/d. **IV: Initial:** 20 mg over 2 min, then may give 40-80 mg q10min until desired response. **Max:** 300 mg.	C >

ANGIOTENSIN II RECEPTOR ANTAGONISTS

Candesartan Cilexetil (Atacand)	**Tab:** 4 mg, 8 mg, 16 mg, 32 mg	**Adults: Initial:** 16 mg qd. **Usual:** 8-32 mg/d, given qd-bid.	C (1st trimester) D (2nd/3rd trimester) v **R** [9]
Eprosartan Mesylate (Teveten)	**Tab:** 400 mg, 600 mg	**Adults: Initial:** 600 mg qd. **Usual:** 400-800 mg/d, given qd-bid.	C (1st trimester) D (2nd/3rd trimester) v **R** [9]
Irbesartan (Avapro)	**Tab:** 75 mg, 150 mg, 300 mg	**Adults: Initial:** 150 mg qd. **Titrate:** May increase to 300 mg qd. **Intravascular Volume/Salt Depletion: Initial:** 75 mg qd.	C (1st trimester) D (2nd/3rd trimester) v [9]
Losartan Potassium (Cozaar)	**Tab:** 25 mg, 50 mg, 100 mg	**Adults: HTN: Initial:** 50 mg qd. **Usual:** 25-100 mg given qd-bid. **HTN w/ LVH: Initial:** 50 mg qd. Add HCTZ 12.5 mg qd and/or increase losartan to 100 mg qd, followed by an increase in HCTZ to 25 mg qd based on BP response.	C (1st trimester) D (2nd/3rd trimester) v **H** [9]

[9] Drugs acting directly on the renin-angiotensin system can cause fetal/neonatal morbidity & death, primarily during 3rd trimester.

NAME	FORM/STRENGTH	DOSAGE	COMMENTS
Olmesartan Medoxomil (Benicar)	**Tab:** 5 mg, 20 mg, 40 mg	**Adults: Monotherapy Without Volume Depletion: Initial:** 20 mg qd. **Titrate:** May increase to 40 mg qd after 2 wks if needed. May add diuretic if BP not controlled. **Intravascular Volume Depletion (eg, w/ diuretics, impaired renal function):** Lower initial dose; monitor closely.	C (1st trimester) D (2nd/3rd trimester) v [9]
Telmisartan (Micardis)	**Tab:** 20 mg, 40 mg, 80 mg	**Adults: Initial:** 40 mg qd. **Usual:** 20-80 mg qd.	C (1st trimester) D (2nd/3rd trimester) v [9]
Valsartan (Diovan)	**Tab:** 40 mg, 80 mg, 160 mg, 320 mg	**Adults: Initial:** 80 or 160 mg qd. **Titrate:** Increase to 320 mg qd or add diuretic (greater effect than increasing dose >80 mg).	C (1st trimester) D (2nd/3rd trimester) v **H R** [9]
ANGIOTENSIN II RECEPTOR ANTAGONISTS/THIAZIDES			
Candesartan/HCTZ (Atacand HCT)	**Tab:** 16-12.5 mg, 32-12.5 mg	**Initial:** If not controlled on 25 mg HCTZ/d or controlled but serum K^+ decreased, 16-12.5 mg tab qd. If not controlled on 32 mg candesartan/d, 32-12.5 mg qd; may increase to 32-25 mg qd.	C (1st trimester) D (2nd/3rd trimester) v **R** [9, 24]
Eprosartan Mesylate/HCTZ (Teveten HCT)	**Tab:** 600-12.5 mg, 600-25 mg	**Adults: Usual (Not Volume Depleted):** 600-12.5 mg qd. May increase to 600-25 mg qd if needed.	C (1st trimester) D (2nd/3rd trimester) v **H R** [9]

Irbesartan/HCTZ (Avalide)	**Tab:** 150-12.5 mg, 300-12.5 mg, 300-25 mg	**Adults: Initial:** 150 mg irbesartan qd. **Max:** 300 mg irbesartan qd. **Elderly:** Start at low end of dosing range. **Intravascular Volume/Salt Depletion: Initial:** 75 mg irbesartan qd. Avoid w/ CrCl ≤30 ml/min.	C (1st trimester) D (2nd/3rd trimester) v **R** [9]
Losartan/HCTZ (Hyzaar)	**Tab:** 50-12.5 mg, 100-12.5, 100-25 mg	**Adults: HTN:** If BP uncontrolled on losartan monotherapy, HCTZ alone or controlled w/ HCTZ 25 mg/d but hypokalemic: 50-12.5 mg tab qd. **Titrate/Max:** If uncontrolled after 3 wks, increase to 2 tabs of 50-12.5 mg qd or 1 tab of 100-25 mg qd. If uncontrolled on losartan 100 mg monotherapy, may switch to 100-12.5 mg qd. **Severe HTN: Initial:** 50-12.5 mg qd. **Titrate/Max:** If inadequate response after 2-4 wks, increase to 1 tab of 100-25 mg qd. **HTN w/ Left Ventricular Hypertrophy: Initial:** Losartan 50 mg qd. If BP reduction inadequate, add HCTZ 12.5 mg or substitute losartan/HCTZ 50-12.5 mg. If additional BP reduction is needed, losartan 100 mg & HCTZ 12.5 mg or losartan/HCTZ 100-12.5 mg may be substituted, followed by losartan 100 mg & HCTZ 25 mg or losartan/HCTZ 100-25 mg.	C (1st trimester) D (2nd/3rd trimester) v **H R** [9, 24]
Olmesartan Medoxomil/HCTZ (Benicar HCT)	**Tab:** 20-12.5 mg, 40-12.5 mg, 40-25 mg	**Adults: Initial:** If not controlled on olmesartan, add HCTZ 12.5 mg qd. May titrate to 25 mg qd after 2-4 wks. If not controlled on HCTZ, add olmesartan 20 mg qd. May titrate to 40 mg after 2-4 wks. **Intravascular Volume Depletion (eg, w/ diuretics, impaired renal function):** Lower initial dose; monitor closely.	C (1st trimester) D (2nd/3rd trimester) v **R** [9]

[9] Drugs acting directly on the renin-angiotensin system can cause fetal/neonatal morbidity & death, primarily during 3rd trimester.
[24] Avoid if CrCl <30 ml/min.

NAME	FORM/STRENGTH	DOSAGE	COMMENTS
Telmisartan/HCTZ (Micardis HCT)	**Tab:** 40-12.5 mg, 80-12.5 mg, 80-25 mg	**Initial:** If not controlled on 80 mg telmisartan, or 25 mg HCTZ/d, or controlled on 25 mg HCTZ/d but serum K^+ decreased, 80-12.5 mg tab qd. **Max:** 160 mg telmisartan-25 mg HCTZ/d.	C (1st trimester) D (2nd/3rd trimester) **H R** [9, 24]
Valsartan/HCTZ (Diovan HCT)	**Tab:** 80-12.5 mg, 160-12.5 mg, 160-25 mg, 320-12.5 mg, 320-25 mg	**Adults: Initial: Uncontrolled on Valsartan Alone:** Switch to 80-12.5 mg, 160-12.5 mg, or 320-12.5 mg tab qd. Increase dose if uncontrolled after 3-4 wks. **Max:** 320 mg valsartan-25 mg HCTZ/d. **Uncontrolled on 25 mg HCTZ/d or Controlled on 25 mg HCTZ/d w/ Hypokalemia:** Switch to 80-12.5 mg or 160-12.5 mg tab qd. Titrate if uncontrolled after 3-4 wks. **Max:** 320 mg valsartan-25 mg HCTZ/d.	C (1st trimester) D (2nd/3rd trimester) v **R** [9, 24]

BETA BLOCKERS

NAME	FORM/STRENGTH	DOSAGE	COMMENTS
Acebutolol HCl (Sectral)	**Cap:** 200 mg, 400 mg	**Adults: Initial:** 400 mg/d given qd-bid. **Usual:** 200-800 mg/d. **Max:** 1200 mg/d.	B v **R**
Atenolol (Tenormin)	**Tab:** 25 mg, 50 mg, 100 mg	**Adults: Initial:** 50 mg qd. **Titrate:** May increase after 1-2 wks. **Max:** 100 mg qd.	D > **R**
Bisoprolol Fumarate (Zebeta)	**Tab:** 5 mg, 10 mg	**Adults: Initial:** 2.5-5 mg qd. **Max:** 20 mg/d.	C > **H R**
Carteolol HCl (Cartrol)	**Tab:** 2.5 mg, 5 mg	**Adults: Initial:** 2.5 mg qd. **Maint:** 2.5-5 mg qd. **Max:** 10 mg/d.	C > **R**

Esmolol HCl (Brevibloc)	**Inj:** 10 mg/ml, 20 mg/ml, 250 mg/ml	**Intra-/Post-op HTN: Adults: Initial: Rapid:** 80 mg IVP, then 150 mcg/kg/min infusion. **Gradual:** 500 mcg/kg/min x 1 min, then 50 mcg/kg/min x 4 min. If inadequate response within 5 min, repeat LD & give maint 100 mcg/kg/min.	C >
Metoprolol Succinate (Toprol-XL)	**Tab,ER:** 25 mg, 50 mg, 100 mg, 200 mg	**Adults: Usual:** 25-100 mg qd. **Titrate:** Increase wkly. **Max:** 400 mg qd.	C >
Metoprolol Tartrate (Lopressor)	**Tab:** 50 mg, 100 mg	**Adults: Initial:** 50 mg bid or 100 mg qd. **Titrate:** Increase qwk. **Usual:** 100-450 mg/d. **Max:** 450 mg/d.	C > [17]
Nadolol (Corgard)	**Tab:** 20 mg, 40 mg, 80 mg, 120 mg, 160 mg	**Adults: Initial:** 40 mg qd. **Titrate:** Increase by 40-80 mg. **Max:** 320 mg/d.	C v **R** [17]
Penbutolol Sulfate (Levatol)	**Tab:** 20 mg	**Adults: Initial/Maint:** 20 mg qd.	C >
Pindolol	**Tab:** 5 mg, 10 mg	**Adults: Initial:** 5 mg bid. **Titrate:** Increase q3-4wks by 10 mg/d. **Max:** 60 mg/d.	B v [18]
Propranolol HCl (Inderal, Inderal LA)	**Cap,ER:** 60 mg, 80 mg, 120 mg, 160 mg; **Tab:** 10 mg, 20 mg, 40 mg, 60 mg, 80 mg	**Adults: Tab: Initial:** 40 mg bid. **Maint:** 120-240 mg qd. **Cap,ER: Initial:** 80 mg qd. **Maint:** 120-160 mg qd. **Peds: Tab: Initial:** 1mg/kg/d. **Usual:** 1-2mg/kg bid. **Max:** 16 mg/kg/d.	C >
Timolol Maleate	**Tab:** 5 mg, 10 mg	**Adults: Initial:** 10 mg bid. **Maint:** 20-40 mg/d. **Max:** 60 mg/d.	C v [18]

[9] Drugs acting directly on the renin-angiotensin system can cause fetal/neonatal morbidity & death, primarily during 3rd trimester.
[17] Abrupt cessation may induce arrhythmia or MI.
[18] Abrupt cessation may exacerbate angina.
[24] Avoid if CrCl <30 ml/min.

BETA BLOCKERS/THIAZIDES

NAME	FORM/STRENGTH	DOSAGE	COMMENTS
Atenolol/Chlorthalidone (Tenoretic)	**Tab:** 50-25 mg, 100-25 mg	**Initial:** 50-25 mg tab qd. **Titrate:** May increase to 100-25 mg tab qd.	◉D ❄> **R**
Bisoprolol/HCTZ (Ziac)	**Tab:** 2.5-6.25 mg, 5-6.25 mg, 10-6.25 mg	**Adults: Initial:** 2.5-6.25 mg tab qd. **Titrate:** Increase q14d up to 20 mg bisoprolol-12.5 mg HCTZ/d.	◉C ❄v **H R**
Nadolol/Bendroflumethiazide (Corzide)	**Tab:** 40-5 mg, 80-5 mg	**Adults: Initial:** 40-5 mg tab qd. **Max:** 80-5 mg tab qd.	◉C ❄v **R**
Timolol Maleate/HCTZ (Timolide)	**Tab:** 10-25 mg	**Adults: Initial/Maint:** 1 tab bid or 2 tabs qd.	◉C ❄v

CALCIUM CHANNEL BLOCKER/HMG COA REDUCTASE INHIBITOR

NAME	FORM/STRENGTH	DOSAGE	COMMENTS
Amlodipine Besylate/Atorvastatin Calcium (Caduet)	**Tab:** 2.5-10 mg, 2.5-20 mg, 2.5-40 mg, 5-10 mg, 5-20 mg, 5-40 mg, 5-80 mg, 10-10 mg, 10-20 mg, 10-40 mg, 10-80 mg	Dosing is based on the appropriate combination of recommendations for the monotherapies. **Amlodipine: Adults: Initial:** 5 mg qd. Titrate over 7-14d. **Max:** 10 mg qd. **Small, Fragile, or Elderly/Hepatic Dysfunction/Concomitant Antihypertensive: Initial:** 2.5 mg qd. **Peds: ≥10 yrs (postmenarchal):** 2.5-5 mg qd. **Atorvastatin:** See under Antilipidemic Agents for dosing.	◉X ❄v **H**

CALCIUM CHANNEL BLOCKERS (DIHYDROPYRIDINES)

NAME	FORM/STRENGTH	DOSAGE	COMMENTS
Amlodipine Besylate (Norvasc)	**Tab:** 2.5 mg, 5 mg, 10 mg	**Adults: Initial:** 5 mg qd. **Max:** 10 mg qd. **Peds: 6-17 yo:** 2.5-5 mg qd.	◉C ❄v **H**
Felodipine (Plendil)	**Tab,ER:** 2.5 mg, 5 mg, 10 mg	**Adults: Initial:** 5 mg qd. **Maint:** 2.5-10 mg qd.	◉C ❄v **H**
Isradipine (DynaCirc, DynaCirc CR)	**Cap:** 2.5 mg, 5 mg; **Tab,ER:** (CR) 5 mg, 10 mg	**Adults: Initial: Cap:** 2.5 mg bid. **Tab,ER:** 5 mg qd. **Titrate:** Increase by 5 mg/d q2-4wks. **Max:** 20 mg/d.	◉C ❄v

Nicardipine (Cardene, Cardene SR)	**Cap:** 20 mg, 30 mg; **Cap,ER:** (SR) 30 mg, 45 mg, 60 mg; **Inj:** 2.5 mg/ml	**Adults: IV: Initial:** 50 ml/h (5 mg/h). **Titrate:** May increase by 25 ml/h (2.5 mg/h) q5-15min. **Max:**150 ml/h (15 mg/h). **Equiv. PO/IV Dose:** 20 mg q8h=0.5 mg/h, 30 mg q8h= 1.2 mg/h, 40 mg q8h=2.2 mg/h. **PO: Cap: Initial:** 20 mg tid. **Usual:** 20-40 mg tid. **Cap,ER: Initial:** 30 mg bid. **Usual:** 30-60 mg bid.	C v **H**
Nifedipine (Adalat CC, Procardia XL)	**Tab,ER:** 30 mg, 60 mg, 90 mg	**Adults: Initial:** (XL) 30-60 mg qd. (CC) 30 mg qd. **Titrate:** Increase over 7-14d. **Max:** (XL) 120 mg/d. (CC) 90 mg/d.	C v (CC) v (XL)
Nisoldipine (Sular)	**Tab,ER:** 10 mg, 20 mg, 30 mg, 40 mg	**Adults: Initial:** 20 mg qd. **Titrate**: Increase by 10 mg qwk or longer interval. **Maint:** 20-40 mg qd. **Max:** 60 mg/d. Avoid high fat meals & grapefruit pre-/post-dosing.	C v **H**

CALCIUM CHANNEL BLOCKERS (NON-DIHYDROPYRIDINES)

Diltiazem HCl (Cardizem, Cardizem CD, Cardizem LA, Cartia XT, Dilacor XR, Diltia XT, Taztia XT, Tiazac)	**Cap,ER:** (Cardizem CD) 120 mg, 180 mg, 240 mg, 300 mg, 360 mg, (Cartia XT) 120 mg, 180 mg, 240 mg, 300 mg, (Dilacor XR/ Diltia XT) 120 mg, 180 mg, 240 mg, (Taztia XT) 120 mg, 180 mg, 240 mg, 300 mg, 360 mg, (Tiazac) 120 mg, 180 mg, 240 mg, 300 mg, 360 mg, 420 mg; **Tab,ER:** (Cardizem LA) 120 mg, 180 mg, 240 mg, 300 mg, 360 mg, 420 mg	**Adults: Cardizem CD/Cartia XT: Initial:** 180-240 mg qd. **Titrate:** Adjust at 2 wk intervals. **Max:** 480 mg/d. **Titrate:** Adjust at 2 wk intervals. **Usual:** 240-360 mg/d. **Dilacor XR/Diltia XT: Initial:** 180-240 mg qd. **Max:** 540 mg/d. **Taztia XT/Tiazac: Initial:** 120-240 mg qd. **Max:** 540 mg/d. **Cardizem LA: Initial:** 180-240 mg qd. Adjust at 2 wk intervals. **Max:** 540 mg qd.	C v

NAME	FORM/STRENGTH	DOSAGE	COMMENTS
Verapamil (Calan, Calan SR, Covera-HS, Isoptin SR, Verelan, Verelan PM)	**Cap,ER:** (Verelan) 120 mg, 180 mg, 240 mg, 360 mg, (Verelan PM) 100 mg, 200 mg, 300 mg; **Tab:** (Calan) 40 mg, 80 mg, 120 mg; **Tab,ER:** (Calan SR, Isoptin SR) 120 mg, 180 mg, 240 mg, (Covera-HS) 180 mg, 240 mg	**Adults: Calan: Initial:** 80 mg tid. **Usual:** 360-480 mg/d. **Calan SR/Isoptin SR: Initial:** 180 mg qam. **Titrate:** Increase to 240 mg qam, then 180 mg bid; or 240 mg + 120 mg qpm, then 240 mg q12h. **Covera-HS: Initial:** 180 mg qhs. **Titrate:** Increase to 240 mg qhs, then 360 mg qhs, then 480 mg qhs. **Verelan:** Usual: 240 mg qam. **Titrate:** Increase by 120 mg qam. **Max:** 480 mg qam. **Verelan PM: Initial:** 200 mg qhs. **Titrate:** Increase to 300 mg qhs, then 400 mg qhs.	C ✽v **H** (Calan, Verelan) **R** (Verelan)

DIURETIC (LOOP)

NAME	FORM/STRENGTH	DOSAGE	COMMENTS
Furosemide (Lasix)	(Generic) **Inj:** 10 mg/ml; **Sol:** 10 mg/ml, 40 mg/5 ml; **Tab:** 20 mg, 40 mg, 80 mg; (Lasix) **Tab:** 20 mg, 40 mg, 80 mg	**Adults: Initial:** 40 mg bid. **Maint:** Adjust according to response.	C ✽> 8
Torsemide (Demadex)	**Inj:** 10 mg/ml; **Tab:** 5 mg, 10 mg, 20 mg, 100 mg	**Adults: Initial:** 5 mg PO/IV qd. **Maint:** May increase to 10 mg PO/IV qd after 4-6 wks.	B ✽>

DIURETICS (INDOLINE)

NAME	FORM/STRENGTH	DOSAGE	COMMENTS
Indapamide (Lozol)	(Lozol) **Tab:** 1.25 mg; (Generic) **Tab:** 1.25 mg, 2.5 mg	**Adults: Initial:** 1.25 mg qam. **Titrate:** After 4 wks, increase to 2.5 mg qd; after another 4 wks, increase to 5 mg qd.	B ✽v

DIURETICS (POTASSIUM SPARING)

Amiloride HCl (Midamor)	**Tab:** 5 mg	**Adults: Initial:** 5 mg qd. **Titrate:** Increase to 10 mg/d. If hyperkalemia persists, may increase to 15 mg/d then to 20 mg/d **Maint:** May be on an intermittent basis.	◙B ❉v
Spironolactone (Aldactone)	**Tab:** 25 mg, 50 mg, 100 mg	**Adults: Initial:** 50-100 mg/d as single or divided doses. **Maint:** After 2 wks, adjust by response.	◙C ❉v [16]
Triamterene (Dyrenium)	**Cap:** 50 mg, 100 mg	**Adults: Initial:** 100 mg bid. **Max:** 300 mg/d.	◙C ❉v

DIURETICS (POTASSIUM SPARING/THIAZIDE)

Amiloride/HCTZ (Moduretic)	**Tab:** 5-50 mg	**Adults: Initial:** 1 tab qd. **Maint:** May be given on intermittent basis. **Max:** 2 tabs qd.	◙B ❉v
Spironolactone/HCTZ (Aldactazide)	**Tab:** 25-25 mg, 50-50 mg	**Adults:** 50-100 mg/d per component qd or in divided doses.	◙C ❉v Not for initial therapy. [16]
Triamterene/HCTZ (Dyazide, Maxzide)	**Cap:** (Dyazide) 37.5-25 mg; **Tab:** (Maxzide) 37.5-25 mg, 75-50 mg	**Adults: Usual:** (37.5-25 mg cap/tab) 1-2 caps or tabs qd. (75-50 mg tab) 1 tab qd.	◙C ❉v

DIURETICS (QUINAZOLINE)

Metolazone (Mykrox, Zaroxolyn)	**Tab:** (Mykrox) 0.5 mg, (Zaroxolyn) 2.5 mg, 5 mg, 10 mg	**Adults: Mykrox: Initial:** 0.5 mg qam. **Titrate/Max:** 1 mg qam. **Zaroxolyn:** 2.5-5 mg qd.	◙B ❉v Rapid and slow formulations are not equivalent.

[8] Excess amounts may lead to water & electrolyte depletion.
[16] Tumorigenic in chronic toxicity studies. Avoid unnecessary use.

NAME	FORM/STRENGTH	DOSAGE	COMMENTS
DIURETICS (THIAZIDE)			
Chlorothiazide (Diuril)	**Susp:** 250 mg/5 ml; **Tab:** 250 mg, 500 mg	**Adults: Initial:** 0.5-1 gm qd or in divided doses. **Max:** 2 gm/d. **Peds: Usual:** 10-20 mg/kg/d given qd-bid. **Max: 2-12 yo:** 1 gm/d. **≤2 yo:** 375 mg/d. **<6 mths:** 15 mg/kg bid.	◙C ✽v
Hydrochlorothiazide	**Cap:** 12.5 mg; **Tab:** 25 mg, 50 mg, 100 mg	**Adults: Initial:** 12.5 mg qd. **Max:** 50 mg/d.	◙B ✽v
VASODILATORS (PERIPHERAL)			
Hydralazine	**Inj:** 20 mg/ml; **Tab:** 10 mg, 25 mg, 50 mg, 100 mg	**Adults: PO: Initial:** 10 mg qid x 2-4d. **Titrate:** Increase to 25 mg qid x 3-5d, then 50 mg qid. **Max:** 300 mg/d. **IM/IV:** 20-40 mg, repeat as necessary. **Peds: Initial:** 0.75 mg/kg/d given qid. **Titrate:** Increase gradually over 3-4 wks. **Max:** 7.5 mg/kg/d or 200 mg/d.	◙C ✽>
Minoxidil (Loniten)	**Tab:** 2.5 mg, 10 mg	**Adults & Peds: >12 yo: Initial:** 5 mg qd. **Maint:** 10-40 mg qd. **Max:** 100 mg/d. **<12 yo: Initial:** 0.2 mg/kg qd. **Maint:** 0.25-1 mg/kg/d. **Max:** 50 mg/d.	◙C ✽v Pericardial effusion. Exacerbates angina.

Vasopressors

NAME	FORM/STRENGTH	DOSAGE	COMMENTS
Ephedrine Sulfate	**Inj:** 50 mg/ml	**Adults:** 25-50 mg SC/IM/IV. **Peds:** 3 mg/kg/d or 100 mg/m²/d divided into 4-6 doses.	◙C ✽>
Epinephrine (Adrenalin)	**Inj:** 1 mg/ml (1:1000)	**Cardiac Resuscitation:** 0.5 ml (0.5 mg) diluted to 10 ml w/ NaCl given IV/Intracardially.	◙C ✽>

Acne Preparations

ANTI-INFECTIVES

Clindamycin (Cleocin T, Evoclin)	**Foam:** (Evoclin) 1%; **Gel, Lot, Sol, Swab:** (Cleocin T) 1%	**Adults & Peds: ≥12 yo:** (Cleocin T) Apply to affected area bid. (Evoclin) Apply to affected area qd.	●B ❁v (Cleocin T) ❁> (Evoclin)
Erythromycin (A/T/S)	**Gel:** 2%; **Sol:** 2%	**Adults: Gel:** Apply to affected area qd-bid. **Sol:** Apply to affected area bid.	**Gel:** ●B ❁v **Sol:** ●C ❁>
Erythromycin (Akne-Mycin)	**Oint:** 2%	**Adults:** Apply to affected area bid (qam & qpm).	●N ❁>
Erythromycin (Emgel)	**Gel:** 2%	**Adults:** Apply to affected area qd-bid.	●B ❁v
Erythromycin (Erycette)	**Swab:** 2%	**Adults:** Apply to affected area bid (qam & qpm).	●B ❁>
Sodium Sulfacetamide/Sulfur (Plexion, Sulfacet-R)	**Lot:** (Sulfacet-R) 10%-5%; **Cleanser/Susp:** (Plexion) 10%-5%	**Adults & Peds: ≥12 yo: Lot/Susp** Apply qd-tid. **Cleanser:** Wash qd-bid.	●C ❁>
Sodium Sulfacetamide/Sulfur (Rosac)	**Cre:** 10%-5%	**Adults & Peds: ≥12 yo:** Apply thin film qd-tid.	●C ❁>
Sodium Sulfacetamide/Sulfur (Rosula)	**Cleanser, Gel:** 10%-5%	**Adults & Peds: ≥12 yo: Gel:** Apply thin film qd-tid. **Cleanser:** Wash for 10-20 sec qd-bid.	●C ❁>

NAME	FORM/STRENGTH	DOSAGE	COMMENTS
Sodium Sulfacetamide/Urea (Rosula NS)	**Swab**: 10%-10%	**Adults & Peds: ≥12 yo:** Apply to affected area qd-bid.	◉C ❋>
Tetracycline HCl (Sumycin)	**Cap:** 250 mg, 500 mg; **Susp:** 125 mg/5 ml	**Severe Acne: Adults & Peds: >8 yo:** 1 gm/d in divided doses. **Maint:** After improvement, 125-500 mg/d.	◉D ❋v **R**
DICARBOXYLIC ACID			
Azelaic Acid (Azelex)	**Cre:** 20%	**Adults & Peds: ≥12 yo:** Apply to affected area bid (qam & qpm).	◉B ❋>
Azelaic Acid (Finacea)	**Gel:** 15%	**Adults:** Wash & dry skin. Apply to affected area bid (qam & qpm) x up to 12 wks.	◉B ❋>
ESTROGEN/PROGESTIN COMBINATION			
Ethinyl Estradiol/Norethindrone (Estrostep)	**Tab:** (Phase 1) 35 mcg-1 mg; (Phase 2) 30 mcg-1 mg; (Phase 3) 20 mcg-1 mg	**Women: ≥15 yo:** 1 tab qd. See PI for initiation instructions.	◉X ❋v
Ethinyl Estradiol/Norgestimate (Ortho Tri-Cyclen)	**Tab:** (Phase 1) 35 mcg-0.18 mg; (Phase 2) 35 mcg-0.215 mg; (Phase 3) 35 mcg-0.25 mg	**Women: ≥15 yo:** 1 tab qd. Start 1st Sunday after menses begin or 1st day of menses.	◉X ❋v

KERATOLYTIC/ANTI-INFECTIVES

Benzoyl Peroxide/Clindamycin (BenzaClin)	**Gel:** 5%-1%	**Adults & Peds: ≥12 yo:** Apply to affected area bid.	◙C ❊v
Benzoyl Peroxide/Clindamycin (Duac)	**Gel:** 5%-1%	**Adults & Peds: ≥12 yo:** Apply qpm.	◙C ❊v
Benzoyl Peroxide/Erythromycin (Benzamycin)	**Gel:** 5%-3%	**Adults & Peds: ≥12 yo:** Apply to affected area bid (qam & qpm).	◙C ❊>

KERATOLYTICS

Benzoyl Peroxide (Benzac AC, Benzac AC Wash, Brevoxyl)	**Gel:** (Benzac AC) 2.5%, 5%, 10%; (Brevoxyl) 4%, 8%; **Lot (Cleanser/Wash):** (Brevoxyl) 4%, 8% **Sol:** (Benzac AC Wash) 2.5%, 5%, 10%	**Adults: Gel:** (Benzac AC) Apply to clean area qd-bid. **Sol:** (Benzac AC Wash) Wash area qd-bid; rinse & dry. **≥12 yo: Gel:** (Brevoxyl) Apply to clean area qd-bid. **Lot:** (Brevoxyl) Wash area qd x 1st wk, then bid as tolerated.	◙C ❊>
Benzoyl Peroxide (Zoderm)	**Cleanser, Cre, Gel:** 4.5%, 6.5%, 8.5%	**Adults: Cleanser:** Wash & rinse affected area qd-bid. **Cre, Gel** Apply to cleansed area qd-bid.	◙C ❊>

RETINOID-LIKE AGENTS

Adapalene (Differin)	**Cre, Gel, Sol:** 0.1%	**Adults & Peds: ≥12 yo:** Apply to affected area qhs. Avoid eyes, lips & mucous membranes.	◙C ❊>

RETINOIDS

NAME	FORM/STRENGTH	DOSAGE	COMMENTS
Isotretinoin (Accutane, Sotret)	**Cap:** (Accutane) 10 mg, 20 mg, 40mg; (Sotret) 10 mg, 20 mg, 30 mg, 40 mg	**Adults & Peds: ≥12 yo: Initial:** 0.5-1 mg/kg/d given bid x 15-20 wks w/ food. Repeat if needed after 2 mths off of drug.	◉X ❁v [52]
Tazarotene (Tazorac)	**Cre:** 0.1%; **Gel:** 0.1%	**Adults & Peds: ≥12 yo:** Apply to affected area qpm.	◉X ❁>
Tretinoin (Avita)	**Cre:** 0.025%; **Gel:** 0.025%	**Adults:** Apply to affected area qpm.	◉C ❁>
Tretinoin (Retin-A, Retin-A Micro)	**Cre:** 0.025%, 0.05%, 0.1%; **Gel:** 0.01%, 0.025%, (Micro) 0.04%, 0.1%; **Sol:** 0.05%	**Retin-A: Adults:** Apply to affected area qhs. **Retin-A Micro: Adults & Peds: ≥12 yo:** Apply to affected area qhs.	◉C ❁>

Anti-Infective Agents

ANTIBACTERIALS

NAME	FORM/STRENGTH	DOSAGE	COMMENTS
Bacitracin (Baciguent)	**Oint:** 500 U/gm	**Adults & Peds:** Apply small amount qd-tid.	◉N ❁>
Gentamicin (Garamycin)	**Cre, Oint:** 0.1%	**Adults & Peds: >1 yo:** Apply to lesions tid-qid.	◉N ❁>
Metronidazole (MetroCream, MetroGel, MetroLotion, Noritate)	**Cre:** (Noritate) 1%; **Cre, Lot:** 0.75%; **Gel:** 0.75%, 1%	**Rosacea: Adults:** (MetroCream, MetroGel 0.75%, MetroLotion) Wash affected area then apply qam & qpm. (MetroGel 1%, Noritate) Wash affected area then apply qd.	◉B ❁v

Mupirocin (Bactroban, Bactroban Nasal)	**Cre, Oint:** 2%; **Oint:** (Nasal) 2%	***S.aureus/S.pyogenes:* Adults & Peds ≥2 mths: Oint:** Apply tid. **≥3 mths: Cre:** Apply tid x 10d. **Nasal Colonization w/ MRSA: ≥12 yrs:** Apply nasal oint 1/2 tube per nostril bid x 5d.	◙B ❋v
Neomycin	**Oint:** 3.5 mg/gm	**Adults & Peds:** Apply small amount qd-tid.	◙N ❋>
Polymyxin B Sulfate/ Bacitracin Zinc (Polysporin)	**Oint:** 10,000 U-500 U; **Pow:** 10,000 U-500 U	**Prevent Infection in Minor Cuts, Scrapes, & Burns: Adults & Peds:** Apply to affected area qd-tid.	◙N ❋>
Polymyxin B Sulfate/ Bacitracin Zinc/Neomycin (Neosporin)	**Oint:** 5,000 U-400 U-3.5 mg/gm	**Prevent Infection in Minor Cuts, Scrapes, & Burns: Adults & Peds:** Apply to affected area qd-tid.	◙N ❋>
Sodium Sulfacetamide/Sulfur (Plexion, Sulfacet-R)	**Lot:** (Sulfacet-R) 10%-5%; **Cleanser/Susp:** (Plexion) 10%-5%	**Adults & Peds: ≥12 yo: Rosacea: Lot** Apply qd-tid. **Seborrheic Dermatitis: Lot/Susp:** Apply qd-tid. **Cleanser:** Wash qd-bid.	◙C ❋> CI in kidney disease.
Sodium Sulfacetamide/Sulfur (Rosula)	**Cleanser, Gel:** 10%-5%	**Seborrheic Dermatitis: Adults & Peds: ≥12 yo: Gel** Apply thin film qd-tid. **Cleanser:** Wash for 10-20 sec qd-bid.	◙C ❋>

ANTIFUNGALS

Butenafine (Mentax)	**Cre:** 1%	**Adults & Peds: ≥12 yo: Interdigital Tinea Pedis:** Apply bid x 7d or qd x 4 wks. **Tinea Corporis/Tinea Cruris/Tinea Versicolor:** Apply qd x 2 wks.	◙B ❋>

52 Not for use by females who are or may become pregnant, or if breastfeeding. Birth defects documented. Approved for marketing only under iPLEDGE. Prescriber and patient must be registered with iPLEDGE.

NAME	FORM/STRENGTH	DOSAGE	COMMENTS
Ciclopirox (Loprox)	**Cre, Gel, Lot:** 0.77%; **Shampoo:** 1%	**Adults: Seborrheic Dermatitis: Shampoo:** Apply about 5 ml (up to 10 ml for long hair) to wet scalp. Lather & rinse off after 3 min. Repeat 2x/wk x 4 wks, at least 3d apart. **≥10 yo: Tinea Pedis/Tinea Cruris/Tinea Corporis/Cutaneous Candidiasis/Tinea Versicolor: Cre/Gel/Lot:** Apply qam & qpm x 4 wks. Avoid gel or shampoo in peds <16 yo.	B >
Clotrimazole (Lotrimin)	**Cre, Lot, Sol:** 1%	**Candidiasis/Tinea Versicolor: Adults & Peds:** Apply qam & qpm.	B >
Econazole (Spectazole)	**Cre:** 1%	**Adults & Peds: Tinea Cruris/Tinea Corporis/Tinea Versicolor:** Apply qd x 2 wks. **Tinea Pedis:** Apply qd x 4 wks. **Candidiasis:** Apply qam & qpm x 2 wks.	C >
Ketoconazole	**Cre:** 2%	**Adults: Tinea Cruris/Tinea Corporis/Tinea Versicolor/ Cutaneous Candidiasis:** Apply qd x 2 wks. **Tinea Pedis:** Apply qd x 6 wks. **Seborrheic Dermatitis:** Apply bid x 4 wks.	C v
Ketoconazole (Nizoral, Nizoral A-D)	**Shampoo:** (A-D) 1%, (Nizoral) 2%	**Tinea Versicolor (2%): Adults:** Apply to damp skin of affected area, lather & rinse off after 5 min. **Dandruff (1%): Adults & Peds: >12 yo:** Apply to wet hair q3-4d x up to 8 wks if needed.	C >
Miconazole (Monistat-Derm)	**Cre:** 2%	**Adults: Tinea Cruris/Tinea Corporis/Cutaneous Candidiasis:** Apply qam & qpm x 2 wks. **Tinea Pedis:** Apply qam & qpm x 4 wks. **Tinea Versicolor:** Apply qd x 2 wks.	N >

Naftifine (Naftin)	**Cre, Gel:** 1%	**Tinea Pedis/Tinea Cruris/Tinea Corporis: Adults: Cre:** Apply qd. **Gel:** Apply qam & qpm.	◙B ❈>
Nystatin (Nystop)	**Pow:** 100,000 U/gm	**Candida Species: Adults & Peds:** Apply to lesions bid-tid.	◙N ❈>
Oxiconazole (Oxistat)	**Cre, Lot:** 1%	**Adults: Tinea Cruris/Tinea Corporis: Cre/Lot:** Apply qd-bid x 2 wks. **Tinea Pedis: Cre/Lot:** Apply qd-bid x 4 wks. **Tinea Versicolor: Cre:** Apply qd x 2 wks. **Peds: ≥12 yo: Cre:** Same as adult dose.	◙B ❈>
Sertaconazole Nitrate (Ertaczo)	**Cre:** 2%	**Interdigital Tinea Pedis: Adults & Peds: ≥12 yo:** Apply bid x 4 wks. Re-evaluate if no improvement after 2 wks.	◙C ❈>
Sulconazole (Exelderm)	**Cre, Sol:** 1%	**Adults: Tinea Corporis/Tinea Cruris/Tinea Versicolor:** Apply to affected area qd-bid x 3 wks. **Tinea Pedis:** Apply to affected area bid x 4 wks.	◙C ❈>
Terbinafine (Lamisil AT)	**Cre:** 1%	**Adults & Peds: ≥12 yo: Tinea Pedis:** Apply to area bid x 1 wk (interdigital) or x 2 wks (bottom/sides of foot). **Tinea Cruris/Tinea Corporis:** Apply to area qd x 1 wk. Wash & dry area before applying.	◙N ❈>
Tolnaftate (Tinactin)	**Cre, Pow, Sol, Spr:** 1%	**Tinea Pedis/Tinea Cruris/Tinea Corporis/Tinea Versicolor: Adults & Peds:** Apply bid x 2-3 wks, up to 4-6 wks.	◙N ❈>

NAME	FORM/STRENGTH	DOSAGE	COMMENTS
ANTIVIRALS			
Acyclovir (Zovirax)	**Cre, Oint:** 5%	**Herpes Genitalis/Herpes Labialis: Adults: Oint:** Apply q3h, 6x/d x 7d. Initiate w/ 1st sign/symptom. **Herpes Labialis: Adults & Peds: ≥12 yo: Cre:** Apply 5x/d x 4d.	◉B ✿>
Imiquimod (Aldara)	**Cre:** 5%	**Actinic Keratosis: Adults:** Apply 2x/wk qhs to area on face/scalp (but not both concurrently). Wash off after 8h. **Max:** 16 wks of therapy. **Genital/Perianal Warts (Condyloma Acuminata): Adults & Peds: ≥12 yo:** Apply 3x/wk qhs. Wash off after 6-10h. Use until warts clear. **Max:** 16 wks of therapy. Do not occlude treatment area.	◉C ✿>
Penciclovir (Denavir)	**Cre:** 1%	**Recurrent Herpes Labialis (Cold Sores): Adults:** Apply q2h w/a x 4d. Start w/ earliest sign or symptom.	◉B ✿v
Podofilox (Condylox)	**Gel, Sol:** 0.5%	**External Genital Warts (Condyloma Acuminata) (Gel/Sol), Perianal Warts (Gel): Adults:** Apply q12h x 3d, then withhold x 4d. May repeat up to 4 treatment cycles. **Max:** 0.5 gm/d or 0.5 ml/d & <10 cm^2 of wart tissue.	◉C ✿v

Anti-Infective Combinations

ANTIBIOTIC/ANTI-INFLAMMATORY AGENTS

NAME	FORM/STRENGTH	DOSAGE	COMMENTS
Clotrimazole/ Betamethasone (Lotrisone)	**Cre, Lot:** 1%-0.05%	**Adults: ≥17 yo: Tinea Cruris/Tinea Corporis:** Apply bid x 2 wks. **Tinea Pedis:** Apply bid x 4 wks.	◉C ✿>
Hydrocortisone/Iodoquinol (Alcortin)	**Gel:** 2%-1%	**Adults & Peds: ≥12 yrs:** Apply to affected area(s) tid-qid.	◉C ✿v

Neomycin/Polymyxin B/ Bacitracin/Hydrocortisone (Cortisporin)	**Oint:** 3.5 mg-5,000 U-400 U-1%	**Adults:** Apply to affected area bid-qid up to 7d.	C >
Neomycin/Polymyxin B/ Hydrocortisone (Cortisporin)	**Cre:** 3.5 mg-10,000 U-0.5%	**Adults:** Apply to affected area bid-qid up to 7d.	C >
Nystatin/Triamcinolone (Mycolog II)	**Cre, Oint:** 100,000 U-1 mg/gm	**Adults & Peds:** Apply to affected area bid.	C >

Antipruritics/Anti-Inflammatory Agents

HISTAMINE RECEPTOR BLOCKER & COMBINATIONS

Calamine/Pramoxine HCl (Caladryl)	**Cre, Lot:** 8%-1%	**Adults & Peds:** **≥2 yo:** Apply tid-qid.	N >
Diphenhydramine/ Zinc Acetate (Benadryl)	**Cre:** 2%-0.1%; **Gel:** 2%-0.1%, 2%-1%	**Adults & Peds:** **≥2 yo:** **Cre:** Apply 1% tid-qid. **≥6 yo:** **Gel:** Apply 1% tid-qid. **≥12 yo:** **Cre/Gel:** Apply 2% tid-qid.	N >
Doxepin (Zonalon)	**Cre:** 5%	**Adults:** Apply a thin film qid up to 8d.	B v
Pramoxine HCl/Zinc Acetate (Caladryl Clear)	**Lot:** 1%-0.1%	**Adults & Peds:** **≥2 yo:** Apply tid-qid.	N >

TOPICAL CORTICOSTEROIDS—RELATIVE POTENCY AND DOSAGE

DRUG	DOSAGE FORM (S)	STRENGTH (%)	POTENCY	FREQUENCY
Alclometasone Dipropionate (Aclovate)	Cre, Oint	0.05	Low	bid/tid
Amcinonide (Cyclocort)	Cre, Lot, Oint	0.1	High	bid/tid
Augmented Betamethasone Dipropionate Diprolene, Diprolene AF)	Gel, Oint	0.05	Very High	qd/bid
	Cre, Lot	0.05	High	qd/bid
Betamethasone Dipropionate (Diprosone, Alphatrex)	Cre, Lot, Oint	0.05	High	qd/bid
Betamethasone Valerate (Betatrex, Beta-Val, Betaderm)	Cre, Lot, Oint	0.1	Medium	qd/tid
Betamethasone Valerate (Luxiq)	Foam	0.12	Medium	bid
Clobetasol Propionate (Clobex, Cormax, Olux, Temovate)	Cre, Foam, Gel Lot, Oint, Sol	0.05	Very High	bid
	Shampoo (Clobex)	0.05	Very High	qd
Clocortolone Pivalate (Cloderm)	Cre	0.1	Low	tid
Desonide (DesOwen, Tridesilon)	Cre, Lot, Oint	0.05	Low	bid/tid
Desoximetasone (Topicort)	Cre	0.05	Medium	bid
	Gel	0.05	High	bid
	Cre, Oint	0.25	High	bid
Diflorasone Diacetate (Florone, Florone E, Psorcon)	Cre, Oint (Florone)	0.05	High	qd/qid
	Cre, Oint (Psorcon)	0.05	Very High	qd/tid

Fluocinolone Acetonide (Capex, Derma-Smoothe/FS, Synalar)	Cre, Oint	0.025	Medium	bid/qid
	Oil	0.01	Medium	qd/tid
	Shampoo (Capex)	0.01	Medium	qd
	Sol	0.01	Medium	bid/qid
Fluocinonide (Lidex, Lidex-E)	Cre, Gel, Oint, Sol	0.05	High	bid/qid
Flurandrenolide (Cordran, Cordran SP)	Cre, Lot	0.05	Medium	bid/qid
	Tape	4 mcg/cm²	Medium	qd/bid
Fluticasone Propionate (Cutivate)	Cre	0.05	Medium	qd/bid
	Oint	0.005	Medium	bid
Halcinonide (Halog, Halog-E)	Cre, Oint, Sol	0.1	High	qd/tid
Halobetasol Propionate (Ultravate)	Cre, Oint	0.05	Very High	qd/bid
Hydrocortisone (Ala-Scalp HP, Ala-Cort, Cortaid, Hydrocort, Hytone, Nutracort, Texacort, Cetacort)	Cre, Oint	0.5	Low	tid/qid
	Cre, Lot, Oint, Sol	1	Low	tid/qid
	Lot	2	Low	tid/qid
	Cre, Lot, Oint, Sol	2.5	Low	bid/qid
Hydrocortisone Butyrate (Locoid)	Cre, Oint, Sol	0.1	Medium	bid/tid
Hydrocortisone Probutate (Pandel)	Cre	0.1	Medium	qd/bid
Hydrocortisone Valerate (Westcort)	Cre, Oint	0.2	Medium	bid/tid
Mometasone Furoate (Elocon)	Cre, Lot, Oint	0.1	Medium	qd
Prednicarbate (Dermatop E)	Cre, Oint	0.1	Medium	bid

NAME	DOSAGE FORM (S)	STRENGTH (%)	POTENCY	FREQUENCY
Triamcinolone Acetonide (Aristocort A, Kenalog, Triacet)	Cre, Lot, Oint	0.025	Medium	bid/qid
	Cre, Lot, Oint	0.1	Medium	bid/tid
	Cre, Oint	0.5	High	bid/tid
	Spr	0.147 mg/gm	Medium	tid/qid

NAME	FORM/STRENGTH	DOSAGE	COMMENTS
TOPICAL CORTICOSTEROIDS/LOCAL ANESTHETIC AGENTS			
Hydrocortisone Acetate/ Pramoxine HCl (Analpram-HC, ProctoFoam-HC)	**Aer:** 1%-1%; **Cre:** 1%-1%, 1%-2.5%; **Lot:** 1%-2.5%	**Anal Dermatoses: Adults & Peds:** Apply to affected area tid-qid. Use applicator for anal administration w/ ProctoFoam-HC.	●C ❊>
Hydrocortisone Acetate/Pramoxine HCl (Novacort)	**Gel:** 2%-1%	**Corticosteroid-Responsive Dermatoses: Adults & Peds:** Apply to affected area(s) tid-qid. May use occlusive dressings for psoriasis or recalcitrant conditions. D/C dressings if infection develops.	● C ❊>
Lidocaine HCl/Hydrocortisone Acetate (AnaMantle HC)	**Cre:** 3%-0.5%	**Hemorrhoids/Anal Fissures/Pruritus Ani: Adults:** Apply PR bid.	●B ❊>
MISCELLANEOUS			
Pimecrolimus (Elidel)	**Cre:** 1%	**Moderate-Severe Atopic Dermatitis:** **≥2 yrs:** Apply bid. D/C upon resolution.	●C ❊v

Tacrolimus (Protopic)	**Oint:** 0.03%, 0.1%	**Moderate-Severe Atopic Dermatitis: Adults: ≥16 yo:** Apply bid. **Peds: 2-15 yo:** Apply 0.03% ointment bid. Continue x 1 wk after symptoms clear.	◙C ❉v

Psoriasis

ANTIMETABOLITES

Methotrexate	**Inj:** 20 mg, 1 gm, 25 mg/ml; **Tab:** 2.5 mg, 5 mg, 7.5 mg, 10 mg,15 mg	**Adults: Usual:** 10-25 mg/wk PO/IV/IM until adequate response achieved or use 2.5 mg q12h x 3 doses. **Titrate:** May increase gradually. **Max:** 30 mg/wk.	◙X ❉v [19]

COAL TAR AGENTS

Coal Tar (Tegrin)	**Cre:** 5%; **Shampoo:** 7%	**Adults: Cre:** Apply qd-qid. **Shampoo:** Apply 2x/wk.	◙N ❉>

IMMUNOSUPPRESSIVES

Alefacept (Amevive)	**Inj:** (IV) 7.5 mg, (IM) 15 mg	**Adults:** 7.5 mg IV bolus or 15 mg IM once wkly x 12 wks. May retreat x 12 wks if >12 wk interval since 1st course. Adjust dose, D/C, and/or retreat, based on CD4+ T-lymphocyte counts.	◙B ❉v CI with HIV.
Cyclosporine (Neoral)	**Cap:** 25 mg, 100 mg; **Sol:** 100 mg/ml	**Adults: Initial:** 1.25 mg/kg bid x 4 wks. **Maint:** If no improvement, increase q2wks by 0.5 mg/kg/d. **Max:** 4 mg/kg/d.	◙C ❉ Infection. Neoplasia. HTN. Nephrotoxicity. Malignancy risk w/certain psoriasis therapies.

[19] Monitor for bone marrow, lung, liver & kidney toxicities. Serious toxic reactions.

NAME	FORM/STRENGTH	DOSAGE	COMMENTS
Efalizumab (Raptiva)	**Inj:** 125 mg	**Adults: ≥18 yo: Initial:** 0.7 mg/kg SC single dose. **Maint:** 1 mg/kg SC once weekly. **Max:** 200 mg/dose.	C v
PSORALENS			
Methoxsalen (8-MOP)	**Cap:** 10 mg	**Adults: Initial: <30 kg:** 10 mg. **30-50 kg:** 20 mg. **51-65 kg:** 30 mg. **66-80 kg:** 40 mg. **81-90 kg:** 50 mg. **91-115 kg:** 60 mg. **>115 kg:** 70 mg. Take 2h before UVA exposure w/ food or milk. **Titrate:** May increase by 10 mg after 15th treatment under certain conditions. **Max:** Do not treat more often than qod.	C > [20]
Methoxsalen (Oxsoralen-Ultra)	**Cap:** 10 mg	**Adults: Initial: <30 kg:** 10 mg. **30-50 kg:** 20 mg. **51-65 kg:** 30 mg. **66-80 kg:** 40 mg. **81-90 kg:** 50 mg. **91-115 kg:** 60 mg. **>115 kg:** 70 mg. Take 1.5-2h before UVA exposure w/ a low fat meal or milk. **Titrate:** May increase by 10 mg after 15th treatment under certain conditions. **Max:** Do not treat more often than qod.	C v [21]
RETINOIDS			
Acitretin (Soriatane)	**Cap:** 10 mg, 25 mg	**Adults:** 25-50 mg qd w/ food. Individualize dose based on intersubject variation in pharmacokinetics, clinical efficacy, & incidence of side effects. Terminate therapy when lesions resolve. May retreat relapses.	X v CI in pregnancy & up to 3 yrs after d/c med. Females should avoid ethanol.
Tazarotene (Tazorac)	**Cre:** 0.05%, 0.1%; **Gel:** 0.05%, 0.1%	**Adults & Peds: ≥12 yo:** Apply to lesions qpm. Apply gel to no more than 20% of BSA.	X >

STEROIDS, TOPICAL

Clobetasol Propionate (Clobex)	**Lot:** 0.05%; **Sham:** 0.05%; **Spr:** 0.05%	**Adults: ≥18 yrs: Lotion** Apply bid for up to 2 consecutive wks. Reassess after 2 wks; may repeat for additional 2 wks. Limit treatment to 4 wks. **Max:** 50 g/wk or 50 ml/wk. **Shampoo:** Apply thin film daily to dry scalp for up to 4 consecutive wks. Leave in place for 15 min before lathering & rinsing. **Spr:** Spr on affected area(s) bid. Rub in gently & completely. Reassess after 2 wks. Limit treatment to 4 wks. **Max:** 50 g/wk.	C >
Fluocinonide (Vanos)	**Cre:** 0.1%	**Adults:** Apply qd-bid. **Max:** 60 g/wk. Do not exceed 2 wks.	C v

TUMOR NECROSIS FACTOR RECEPTOR BLOCKER

Etanercept (Enbrel)	**Inj:** 25 mg, 50 mg/ml	**Plaque Psoriasis: Adults: Initial:** 50 mg SC twice wkly given 3-4 days apart x 3 mths. May begin w/ 25-50 mg/wk. **Maint:** 50 mg/wk.	B v

VITAMIN D_3 DERIVATIVES & COMBINATIONS

Calcipotriene (Dovonex)	**Cre, Oint, Sol:** 0.005%	**Adults: Sol:** Apply only to lesions on scalp bid x up to 8 wks. Rub in gently & completely. **Oint:** Apply to affected area qd-bid. **Cre:** Apply to affected area bid x up to 8 wks.	C >

[20] Risk of ocular damage, aging skin, & skin cancer. Do not interchange with Oxsoralen-Ultra without re-titration.
[21] Risk of ocular damage, aging skin, & skin cancer. Do not interchange with regular Oxsoralen or 8-Mop. Determine minimum phototoxic dose & phototoxic peak time.

NAME	FORM/STRENGTH	DOSAGE	COMMENTS
Calcipotriene/ Betamethasone Dipropionate (Taclonex)	**Oint:** 0.005%-0.064%	**Psoriasis Vulgaris: Adults:** Apply to affected area(s) qd x up to 4 wks. **Max:** 100 g/wk. Treatment of >30% BSA not recommended. Do not apply to face, axillae, or groin.	C >

Miscellaneous

ALPHA-REDUCTASE INHIBITORS

Finasteride (Propecia)	**Tab:** 1 mg	**Androgenetic Alopecia: Adults:** 1 mg qd.	X v

ORNITHINE DECARBOXYLASE INHIBITOR

Eflornithine (Vaniqa)	**Cre:** 13.9%	**Facial Hair Reduction: Adults & Peds: ≥12 yo:** Apply bid; at least 8h between doses. May wash off after 4h.	C >

PSORALENS

Methoxsalen (Oxsoralen)	**Lot:** 1%	**Vitiligo: Adults & Peds: ≥12 yo:** Apply to small well defined lesions before UVA exposure. Determine treatment intervals by erythema response; generally ≤1 wk.	C >

RETINOID COMBINATION

Fluocinolone/Hydroquinone/ Tretinoin (Tri-Luma)	**Cre:** 0.01%-4%-0.05%	**Moderate-to-Severe Melasma of the Face: Adults:** Wash face & neck w/ mild cleanser. Apply thin film to hyperpigmented areas including 0.5 inch of normal skin surrounding lesion, at least 30 min before hs.	C >
Mequinol/Tretinoin (Solage)	**Sol:** 2%-0.01%	**Solar Lentigines: Adults:** Apply to solar lentigines qam & qpm, at least 8h apart.	X v

RETINOIDS

Tazarotene (Avage)	**Cre:** 0.1%	**Facial Wrinkles/Hyperpigmentation or Hypopigmentation/Lentigines: Adults: ≥17 yo:** Cleanse & dry skin. Apply a pea-sized (1/4 inch or 5 mm diameter) amount to face (including eyelids, if desired) qhs.	◙X ✽>
Tretinoin (Renova)	**Cre:** 0.02%, 0.05%	**Wrinkles/Hyperpigmentation/Facial Skin Roughness: 0.05%: Adults: 18-50 yo:** Apply qpm. **Max:** 48 wks. **Wrinkles: 0.02%: Adults: 18-71 yo:** Apply qpm. **Max:** 52 wks.	◙C ✽> (0.05%) ✽v (0.02%)

VASODILATORS (PERIPHERAL)

Minoxidil (Rogaine)	**Sol:** 5%	**Men:** Apply 1 ml bid to scalp.	◙N ✽>
Minoxidil (Rogaine)	**Sol:** 2%	**Women:** Apply 1 ml bid to scalp.	◙N ✽>

WOUND CARE AGENTS

Castor Oil/Peruvian Balsam/Trypsin (Granulex)	**Spr:** 650-72.5-0.1 mg/0.82 ml	**Adults/Peds:** Spray wound at least bid or more often prn.	◙N ✽>
Chlorophyllin Copper Complex Sodium/Papain/Urea (Panafil)	**Oint:** 0.5%-10%-10%; **Spr:** 0.5%-10%-10%	**Adults:** Clean wound, then apply qd-bid. Cover w/ dressing.	◙N ✽>
Collagenase (Collagenase Santyl)	**Oint:** 250 U/g	**Adults:** Clean & debride wound. Apply oint qd; use more frequently if dressings become soiled.	◙N ✽>

NAME	FORM/STRENGTH	DOSAGE	COMMENTS
Papain/Urea (Accuzyme)	**Oint, Spr:** 830,000 U/gm-10%	**Adults:** Clean wound, then apply qd-bid. Cover w/ dressing. Irrigate wound at each re-dressing.	●N ❋>

EENT/NASAL PREPARATIONS

ANTIHISTAMINES

DRUG	RX/OTC	FORM/STRENGTH	DOSAGE	COMMENTS
Azelastine (Astelin)	RX	**Spr:** 137 mcg/spray	**Seasonal Allergic Rhinitis: Adults & Peds: ≥12 yo:** 2 sprays per nostril bid. **5-11 yo:** 1 spray per nostril bid. **Vasomotor Rhinitis: Adults & Peds: ≥12 yo:** 2 sprays per nostril bid.	●C ❋>
Brompheniramine Maleate (Lodrane 24)	RX	**Cap,ER:** 12 mg	**Adults & Peds: ≥12 yo:** 12-24 mg qd. **6-12 yo:**12 mg qd.	●C ❋v
Carbinoxamine Maleate (Palgic)	RX	**Sol:** 4 mg/5 ml; **Tab:** 4 mg	**Adults & Peds: ≥6 yo: Usual:** 4 mg prn. **Max:** 24 mg/day given q6-8h; **1-6 yo: Usual:** 2 mg prn. May increase to 0.2-0.4 mg/kg/day given q6-8h.	●C ❋v
Cetirizine HCl (Zyrtec)	RX	**Chewtab:** 5mg, 10 mg; **Syr:** 1 mg/ml; **Tab:** 5 mg, 10 mg	**Seasonal or Perennial Allergic Rhinitis/ Urticaria: Adults & Peds ≥6 yo:** 5-10 mg qd. **Syr: 2-5 yo:** 2.5 ml (2.5 mg) qd. **Max:** 5 mg/d. **Perennial Allergic Rhinitis/Urticaria: 6 mo-23 mo:** 2.5 ml (2.5 mg) qd. **12 mo-23 mo:** May increase to max 5 mg/d.	●B ❋v **H R**

Chlorpheniramine Maleate (Chlor-Trimeton)	OTC	**Syr:** 2 mg/5 ml; **Tab:** 4 mg; **Tab,ER:** 8 mg, 12 mg	**Adults & Peds ≥12 yo: Syr/Tab:** 4 mg q4-6h. **Tab,ER:** 8 mg q8-12h or 12 mg q12h. **Max:** 24 mg/d. **6-11 yo: Syr/Tab:** 2 mg q4-6h. **Max:** 12 mg/d.	●N ❁>
Clemastine Fumarate (Tavist)	OTC (Tab 1.34 mg); RX (Tab 2.68 mg, Syr 0.5 mg/ 5 ml)	(Tavist) **Syr:** 0.5 mg/ 5 ml; **Tab:** 1.34 mg, (Generic) **Syr:** 0.5 mg/ 5 ml; **Tab:** 1.34 mg, 2.68 mg	**Adults & Peds ≥12 yo: Tab:** 1.34 mg bid or 2.68 mg qd. **Max:** 8.04 mg/d. **Syr:** 1-2 mg bid. **Max:** 6 mg/d. **6-12 yo: Syr:** 0.5-1 mg bid. **Max:** 3 mg/d.	●B ❁v
Cyproheptadine HCl	RX	**Syr:** 2 mg/5 ml; **Tab:** 4 mg	**Adults: Initial:** 4 mg tid. **Usual:** 4-20 mg/d. **Max:** 0.5 mg/kg/d. **7-14 yo:** 4 mg bid-tid. **Max:** 16 mg/d. **2-6 yo:** 2 mg bid-tid. **Max:** 12 mg/d.	●B ❁v
Desloratadine (Clarinex, Clarinex Reditabs, Clarinex Syrup)	RX	**ODT:** (Reditab) 2.5 mg, 5 mg; **Syr:** 0.5 mg/ml; **Tab:** 5 mg	**Perennial Allergic Rhinitis/Urticaria: Adults & Peds: Tabs: ≥12 yo:** 5 mg qd. **6-11 yo:** 2.5 mg qd. **Syr: ≥12 yo:** 10 ml (5 mg) qd. **6-11 yo:** 5 ml (2.5 mg) qd. **12 mths - 5 yo:** 2.5 ml (1.25 mg) qd. **6-11 mths:** 2 ml (1 mg) qd. **Seasonal Allergic Rhinitis: Adults & Peds: Tabs: ≥12 yrs:** 5 mg qd. **6-11 yo:** 2.5 mg qd. **Syr: ≥12 yo:** 10 ml (5 mg) qd. **6-11 yo:** 5 ml (2.5 mg) qd. **2-5 yo:** 2.5 ml (1.25 mg) qd.	●C ❁v **H R**
Diphenhydramine HCl (Benadryl)	OTC (PO), RX (Inj), OTC/RX (50 mg cap)	**Cap:** 25 mg, 50 mg; **Chewtab:** 12.5 mg; **Inj:** 50 mg/ml; **Syr:** 12.5 mg/5 ml; **Tab:** 25 mg, 50 mg	**Adults: PO:** 25-50 mg q4-6h. **Max:** 300 mg/d **Inj:** 10-50 mg IV or up to 100 mg deep IM. **Max:** 400 mg/d. **6-11 yo: PO:** 12.5-25 mg q4-6h. **Max:** 150 mg/d. **Peds: Inj:** 5 mg/kg/d or 150 mg/m²/d IV/IM in 4 divided doses. **Max:** 300 mg/d.	●B ❁v

NAME	RX/OTC	FORM/STRENGTH	DOSAGE	COMMENTS
Fexofenadine HCl (Allegra)	RX	**Tab:** 30 mg, 60 mg, 180 mg	**Seasonal Allergic Rhinitis: Adults & Peds: ≥12 yo:** 60 mg bid or 180 mg qd. **6-11 yo:** 30 mg bid. **Chronic Idiopathic Urticaria: Adults & Peds: ≥12 yo:** 60 mg bid. **6-11 yo:** 30 mg bid.	C > R
Hydroxyzine HCl (Atarax)	RX	(Atarax) **Syr:** 10 mg/5 ml; (Generic) **Syr:** 10 mg/5 ml; **Tab:** 10 mg,25 mg, 50 mg	**Adults:** 25 mg tid-qid. **≥6 yo:** 50-100 mg/d in divided doses. **<6 yo:** 50 mg/d in divided doses.	N v
Hydroxyzine Pamoate (Vistaril)	RX	**Susp:** 25 mg/5 ml (Generic) **Cap:** 25 mg; 50 mg, 100 mg; **Susp:** 25 mg/5 ml	**Adults:** 25 mg tid-qid. **Ped: ≥6 yo:** 50-100 mg/d in divided doses. **<6 yo:** 50 mg/d in divided doses.	N v
Loratadine (Alavert, Claritin, Claritin Reditabs)	OTC	**ODT:** (Reditab) 10 mg; **Syr:** 1 mg/ml; **Tab:** 10 mg	**Adults & Peds: ≥6 yo: ODT/Syr/Tab:** 10 mg qd. **2-5 yo: Syr:** 5 mg qd.	B > H R
Promethazine HCl (Phenergan)	RX	(Generic) **Inj:** 25 mg/ml, 50 mg/ml; **Sup:** 12.5 mg, 25 mg, 50 mg; **Syr:**6.25 mg/5 ml; **Tab:**12.5 mg, 25 mg, 50 mg; (Phenergan) **Inj:** 25 mg/ml, 50 mg/ml; **Sup:** 12.5 mg, 25 mg, 50 mg; **Tab:** 12.5 mg, 25 mg, 50 mg	**Adults:** 25 mg PO/PR qhs or 12.5 mg ac & qhs; 25 mg IM/IV and repeat in 2h if needed. **Peds: ≥2 yo:** 25 mg or 0.5 mg/lb PO/PR qhs or 6.25-12.5 mg tid; up to 12.5 mg IM/IV.	C v

COUGH & COLD COMBINATIONS

DRUG	RX/OTC	ANTIHISTAMINE	DECONGESTANT	COUGH SUPPRESSANT	OTHER CONTENT	DOSE
Actifed Cold & Sinus Caplets	OTC	Chlorpheniramine Maleate, 2 mg	Pseudoephedrine HCl, 30 mg		Acetaminophen, 500 mg	≥12 yo: 2 q6h.
Advil Cold & Sinus	OTC		Pseudoephedrine HCl, 30 mg		Ibuprofen 200 mg	≥12 yo: 1-2 q4-6h.
Aleve Cold & Sinus	RX		Pseudoephedrine HCl, 120 mg		Naproxen Sodium 220 mg	≥12 yo: 1 q12h.
Allegra-D 12 Hour Extended-Release Tablets	RX	Fexofenadine HCl, 60 mg	Pseudoephedrine HCl, 120 mg			≥12 yo: 1 bid.
Allegra-D 24 Hour Release Tablets	RX	Fexofenadine HCl, 180 mg	Pseudoephedrine HCl, 240 mg			≥12 yo: 1 bid.
Clarinex-D 12 Hour Extended-Release Tablets	RX	Desloratadine, 2.5 mg	Pseudoephedrine Sulfate, 120 mg			≥12 yo: 1 bid.
Clarinex-D 24 Hour Extended-Release Tablets	RX	Desloratadine, 5 mg	Pseudoephedrine Sulfate, 240 mg			≥12 yo: 1 qd.
Claritin-D 12 Hour ≥12 yo: 1 q12h.	OTC	Loratadine, 5 mg	Pseudoephedrine Sulfate,			

DRUG	RX/OTC	ANTIHISTAMINE	DECONGESTANT	COUGH SUPPRESSANT	OTHER CONTENT	DOSE
Tablet			120 mg			
Claritin-D 24 Hour Tablet	OTC	Loratadine, 10 mg	Pseudoephedrine Sulfate, 240 mg			≥12 yo: 1 qd.
Contac Severe Cold & Flu Maximum Strength Caplet	OTC	Chlorpheniramine Maleate, 2 mg	Pseudoephedrine HCl, 30 mg	Dextromethorphan HBr, 15 mg	Acetaminophen, 500 mg	≥12 yo: 2 q6h.
Coricidin HBP Cough/Cold Tablet	OTC	Chlorpheniramine Maleate, 4 mg		Dextromethorphan HBr, 30 mg		≥12 yo: 1 q6h.
DayQuil	OTC		Pseudoephedrine HCl, 30 mg/15 ml	Dextromethorphan HBr, 15 mg/15 ml	Acetaminophen, 325 mg/15 ml	≥12 yo: 2 tsp. q6h.
Delsym Suspension	OTC			Dextromethorphan Polistirex, 30 mg/5 ml		≥12 yo: 2 tsp. 6 to <12 yo: 1 tsp. 2 to <6 yo: 1/2 tsp. May repeat q12h.
Dimetapp Cold & Allergy Elixir	OTC	Brompheniramine Maleate, 1 mg/5 ml	Pseudoephedrine HCl, 15 mg/5 ml			≥12 yo: 4 tsp. 6 to <12 yo: 2 tsp. May repeat q4h. Max: 4 doses/24h.
Drixoral Cold & Allergy Tablet	OTC	Dexbrompheniramine Maleate, 6 mg	Pseudoephedrine Sulfate, 120 mg			≥12 yo: 1 q12h.

Entex PSE Tablet	RX		Pseudoephedrine HCl, 120 mg		Guaifenesin, 600 mg	≥12 yo: 1 q12h. 6 to <12 yo: 1/2 q12h.
Hycodan Syrup	CIII			Hydrocodone Bitartrate, 5 mg/5 ml	Homatropine MBr, 1.5 mg/5 ml	>12 yo: 1 tsp q4-6h. 6-12 yo: 1/2 tsp q4-6h.
Mucinex	OTC				Guaifenesin 600 mg	≥12 yo: 1-2 q12h. Max: 4/24h
Mucinex DM	OTC			Dextromethorphan HBr, 30 mg	Guaifenesin, 600 mg;	≥12 yo: 1-2 q12h. Max: 4/24h
NyQuil	OTC	Doxylamine 6.25 mg/15 ml	Pseudoephedrine HCl, 30 mg/15 ml	Dextromethorphan HBr, 15 mg/15 ml	Acetaminophen 500 mg/15 ml	>12 yo: 2 tsp. q6h.
Phenergan w/ Codeine	CV	Promethazine 6.25 mg/5 ml		Codeine 10 mg/5 ml		≥12 yo: 1-2 tsp. 6 to <12 yo: 2.5-5 ml. 2 to <6 yo: 1.25-2.5 ml. May repeat q4-6h.
Robitussin AC	CV			Codeine 10 mg/5 ml	Guaifenesin 100 mg/5 ml	≥12 yo: 1-2 tsp. q4h. 6 to <12 yo: 1 tsp. q4h. 2 to <6 yo: 1-1.5 mg/kg/d of codeine in 4 divided doses.

DRUG	RX/OTC	ANTIHISTAMINE	DECONGESTANT	COUGH SUPPRESSANT	OTHER CONTENT	DOSE
Robitussin CF	OTC		Pseudoephedrine HCl, 30 mg/5 ml	Dextromethorphan HBr, 10 mg/5 ml	Guaifenesin, 100 mg/5 ml	≥12 yo: 2 tsp. 6 to <12 yo: 1 tsp. 2 to <6 yo: 2.5 ml. May repeat q4h.
Robitussin DM Syrup	OTC			Dextromethorphan HBr, 10 mg/5 ml	Guaifenesin, 100 mg/5 ml	≥12 yo: 2 tsp q4h. 6 to <12 yo: 1 tsp q4h. 2 to <6 yo: 1/2 tsp q4h.
Robitussin PE Syrup	OTC		Pseudoephedrine HCl, 30 mg/5 ml		Guaifenesin, 100 mg/5 ml	≥12 yo: 2 tsp q4h 6 to <12 yo: 1 tsp q4h. 2 to <6 yo: 1/2 tsp q4h.
Ryna-12X Suspension	RX	Pyrilamine Tannate, 30 mg	Phenylephrine Tannate, 5 mg		Guaifenesin, 100 mg	≥6 yo: 1-2 tsp. q12h. 2 to <6 yo: 2.5-5 ml. q12h.
Sudafed Cold & Cough	OTC		Pseudoephedrine HCl, 30 mg	Dextromethorphan HBr, 10 mg	Guaifenesin, 100 mg Acetaminophen, 250 mg	≥12 yo: 2 q4h
TheraFlu Cold & Sore Throat Nighttime Liquid	OTC	Chlorpheniramine Maleate, 4 mg	Pseudoephedrine HCl, 60 mg		Acetaminophen, 650 mg	≥12 yo: 1 pkt q4-6h. Max: 4 pkts/24h.

Triaminic Cold & Cough Liquid	OTC	Chlorpheniramine Maleate, 1 mg/5 ml	Pseudoephedrine HCl, 15 mg/5 ml	Dextromethorphan HBr, 5 mg/5 ml		6 to <12 yo: 2 tsp q4-6h. Max: 4 doses/24h.
Triaminic Cold & Cough Softchews	OTC	Chlorpheniramine Maleate, 1 mg	Pseudoephedrine HCl, 15 mg	Dextromethorphan HBr, 5 mg		6 to <12 yo: 2 tabs q4-6h. Max: 4 doses/24h.
Triaminic Flu, Cough & Fever Liquid	OTC	Chlorpheniramine Maleate, 1 mg/5 ml	Pseudoephedrine HCl, 15 mg/5 ml	Dextromethorphan HBr, 7.5 mg/5 ml	Acetaminophen, 160 mg/5 ml	6 to <12 yo: 2 tsp q6h. Max: 4 doses/24h.
Triaminic Night Time Cough & Cold Liquid	OTC	Chlorpheniramine Maleate, 1 mg/5 ml	Pseudoephedrine HCl, 15 mg/5 ml	Dextromethorphan HBr, 7.5 mg/5 ml		6 to <12 yo: 2 tsp q6h. Max: 4 doses/24h.
Triaminic Cough & Sore Throat Softchews	OTC		Pseudoephedrine HCl 15 mg	Dextromethorphan HBr, 5 mg	Acetaminophen, 160 mg	6 to <12 yo: 2 tabs. 2 to <6 yo: 1 tab. May repeat q4-6h. Max: 4 doses/24h.
Tussi-12 D Suspension	RX	Pyrilamine Tannate, 30 mg	Phenylephrine Tannate, 5 mg	Carbetapentane Tannate, 30 mg		≥6 yo: 1-2 tsp. q12h. 2 to <6 yo: 2.5-5 ml q12h.
Tussionex Pennkinetic Suspension	CIII	Chlorpheniramine Polistirex, 8 mg/5 ml		Hydrocodone Polistirex, 10 mg/5 ml		>12 yo: 1 tsp q12h. 6-12 yo: 1/2 tsp q12h.

DRUG	RX/OTC	ANTIHISTAMINE	DECONGESTANT	COUGH SUPPRESSANT	OTHER CONTENT	DOSE
Tylenol Cold Day Caplet	OTC		Pseudoephedrine HCl, 30 mg	Dextromethorphan HBr, 15 mg	Acetaminophen, 325 mg	≥12 yo: 2 q6h.
Zyrtec-D Tablet	RX	Cetirizine HCl, 5 mg	Pseudoephedrine HCl, 120 mg			≥12 yo: 1 bid.

NAME	FORM/STRENGTH	DOSAGE	COMMENTS
Anticholinergics			
Ipratropium Bromide (Atrovent)	**Spr:** 0.03% (21 mcg/spr), 0.06% (42 mcg/spr)	**Rhinorrhea w/Common Cold: Adults & Peds: ≥12 yo:** 2 spr 0.06% per nostril tid-qid. **5-11 yo:** 2 spr 0.06% per nostril tid. **Allergic/Nonallergic Perennial Rhinitis: Adults & Peds: ≥6 yo:** 2 spr 0.03% per nostril bid-tid.	B >
Corticosteroids			
Beclomethasone (Beconase, Beconase AQ)	**Spr:** 42 mcg/spr	**Allergic/Nonallergic (Vasomotor) Rhinitis: Beconase AQ: Adults & Peds: ≥6 yo:** 1-2 spr per nostril bid. **Beconase: Adults & Peds: ≥12 yo:** 1 spr per nostril bid-qid. **6-12 yo:** 1 spr per nostril tid.	C v
Budesonide (Rhinocort Aqua)	**Spr:** 32 mcg/spr	**Seasonal/Perennial Rhinitis: Adults & Peds: ≥6 yo: Initial:** 1 spr per nostril qd. **Max: ≥12 yo:** 4 spr/nostril/d. **6-12 yo:** 2 spr/nostril/d.	B >

Flunisolide (Nasalide, Nasarel)	**Spr:** 29 mcg/spr	**Seasonal/Perennial Rhinitis: Adults: Initial:** 2 spr per nostril bid. **Titrate:** Increase to 2 spr per nostril tid. **Max:** 16 spr/d. **6-14 yo:** 1 spr per nostril tid or 2 spr per nostril bid. **Max:** 8 spr/d.	◙C ❉>
Fluticasone (Flonase)	**Spr:** 50 mcg/spr	**Seasonal & Perennial Allergic/Nonallergic Rhinitis: Adults: Initial:** 2 spr per nostril qd or 1 spr per nostril bid. **Maint:** 1 spr per nostril qd. **≥4 yo: Initial:** 1-2 spr per nostril qd. **Maint:** 1 spr per nostril qd. **Max:** 2 spr per nostril/d. **Seasonal Allergic Rhinitis: ≥12 yo:** May also dose as 2 spr per nostril qd prn.	◙C ❉>
Mometasone Furoate Monohydrate (Nasonex)	**Spr:** 50 mcg/spr	**Treatment & Prevention of Seasonal Allergic Rhinitis/Treatment of Perennial Allergic Rhinitis: Adults & Peds: ≥12 yo:** 2 spr per nostril qd. **Treatment of Seasonal/Perennial Allergic Rhinitis: Peds: 2-11 yo:** 1 spr per nostril qd. **Nasal Polyps: Adults: ≥18 yo:** 2 spr per nostril bid.	◙C ❉>
Triamcinolone (Nasacort AQ, Nasacort HFA, Tri-Nasal Spray)	**Spr:** (Nasacort AQ/ Nasacort HFA) 55 mcg/spr; (Tri-Nasal) 50 mcg/spr	**Allergic/Nonallergic Rhinitis: Nasacort AQ: ≥12 yo: Initial/Max:** 2 spr per nostril qd. **Maint:** 1 spr per nostril qd. **6-12 yo: Initial:** 1 spr per nostril qd. **Max:** 2 spr per nostril qd. **Nasacort HFA: ≥6 yo: Initial:** 2 spr per nostril qd. **Max: ≥12 yo:** 4 spr per nostril qd. **Tri-Nasal Spr:** 2 spr per nostril qd. **Max:** 8 spr/d.	◙C ❉>

NAME	FORM/STRENGTH	DOSAGE	COMMENTS

Decongestant Agents

NAME	FORM/STRENGTH	DOSAGE	COMMENTS
Oxymetazoline (Afrin, Neo-Synephrine, Vicks Sinex 12-Hour)	**Drops:** 0.05%; **Spr:** 0.05%	**Nasal Congestion: Adults & Peds: ≥6 yo: Usual:** 2-3 gtts/spr q10-12h. **Max:** 2 doses/24h.	◙N ❋>
Phenylephrine (Vicks Sinex)	**Spr:** 0.5%	**Nasal Congestion: Adults & Peds: ≥12 yo:** 2-3 spr per nostril q4h prn.	◙N ❋>

EENT/OPHTHALMOLOGY

Anesthetics

NAME	FORM/STRENGTH	DOSAGE	COMMENTS
Proparacaine (Alcaine, Ocu-Caine, Ophthetic, Parcaine)	**Sol:** 0.5%	**Adults: Foreign Bodies/Sutures:** 1-2 gtts pre-op. **Deep Ophthalmic Anesthesia:** 1 gtt q5-10min x 5-7 doses.	◙C ❋>
Tetracaine (Pontocaine, Tetcaine)	**Sol:** 0.5%	**Adults: Foreign Bodies/Sutures:** 1-2 gtts before operating/suture removal. **Tonometry:** 1-2 gtts before measurement. **Cataract Extraction:** 1 gtts q5-10min x 5-7 doses.	◙N ❋>

Antibiotic Agents

NAME	FORM/STRENGTH	DOSAGE	COMMENTS
Bacitracin	**Oint:** 500 U/gm	**Adults:** Apply 1/4 inch qd-tid.	◙N ❋>
Bacitracin Zinc/Neomycin Sulfate/Polymyxin B Sulfate (Neosporin)	**Oint:** 400 U-3.5 mg-10,000 U/gm	**Adults:** Apply q3-4h x 7-10d.	◙C ❋>

Bacitracin Zinc/Polymyxin B Sulfate (Polysporin)	**Oint:** 500 U-10,000 U/gm	**Adults:** Apply q3-4h x 7-10d.	◙C ❁>
Chloramphenicol (Chloroptic, Ocu-Chlor)	**(Chloroptic) Oint:** 1%; **Sol:** 0.5%; **(Ocu-Chlor) Oint:** 1%	**Adults: Oint:** 1/2 inch q3h x 48h, then increase frequency. Treat x 7d; continue x 48h after normal. **Max:** 3 wks. **Sol:** 1-2 gtts 4-6x/d x 72h. May increase interval after 48h. Continue x 48h after normal.	◙C ❁v Bone marrow hypoplasia including aplastic anemia & death.
Ciprofloxacin HCl (Ciloxan)	**Oint, Sol:** 0.3%	**Bacterial Conjunctivitis: Sol: Adults & Peds: ≥1 yo:** 1-2 gtts q2h w/a x 2d, then 1-2 gtts q4h w/a x 5d. **Oint: Adults & Peds: ≥2 yo:** 1/2 in tid x 2d, then bid x 5d. **Corneal Ulcers: Sol: Adults & Peds: ≥2 yo:** 2 gtts q15 min x 6h, then 2 gtts q30min on Day 1, then 2 gtts q1h on Day 2, then 2 gtts q4h on Days 3-14.	◙C ❁>
Gatifloxacin (Zymar)	**Sol:** 0.3%	**Adults & Peds: ≥1 yo:** 1 gtt q2h w/a, up to 8x/d for 2d; then 1 gtt up to qid w/a for 5d.	◙C ❁>
Gentamicin Sulfate (Garamycin, Genoptic, Gentak, Ocu-mycin)	**Oint, Sol:** 0.3%	**Adults & Peds: Usual:** 1/2 inch bid-tid or 1-2 gtts q4h. **Severe Infection:** 2 gtts q1h.	◙C ❁>
Gramicidin/Neomycin Sulfate/Polymyxin B Sulfate (AK-Spore, Neocidin, Neosporin)	**Sol:** 0.025 mg-1.75 mg-10,000 U/ml	**Adults: Usual:** 1-2 gtts q4h x 7-10d. **Severe Infection:** 2 gtts q1h.	◙C ❁>
Levofloxacin (Quixin)	**Sol:** 0.5%	**Conjunctivitis: Adults & Peds: ≥1 yo: Days 1-2:** 1-2 gtts q2h w/a up to 8x/d. **Days 3-7:** 1-2 gtts q4h w/a up to qid.	◙C ❁>

NAME	FORM/STRENGTH	DOSAGE	COMMENTS
Moxifloxacin HCl (Vigamox)	**Sol:** 0.5%	**Adults & Peds:** 1 gtt tid x 7d.	C >
Norfloxacin (Chibroxin)	**Sol:** 0.3%	**Adults & Peds: ≥1 yo: Usual:** 1-2 gtts qid up to 7d. **Severe Infection:** 1-2 gtts q2h w/a on Day 1, then qid up to 7d.	C v
Ofloxacin (Ocuflox)	**Sol:** 0.3%	**Adults & Peds: ≥1 yo: Bacterial Conjunctivitis:** 1-2 gtts q2-4h x 2d, then 1-2 gtts qid x 5d. **Bacterial Corneal Ulcer:** 1-2 gtts q30min w/a & 1-2 gtts 4-6h after retiring x 2d, then 1-2 gtts q1h w/a x 5-7d, then 1-2 gtts qid x 2d.	C v
Polymyxin B Sulfate/Trimethoprim Sulfate (Polytrim)	**Sol:** 10,000 U-1 mg/ml	**Adults & Peds: ≥2 mth:** Usual: 1 gtt q3h x 7-10d. **Max:** 6 doses/d.	C >
Sulfacetamide Sodium (AK-Sulf, Bleph-10, Ocu-Sul, Sodium Sulamyd)	**Oint:** 10%; **Sol:** 10%, 15%, 30%	**Adults: Initial:** Apply 1/2 inch qid & qhs or 1-2 gtts q2-3h w/a x 7-10d. **Maint:** Increase dose interval as condition responds. **Trachoma:** 2 gtts q2h w/ systemic administration.	C v
Tobramycin (Tobrasol, Tobrex, Tomycine)	**Oint:** 0.3%; **Sol:** 0.3%	**Adults: Usual:** 1/2 inch bid-tid or 1-2 gtts q4h. **Severe Infection:** 1/2 inch q3-4h or 2 gtts q1h until improvement.	B v

Antibiotic/Corticosteroid Combinations

Bacitracin Zinc/ Hydrocortisone/Neomycin Sulfate/Polymyxin B Sulfate (Cortisporin)	**Oint:** 400 U-1%-3.5 mg-10,000 U/gm	**Adults:** Apply q3-4h, depending on severity.	C v
Dexamethasone/Neomycin Sulfate/Polymyxin B Sulfate (AK-Trol, Maxitrol, Poly-Dex)	**Oint, Susp:** 1 mg-3.5 mg-10,000 U/gm or ml	**Adults: Oint:** Apply up to tid-qid or use susp hs. **Susp:** 1-2 gtts 4-6x/d. **Severe Infection:** 1-2 gtts q1h; taper to 4-6x/d.	C >
Dexamethasone/Tobramycin (TobraDex)	**Oint:** 0.1%-0.3%; **Susp:** 0.1%-0.3%	**Adults & Peds: ≥2 yo: Oint:** Apply 1/2 inch up to tid-qid. **Susp:** 1-2 gtts q2h x 24-48h, then 1-2 gtts q4-6h thereafter.	C >
Fluorometholone/ Sulfacetamide Sodium (FML-S Liquifilm)	**Susp:** 0.1%-10%	**Adults:** 1 gtt qid.	C v
Gentamicin Sulfate/ Prednisolone Acetate (Pred-G)	**Oint:** 0.3%-0.6%; **Susp:** 0.3%-1%	**Adults: Usual:** Apply 1/2 inch qd-tid or 1 gtt bid-qid. May give gtts q1h x 1st 24-48h.	C v
Loteprednol/Tobramycin (Zylet)	**Susp:** 2.5 ml, 5 ml, 10 ml	**Adults: Initial:** 1-2 gtts q4-6h. **Max:** 1-2 gtts q1-2h.	C >
Neomycin Sulfate/ Polymyxin B Sulfate/ Hydrocortisone (Cortisporin)	**Susp:** 1%-3.5 mg-10,000 U/ml	**Adults:** 1-2 gtts q3-4h, depending on severity.	C v

NAME	FORM/STRENGTH	DOSAGE	COMMENTS
Neomycin Sulfate/ Polymyxin B Sulfate/ Prednisolone Acetate (Poly Pred)	**Susp:** 0.35%-10,000 U-0.5%/ml	**Adults:** 1-2 gtts q3-4h. **Acute Infection:** 1-2 gtts q30min. Reduce dose as infection resolves.	◙N ❀>
Prednisolone Acetate/ Sulfacetamide Sodium (AK-Cide, Blephamide, Metimyd, Ocu-Lone C)	**Oint, Susp:** (Blephamide) 0.2%-10%, (Metimyd) 0.5%-10%; **Oint:** (AK-Cide, Ocu-Lone C) 0.5%-10%	**Adults & Peds: ≥6 yo: Initial:** Apply 1/2 inch 3-4x/d & 1-2x/qpm or instill 2 gtts q4h & qhs. Reduce dose when condition improves.	◙C ❀v
Prednisolone Sodium Phosphate/Sulfacetamide Sodium (Vasocidin)	**Sol:** 0.25%-10%	**Adults & Peds: ≥6 yo:** 2 gtts q4h.	◙C ❀v

Corticosteroids

NAME	FORM/STRENGTH	DOSAGE	COMMENTS
Dexamethasone (Maxidex)	**Susp:** 0.1%	**Adults:** 1-2 gtts q4-6h. **Severe Disease:** 1-2 gtts q1h, & taper to d/c.	◙C ❀v
Dexamethasone Sodium Phosphate (Decadron, Ocu-Dex)	**Oint:** 0.05%; **Sol:** 0.1%	**Adults: Initial:** Apply oint tid-qid or instill 1-2 gtts q1h w/a & q2h during night. With improvement, apply oint qd-bid or instill 1 gtt 3-6x/d. **Ear:** 3-4 gtts bid-tid w/ gradual dose reduction.	◙C ❀v
Fluorometholone (Fluor-Op, FML)	**Oint:** 0.1%; **Susp:** 0.1%, 0.25%	**Adults & Peds: ≥2 yo:** 1 gtt bid-qid or 1/2 inch oint qd-tid x 24-48h.	◙C ❀v
Loteprednol Etabonate (Alrex, Lotemax)	**Susp:** (Alrex) 0.2%, (Lotemax) 0.5%	**Adults:** (Lotemax) 1-2 gtts qid, may increase to 1 gtt q1h during 1st wk. **Post-Op:** 1-2 gtts qid starting 24h post-op. Continue x 2 wks. (Alrex) 1 gtt qid.	◙C ❀v

Prednisolone Acetate (Econopred Plus, Ocu-Pred A, Pred Forte, Pred Mild)	**Susp:** 0.12%, 0.125%, 1%	**Adults:** 1-2 gtts bid-qid. May increase frequency during 1st 24-48h.	▣C ✽v
Prednisolone Sodium Phosphate (AK Pred, Inflamase)	**Sol:** (Inflamase) 0.125%, 1%, (AK-Pred) 1%	**Adults:** 1-2 gtts q1h w/a & q2h at night. With improvement, 1 gtt q4h, then 1 gtt tid-qid.	▣C ✽>

Fungal Infection

Natamycin (Natacyn)	**Susp:** 5%	**Adults: Keratitis:** 1 gtt q1-2h x 3-4d, then 1 gtt 6-8x/d x 14-21d. **Blepharitis/Conjunctivitis:** 1 gtt 4-6x/d.	▣C ✽>

Glaucoma

ADRENERGIC AGONISTS

Dipivefrin (Propine)	**Sol:** 0.1%	**Adults: Usual:** 1 gtt q12h.	▣B ✽>

ALPHA ADRENERGIC AGONISTS

Apraclonidine HCl (Iopidine)	**Sol:** 0.5%, 1%	**Adults: 0.5%:** 1-2 gtts tid. **1%:** 1 gtt 1h pre-op & 1 gtt post-op.	▣C ✽v (1%) ✽> (0.5%)

BETA BLOCKERS

Betaxolol (Betoptic S)	**Susp:** 0.25%	**Adults:** 1-2 gtts bid.	▣C ✽>
Carteolol HCl (Ocupress)	**Sol:** 1%	**Adults:** 1 gtt bid.	▣C ✽>

NAME	FORM/STRENGTH	DOSAGE	COMMENTS
Levobunolol HCl (Betagan, Betagan C Cap)	**Sol:** (Betagan C Cap) 0.25%, (Betagan) 0.5%	**Adults: Usual:** (0.5%) 1-2 gtts qd. (0.25%) 1-2 gtts bid. **Severe/Uncontrolled:** (0.5%) 1-2 gtts bid.	C >
Metipranolol (Optipranolol)	**Sol:** 0.3%	**Adults:** 1 gtt bid.	C v
Timolol Maleate (Istalol)	**Sol:** 0.5%	**Adults:** 1 gtt in affected eye qam.	C v
Timolol Maleate (Timoptic, Timoptic-XE)	**Sol:** 0.25%, 0.5%; **Sol, gel forming:** (XE) 0.25%, 0.5%	**Adults: Timoptic:** 1 gtt 0.25% bid, may increase to 1 gtt 0.5% bid. **Maint:** 1 gtt 0.25%/0.5% qd. **Timoptic-XE:** 1 gtt 0.25%/0.5% qd. **Max:** 1 gtt 0.5% qd.	C v

CARBONIC ANHYDRASE INHIBITOR/BETA BLOCKER

NAME	FORM/STRENGTH	DOSAGE	COMMENTS
Dorzolamide/ Timolol Maleate (Cosopt)	**Sol:** 2%-0.5%	**Adults:** 1 gtt bid.	C v

CARBONIC ANHYDRASE INHIBITORS

NAME	FORM/STRENGTH	DOSAGE	COMMENTS
Acetazolamide (Diamox Sequels)	**Cap,ER:** 500 mg	**Adults: Glaucoma:** 500 mg qam & qpm.	C v
Brinzolamide (Azopt)	**Susp:** 1%	**Adults:** 1 gtt tid.	C v
Dichlorphenamide (Daranide)	**Tab:** 50 mg	**Adults: Initial:** 100-200 mg, then 100 mg q12h until response. **Maint:** 25-50 mg qd-tid.	C >
Dorzolamide (Trusopt)	**Sol:** 2%	**Adults & Peds:** 1 gtt tid.	C v
Methazolamide (Neptazane)	**Tab:** 25 mg, 50 mg	**Adults:** 50-100 mg bid-tid.	C v

CHOLINERGIC AGONISTS

Carbachol (Isopto Carbachol)	**Sol:** 1.5%, 2.25%, 3%	**Adults:** 2 gtts up to tid.	◙C ❁>
Echothiophate Iodide (Phospholine Iodide)	**Sol:** 0.03%, 0.06%, 0.125%, 0.25%	**Adults: Early Chronic Simple Glaucoma:** (0.3%) 1 gtt qam & qhs. **Advanced Chronic Simple Glaucoma/ Glaucoma 2° to Cataract Surgery: Initial:** (0.3%) 1 gtt qam & qhs. **Titrate:** Increase to higher strength as needed. **Peds: Accommodative Esotropia: Diagnosis:** (0.125%) 1 gtt qhs x 2-3 wks. **Treatment:** Decrease to 1 gtt (0.125%) qod or (0.6%) 1 gtt qd. **Titrate:** Decrease strength gradually. **Max:** (0.125%) 1 gtt qd.	◙C ❁v
Pilocarpine (Isopto Carpine, Pilopine HS)	**Gel:** (Pilopine HS) 4%; **Sol:** (Generic) 0.5%, 1%, 2%, 3%, 4%, 6%, (Isopto Carpine) 1%, 2%, 4%	**Usual: Sol:** 2 gtts tid-qid. **Gel:** Apply 1/2 inch ribbon qhs.	◙C ❁>

PROSTAGLANDIN ANALOGUES

Bimatoprost (Lumigan)	**Sol:** 0.03%	**Adults: Usual/Max:** 1 gtt qpm.	◙C ❁>
Latanoprost (Xalatan)	**Sol:** 0.005%	**Adults: Usual/ Max:** 1 gtt qpm.	◙C ❁>
Travaprost (Travatan)	**Sol:** 0.004%	**Adults:** 1 gtt qpm.	◙C ❁>

NAME	FORM/STRENGTH	DOSAGE	COMMENTS
SYMPATHOMIMETICS			
Brimonidine (Alphagan, Alphagan P)	**Sol:** (Alphagan) 0.2%, (Alphagan P) 0.1%, 0.15%	**Adults & Peds: ≥2 yo:** 1 gtt tid (q8h). Separate other topical products that lower IOP by at least 5 min.	◉B ❀v

Mydriatics/Cycloplegics

NAME	FORM/STRENGTH	DOSAGE	COMMENTS
ANTICHOLINERGICS			
Atropine Sulfate	**Oint:** 1%; **Sol:** 1%	1-2 gtts tid or small amount of oint qd-bid.	◉C ❀>
Cyclopentolate HCl (Cyclogyl, Cylate, Ocu-Pentolate)	**Sol:** 0.5%, 1%, 2%	**Adults:** 1-2 gtts, may repeat in 5-10 min. **Peds:** 1-2 gtts, may repeat in 5-10 min w/ 0.5%-1%.	◉C ❀>
Cyclopentolate HCl/ Phenylephrine (Cyclomydril)	**Sol:** 0.2%-1%	**Adults & Peds:** 1 gtt q5-10min, up to 3x.	◉N ❀>
Homatropine HBr (Isopto Homatropine)	**Sol:** 2%, 5%	**Refraction:** 1-2 gtts, may repeat in 5-10 min. **Uveitis:** 1-2 gtts up to q3-4h. Only use 2% in peds.	◉C ❀>
Scopolamine HBr (Isopto Hyoscine)	**Sol:** 0.25%	**Refraction:** 1-2 gtts 1h prior to refracting. **Uveitis:** 1-2 gtts up to 4x/d.	◉N ❀>
Tropicamide (Mydral, Mydriacyl, Ocu-Tropic, Tropicacyl)	**Sol:** 0.5%, 1%	**Refraction:** (1%) 1-2 gtts, may repeat in 5 min. **Fundal Exam:** (0.5%) 1-2 gtts 15-20 min before exam.	◉N ❀>

Phenylephrine (Neo-Synephrine)	**Sol:** 2.5%, 10%; **Sol, viscous:** 10%	**Glaucoma/Vasocontriction/Pupil Dilation:** (10%) 1 gtt. **Uveitis:** (10%) 1 gtt. May continue the following day. **Surgery:** (2.5%/10%) 30-60 min pre-op. **Refraction: Adults & Peds:** (2.5%) 1 gtt after cyclopegic. **Ophtho Exam:** (2.5%) 1 gtt. **Diagnostic Procedure:** (2.5%) 1 gtt.	◙C ❃> 10% is CI in infants.

NSAIDs

Bromfenac (Xibrom)	**Sol:** 0.09%	**Adults: Cataract Extraction:** 1 gtt bid, begin 24h post-op x 2wks.	◙C ❃>
Diclofenac Sodium (Voltaren)	**Sol:** 1%	**Adults: Cataract Extraction:** 1 gtt qid, begin 24h post-op x 2wks. **Corneal Refractive Surgery:** 1-2 gtts within 1h pre-op, & 15 min post-op. Continue qid up to 3d.	◙C ❃> Avoid in late pregnancy.
Flurbiprofen Sodium (Ocufen)	**Sol:** 0.03%	**Inhibit Intraoperative Miosis: Adults:** 1 gtts q30min x 4 doses, beginning 2h prior to surgery.	◙C ❃v
Ketorolac Tromethamine (Acular, Acular PF)	**Sol:** 0.5%	**Adults & Peds: ≥3 yo: Acular: Ocular Itching:** 1 gtt qid. **Post-Op Inflammation:** 1 gtt qid. Begin 24h post-op & continue x 2wks. **Acular PF: Pain/Photophobia:** 1 gtt post-op qid prn up to 3d.	◙C ❃>
Nepafenac (Nevanac)	**Susp:** 0.1%	**Cataract Surgery: Adults:** 1 drop tid, start 24 h prior to surgery, continue on day of surgery & for 2 wks post-op.	◙C ❃>

Ocular Decongestant/Allergic Conjunctivitis

NAME	FORM/STRENGTH	DOSAGE	COMMENTS
H_1 ANTAGONIST/MAST CELL STABILIZERS			
Ketotifen Fumarate (Zaditor)	**Sol:** 0.025%	**Adults & Peds: ≥3 yo:** 1 gtt bid, q8-12h.	◙C ✽>
Olopatadine HCl (Patanol)	**Sol:** 0.1%	**Adults & Peds: ≥3 yo:** 1-2 gtts bid, q6-8h.	◙C ✽>
H_1 RECEPTOR ANTAGONISTS			
Azelastine (Optivar)	**Sol:** 0.05%	**Adults & Peds: ≥3 yo:** 1 gtt bid.	◙C ✽>
Epinastine HCl (Elestat)	**Sol:** 0.05%	**Adults & Peds: ≥3 yo:** 1 gtt in each eye bid.	◙C ✽>
Levocabastine (Livostin)	**Susp:** 0.05%	**Adults & Peds: ≥12 yo:** 1 gtt qid.	◙C ✽>
MAST CELL STABILIZERS			
Cromolyn Sodium (Crolom, Opticrom)	**Sol:** 4%	**Adults & Peds: ≥4 yo:** 1-2 gtts 4-6x/d.	◙B ✽>
Lodoxamide Tromethamine (Alomide)	**Sol:** 0.1%	**Adults & Peds: >2 yo:** 1-2 gtts qid up to 3 mths.	◙B ✽>
Nedocromil Sodium (Alocril)	**Sol:** 2%	**Adults & Peds: ≥3 yo:** 1-2 gtts bid.	◙B ✽>
SYMPATHOMIMETIC/H_1 ANTAGONISTS			
Naphazoline HCl/ Pheniramine Maleate (Naphcon-A)	**Sol:** 0.3%-0.025%	**Adults & Peds: ≥6 yo:** 1-2 gtts up to qid.	◙N ✽>

SYMPATHOMIMETICS

Naphazoline (AK-Con, Albalon, Allersol, Ocu-zoline)	**Sol:** 0.1%	**Adults:** 1-2 gtts q3-4h prn.	C >,

Viral Infection

Trifluridine (Viroptic)	**Sol:** 1%	**Adults & Peds: ≥6 yo: Usual:** 1 gtt q2h w/a until re-epithelialization. **Max:** 9 gtts/d. **Following Re-epithelialization:** 1 gtt q4h w/a, min 5 gtts/d x 7d.	C v
Vidarabine (Vira-A)	**Oint:** 3%	**Adults & Peds: ≥2 yo: Usual:** Apply 1/2 in 5x/d q3h x 7d until re-epithelialization. **Following Re-epithelialization:** Apply 1/2 inch bid x 7d.	C v

Miscellaneous

Cyclosporine (Restasis)	**Emulsion:** 0.05%	**Keratoconjunctivitis sicca: Adults:** 1 gtt bid, q12h.	C >
Dapiprazole (Rev-Eyes)	**Sol:** 0.5%	**Reversal of Diagnostic Mydriasis: Adults:** 2 gtts, repeat after 5 min.	B >

MISCELLANEOUS

Pegaptinab Sodium (Macugen)	**Inj:** 0.3 mg	**Macular Degeneration: Adults:** 0.3 mg by intravitreous injection once every 6 wks.	B >

NAME	FORM/STRENGTH	DOSAGE	COMMENTS
EENT/OTIC PREPARATIONS			

Anesthetics

NAME	FORM/STRENGTH	DOSAGE	COMMENTS
Antipyrine/Benzocaine (Aurodex, Auroto, Dolotic)	**Sol:** 54-14 mg/ml	**Otitis Media:** Fill ear canal, then insert moistened pledget. Repeat q1-2h until relief. **Cerumen Removal:** Instill tid x 2-3d, then insert moistened pledget.	●C ❁>
Benzocaine (Americaine Otic)	**Sol:** 20%	**Adults & Peds: ≥1 yo:** Instill 4-5 gtts in external auditory canal, then insert cotton pledget into meatus. May repeat q1-2h.	●C ❁>

Antibacterial/Antifungal Combinations

NAME	FORM/STRENGTH	DOSAGE	COMMENTS
Acetic Acid/ Aluminum Acetate (Borofair, Domeboro)	**Sol:** 2%-0.79%	**Adults:** 4-6 gtts into ear, repeat q2-3h.	●N ❁>
Acetic Acid (Vosol)	**Sol:** 2%	**Adults:** Insert saturated wick in ear & keep moist x 24h, remove wick & instill 5 gtts tid-qid. **Peds:** Insert wick & keep moist x 24h, remove wick & instill 3-4 gtts tid-qid.	●N ❁>

Antibacterial/Corticosteroid Combinations

NAME	FORM/STRENGTH	DOSAGE	COMMENTS
Acetic Acid/Hydrocortisone (Acetasol HC, Oticot HC, Vosol HC)	**Sol:** 2%-1%	**Adults:** Insert cotton saturated w/med & keep moist w/ 3-5 gtts q4-6h x 24h, then remove. Continue to instill 5 gtts tid-qid. **Peds:** Insert cotton saturated w/ med & keep moist w/ 3-4 gtts q4-6h x 24h, then remove. Continue to instill 3-4 gtts tid-qid.	●N ❁>

Ciprofloxacin HCl/ Dexamethasone (Ciprodex)	**Susp:** 0.3%-0.1%	**Adults & Peds: ≥6 mths:** 4 gtts bid x 7d.	◙C ❋v
Ciprofloxacin HCl/ Hydrocortisone (Cipro HC Otic)	**Susp:** 0.2%-1%	**Adults & Peds: ≥1 yo:** 3 gtts bid x 7d.	◙C ❋v
Colistin Sulfate/ Hydrocortisone Acetate/ Neomycin Sulfate/ Thonzonium Bromide (Coly-Mycin S, Cortisporin-TC)	**Susp:** 3-10-3.3-0.5 mg/ml	**Adults:** 4-5 gtts tid-qid. **Peds:** 3-4 gtts tid-qid.	◙N ❋>
Neomycin Sulfate/ Polymyxin B Sulfate/ Hydrocortisone (Cortisporin)	**Sol, Susp:** 1%-0.35%-10,000 U/ml	**Adults:** 4 gtts tid-qid up to 10d. **Peds:** 3 gtts tid-qid up to 10d.	◙C ❋>

Antibiotic Agents

Chloramphenicol	**Sol:** 0.5%	**Adults:** 2-3 gtts tid.	◙N ❋>
Ofloxacin (Floxin Otic, Floxin Otic Singles)	**Sol:** 0.3%	**Otitis Externa: Peds: 6 mths-13 yo:** 5 gtts or 1 single-dispensing container (SDC) qd x 7d. **≥13 yo:** 10 gtts or 2 SDCs qd x 7d. **Acute Otitis Media w/ Tympanostomy Tubes: Peds: 1-12 yo:** 5 gtts or 1 SDC bid x 10d. **Chronic Suppurative Otitis Media w/ Perforated Tympanic Membranes: Adults & Peds: ≥12 yo:** 10 gtts or 2 SDCs bid x 14d.	◙C ❋v

NAME	FORM/STRENGTH	DOSAGE	COMMENTS
Surfactants			
Triethanolamine Polypeptide (Cerumenex)	**Sol:** 10%	**Adults:** Fill ear canal & insert cotton plug x 15-30 min. Flush w/ warm water. May repeat.	◉C ✽>
ENDOCRINE/METABOLIC			
Androgens			
Danazol (Danocrine)	**Cap:** 50 mg, 100 mg, 200 mg	**Adults: Hereditary Angioedema: Initial:** 200 mg bid-tid. After favorable response, decrease up to 50% at intervals of ≥1-3 mths depending on frequency of attacks. Increase up to 200 mg if attack occurs.	◉X ✽v CI in nursing. Begin during menses. [25]
Methyltestosterone CIII (Android, Testred)	**Cap:** 10 mg	**Adults: Androgen-Deficient Males:** 10-50 mg/d. **Breast Cancer in Females:** 50-200 mg/d. **Peds: Delayed Puberty:** Use lower range of 10-50 mg/d x 4-6mths.	◉X ✽v
Oxandrolone CIII (Oxandrin)	**Tab:** 2.5 mg, 10 mg	**Adults: Usual:** 2.5-20 mg/day given bid-qid x 2-4wks. **Peds:** ≤0.1 mg/kg/d. Repeat intermittently as indicated. **Elderly:** 5 mg bid.	◉X ✽v
Testosterone CIII (Androderm, Androgel, Testim, Testoderm, Testoderm TTS)	**Gel:** (Androgel) 1%, (Testim) 1%; **Patch:** (Androderm) 2.5 mg/24 h, 5 mg/24 h; (Testoderm) 4 mg/24 h, 6 mg/ 24 h; (Testoderm TTS) 5 mg/24 h	**Adults: Patch:** (Androderm) **Initial:** 5 mg qhs x 24h on back, abdomen, upper arm, or thigh. **Maint:** 2.5-7.5 mg/d. **Initial:** (Testoderm) 6 mg/d. Apply to scrotal skin x 22-24h. (Testoderm TTS) 1 patch q24h on arm, back or upper buttocks. **Gel:** (Androgel) **Initial:** Apply 5 g qd on shoulders & upper arms and/or abdomen. **Titrate:** May increase to 7.5 g qd, then 10 g qd. (Testim) **Initial:** Apply 5 g qd in am to shoulder or upper arm. **Titrate:** May increase to 10 g qd. **≥15 yrs: Patch:** (Androderm) **Initial:** 5 mg/d. **Maint:** 2.5-7.5 mg/d.	◉X ✽v

[25] Benign intracranial HTN. Thromboembolic events.

Testosterone CIII (Striant)	**Tab,Buccal:** 30 mg	**Adults:** 30 mg q12h to gum region above incisor tooth on either side of mouth. Rotate sites w/ each application. Hold in place for 30 sec.	◙X ❁v
Testosterone Cypionate CIII (Depo-Testosterone)	**Inj:** 100 mg/ml, 200 mg/ml	**Adults & Peds: ≥12 yo:** 50-400 mg IM q2-4wks.	◙X ❁v
Testosterone Enanthate CIII (Delatestryl, Everone)	**Inj:** 200 mg/ml	**Adults & Peds: Male Hypogonadism: Usual:** 50-400 mg IM q2-4wks. **Delayed Puberty:** 50-200 mg q2-4wks for a limited duration (eg, 4-6 mths). Caution in children.	◙X ❁v
Testosterone Propionate CIII	**Inj:** 100 mg/ml	**Adults & Peds: Usual:** 25-50 mg IM BIW-TIW.	◙X ❁v

Antidiabetic Agents

INSULIN FORMULATIONS

TYPE OF INSULIN	BRAND (MANUFACTURER)	ONSET* (HRS)	PEAK* (HRS)	DURATION* (HRS)	COMMON PITFALLS**
Rapid-acting					Hypoglycemia occurs if lag time is too long or the patient exercises within 1 hr of dose; with high-fat meals, the dose should be adjusted downward.
Lispro	**Humalog** (Lilly)	<0.25	0.5 to 1.5	3 to 5	
Aspart	**Novolog** (Novo Nordisk)	<0.25	0.5 to 1	3 to 5	
Short-acting					Lag time is not used appropriately; the insulin should be given 20 to 30 minutes before the patient eats.
Regular	**Humulin R**† (Lilly)	0.5 to 1	2 to 4	4 to 12	
	Novolin R (Novo Nordisk)	0.5 to 1	2 to 5	8	

TYPE OF INSULIN	BRAND (MANUFACTURER)	ONSET* (HRS)	PEAK* (HRS)	DURATION* (HRS)	COMMON PITFALLS
Intermediate-acting NPH (Isophane)	**Humulin N** (Lilly) **Novolin N** (Novo Nordisk)	1 to 3	6 to 12	18 to 24	In many patients, breakfast injection does not last until the evening meal; administration with the evening meal does not meet insulin needs on awakening.
Long-acting Glargine	**Lantus** (Sanofi-Aventis)	1	Flat	24	Administer once daily at the same time every day.
Combinations Isophane susp (70%)/ regular (30%)	**Humulin 70/30** (Lilly) **Novolin 70/30** (Novo Nordisk)	0.5 to 1	4 to 6	24	See individual comments
Isophane susp (50%)/ regular (50%)	**Humulin 50/50** (Lilly)	0.5 to 1	3 to 5	24	See individual comments
Lispro protamine (75%)/ lispro (25%)	**Humalog Mix 75/25** (Lilly)	≤0.25	0.5 to 4	24	See individual comments
Aspart protamine (70%)/ aspart (30%)	**Novolog Mix 70/30** (Novo Nordisk)	≤0.25	1 to 4	24	See individual comments

*Approximate parameters following SC injection of an average patient dose; insulin concentration: 100U/mL.

**Source: Hirsch, IB. Type 1 Diabetes Mellitus and the Use of Flexible Insulin Regimens. *Am Fam Physician*. November 1999;60(8):2343-2352,2355-2356.

†Also available 500U/mL for insulin-resistant patients (rapid onset; up to 24 hour duration).

NAME	FORM/STRENGTH	DOSAGE	COMMENTS
BIGUANIDES			
Metformin HCl (Fortamet, Glucophage, Glucophage XR, Glumetza, Riomet)	**Sol:** (Riomet) 500 mg/5 ml; **Tab:** (Glucophage) 500 mg, 850 mg, 1000 mg; **Tab,ER:** (Fortamet) 500 mg, 1000 mg. (Glucophage XR) 500 mg, 750 mg. (Glumetza) 500 mg, 1000 mg	**Adults: Sol/Tab: Initial** 500 mg bid or 850 mg qd w/ meals. **Titrate:** Increase by 500 mg qwk, or 850 mg q2wks, or from 500 mg bid to 850 mg bid after 2 wks. **Max:** 2550 mg/d. **With Insulin: Initial:** 500 mg qd. **Titrate:** 500 mg qwk. **Max:** 2500 mg/d. Decrease insulin dose by 10-25% when FPG <120 mg/dl. **Tab,ER: Glucophage XR: With/Without Insulin: Initial:** 500 mg qd w/ evening meal. **Titrate:** Increase by 500 mg qwk. **Max:** 2000 mg/d. **Fortamet: Initial:** 500-1000 mg qd w/ evening meal. **With Insulin: Initial:** 500 mg qd. **Titrate:** May increase by 500 mg/wk. **Max:** 2500 mg/d. Decrease insulin dose by 10-25% when FPG <120 mg/dl. **Glumetza:** Take w/ evening meal. **Initial:** 1000 mg qd. **With Insulin: Initial:** 500 mg qd. **Titrate:** May increase by 500 mg/wk. **Max:** 2000 mg/d. Decrease insulin dose by 10-25% if FPG <120 mg/dL. **Peds: 10-16 yo: Sol/Tab: Initial:** 500 mg bid w/ meals. **Titrate:** Increase by 500 mg qwk. **Max:** 2000 mg/d in divided doses.	B v **H R** Lactic acidosis reported (rare).
GLUCOSIDASE INHIBITORS			
Acarbose (Precose)	**Tab:** 25 mg, 50 mg, 100 mg	**Adults: Initial:** 25 mg tid w/ meals. **Titrate:** Adjust at 4-8 wk intervals. **Maint:** 50-100 mg tid. **Max: ≤60 kg:** 50 mg tid. **>60 kg:** 100 mg tid.	B v **R**

NAME	FORM/STRENGTH	DOSAGE	COMMENTS
Miglitol (Glyset)	**Tab:** 25 mg, 50 mg, 100 mg	**Adults: Initial:** 25 mg tid w/ meals. **Titrate:** Increase after 4-8 wks to 50 mg tid x approx. 3 mths, then may further increase to 100 mg tid. **Maint:** 50-100 mg tid. **Max:** 100 mg tid.	◉B ✽v **R**
INCRETIN MIMETIC			
Exenatide (Byetta)	**Inj:** 250 mcg/ml	**Adults:** 5 mcg SC bid, 60 min before qam & qpm meals. **Titrate/Max:** 10 mcg bid after 1 mth. Reduction of sulfonylurea dose may be considered to reduce risk of hypoglycemia.	◉C ✽> **R**
MEGLITINIDES			
Nateglinide (Starlix)	**Tab:** 60 mg, 120 mg	**Adults:** 120 mg tid 1-30 min ac. May use 60 mg tid for near goal HbA_{1c}. Skip dose if meal is skipped.	◉C ✽v
Repaglinide (Prandin)	**Tab:** 0.5 mg, 1 mg, 2 mg	**Adults: Initial: Treatment-Naive or HbA_{1c} <8%**: 0.5 mg w/ each meal. **Previous Oral Antidiabetic Therapy/Combination Therapy & HbA_{1c} ≥8%**: 1-2 mg w/ meals. **Titrate:** May adjust wkly by doubling preprandial dose up to 4 mg (bid-qid). **Maint:** 0.5-4 mg w/ meals. **Max:** 16 mg/d. Take within 15-30 min ac. Skip dose if skip meal & add dose if add meal.	◉C ✽v **H R**

SULFONYLUREA/BIGUANIDE

Glipizide/Metformin HCl (Metaglip)	**Tab:** 2.5/250 mg, 2.5/500 mg, 5/500 mg	**Adults: Initial:** 2.5/250 mg qd w/ meals. If FBG 280-320 mg/dL, give 2.5/500 mg bid. **Titrate:** Increase by 1 tab/d q2wks. **Max:** 10/2000 mg/d. **2nd-Line Therapy: Initial:** 2.5/500 mg or 5/500 mg bid w/ meals. **Titrate:** Increase by ≤5/500 mg/d. **Max:** 20/2000 mg/d.	C v **H R** Lactic acidosis reported (rare).
Glyburide/Metformin HCl (Glucovance)	**Tab:** 1.25-250 mg, 2.5-500 mg, 5-500 mg	**Adults: Initial:** 1.25-250 mg qd-bid w/ meals. **Titrate:** Increase by 1.25-250 mg/d q2wks. **Max:** 10-2000 mg/d. **2nd Line Therapy: Initial:** 2.5-500 mg or 5-500 mg bid w/ meals. **Titrate:** Increase by ≤5-500 mg/d. **Max:** 20-2000 mg/d.	B v **H R** Lactic acidosis reported (rare).

SULFONYLUREAS-1ST GENERATION

Chlorpropamide (Diabinese)	**Tab:** 100 mg, 250 mg	**Adults: Initial:** 250 mg qd w/ breakfast. **Titrate:** After 5-7d, adjust by 50-125 mg/d q3-5d. **Maint:** 100-500 mg qd. **Max:** 750 mg/d.	C v **H R**
Tolazamide (Tolinase)	**Tab:** 100 mg, 250 mg, 500 mg	**Adults: Initial:** 100-250 mg qd w/breakfast. **Titrate:** May increase by 100-250 mg/wk. **Maint:** 100-1000 mg/d. **Max:** 1000 mg/d. Divide dose if >500 mg.	C v **H R**
Tolbutamide (Tol-Tab)	**Tab:** 500 mg	**Adults: Usual/Initial:** 1-2 gm qd 30 min ac. **Maint:** 0.25-3 gm/d. **Max:** 3 gm/d.	C v **H R**

NAME	FORM/STRENGTH	DOSAGE	COMMENTS
SULFONYLUREAS-2ND GENERATION			
Glimepiride (Amaryl)	**Tab:** 1 mg, 2 mg, 4 mg	**Adults: Initial:** 1-2 mg qd w/ breakfast. **Titrate:** Increase ≤2 mg at 1-2 wk intervals. **Maint:** 1-4 mg qd. **Max:** 8 mg/d.	◙C ❋v **H R**
Glipizide (Glucotrol, Glucotrol XL)	**Tab:** 5 mg, 10 mg; **Tab,ER:** 2.5 mg, 5 mg, 10 mg	**Adults: Glucotrol XL: Initial/Combination Therapy:** 5 mg qd w/ breakfast. **Usual:** 5-10 mg qd. **Max:** 20 mg/d. **Glucotrol: Initial:** 5 mg qd 30 min ac. **Titrate:** Increase by 2.5-5 mg; divide if above 15 mg. **Max:** 40 mg/d.	◙C ❋v **H R**
Glyburide (Diabeta, Micronase)	**Tab:** 1.25 mg, 2.5 mg, 5 mg	**Adults: Initial:** 2.5-5 mg qd w/ breakfast. **Titrate:** Increase by no more than 2.5 mg at wkly intervals, give bid if >10 mg/d. **Maint:** 1.25-20 mg/d. **Max:** 20 mg/d.	◙B (Micronase) ◙C (Diabeta) ❋v **H R**
Glyburide, Micronized (Glycron, Glynase Pres-Tab)	**Tab:** 1.5 mg, 3 mg, 4.5 mg, 6 mg	**Adults: Initial:** 1.5-3 mg qd w/ breakfast. **Titrate:** Increase by no more than 1.5 mg at wkly intervals; >6 mg may give bid. **Maint:** 0.75-12 mg/d. **Max:** 12 mg/d.	◙B ❋v **H R**
THIAZOLIDINEDIONE/BIGUANIDE			
Rosiglitazone Maleate/Metformin HCl (Avandamet)	**Tab:** 1-500 mg, 2-500 mg, 4-500 mg, 2-1000 mg, 4-1000 mg	**Adults: Prior Metformin 1 gm/d: Initial:** 2-500 mg tab bid. **Prior Metformin 2 gm/d: Initial:** 2-1000 mg tab bid. **Prior Rosiglitazone 4 mg/d: Initial:** 2-500 mg tab bid. **Prior Rosiglitazone 8 mg/d:** 4-500 mg tab bid. **Titrate:** May increase by 4 mg rosiglitazone and/or 500 mg metformin. **Max:** 8-2000 mg/d. Take w/ meals.	◙C ❋v **H R** Monitor liver enzymes.

THIAZOLIDINEDIONE/SULFONYLUREA

Rosiglitazone Maleate/Glimepiride (Avandaryl)	**Tab:** 4-1 mg, 4-2 mg, 4-4 mg	**Adults: Prior Sulfonylurea Monotherapy or Inital Response To Rosiglitazone Alone Requiring Additional Control:** 4-1 mg or 4-2 mg qd w/ first meal of day. **Switching From Prior Combination Therapy:** Same dose already taken of each component. **Prior Thiazolidinedione Monotherapy:** Titrate dose. After 1-2 wks w/ inadequate control, increase glimepiride component in no more than 2 mg increments at 1-2 wk intervals. **Max:** 8-4 mg qd. **Prior Sulfonylurea Monotherapy:** May take 2-3 mths for full effect of rosiglitazone; do not exceed 8 mg of rosiglitazone daily. **Titrate:** May increase glimepiride component. **Elderly/Debilitated/Malnourished/Renal, Hepatic or Adrenal Insufficiency: Initial:** 4-1 mg qd. Titrate carefully.	◙C ❋v **H R** Monitor liver enzymes.

THIAZOLIDINEDIONES

Pioglitazone (Actos)	**Tab:** 15 mg, 30 mg, 45 mg	**Adults: Initial:** 15-30 mg qd. **Max:** 45 mg/d. **Combination Therapy w/ Insulin:** Decrease insulin by 10-25% if hypoglycemic or FPG <100 mg/dL; individualize further adjustments based on glucose lowering response.	◙C ❋v **H** Monitor liver enzymes.

NAME	FORM/STRENGTH	DOSAGE	COMMENTS
Rosiglitazone Maleate (Avandia)	**Tab:** 2 mg, 4 mg, 8 mg	**Adults: ≥18 yo: Initial:** 2 mg bid or 4 mg qd. **Titrate:** May increase after 8-12 wks to 4 mg bid or 8 mg qd. **Max:** 8 mg/d as monotherapy or w/ metformin, sulfonylureas, or sulfonylureas plus metformin; 4 mg/d w/ insulin. **Combination Therapy With Insulin:** Decrease insulin by 10-25% if hypoglycemic or FPG <100 mg/dL; individualize further adjustments based on glucose lowering response.	●C ❃v **H** Monitor liver enzymes.

Antithyroid Agents

Methimazole (Tapazole)	**Tab:** 5 mg, 10 mg	**Adults: Initial:** 5 mg q8h for mild hyperthyroidism; 30-40 mg/d given q8h for moderately severe hyperthyroidism, 20 mg q8h for severe hyperthyroidism. **Maint:** 5-15 mg/d. **Peds: Initial:** 0.4 mg/kg/d divided q8h. **Maint:** 1/2 of initial dose.	●D ❃v CI in nursing.
Propylthiouracil (PTU)	**Tab:** 50 mg	**Adults:** 100 mg q8h, 400 mg/d as q8h for severe hyperthyroidism/large goiters, up to 600-900 mg/d if needed. **Maint:** 100-150 mg/d. **Peds: 6-10 yo: Initial:** 50-150 mg/d. **≥10 yo:** 150-300 mg/d. **Maint:** Determine dose by response.	●D ❃v CI in nursing.

SYSTEMIC CORTICOSTEROIDS

CORTICOSTEROID	EQUIVALENT POTENCY	MINERALOCORTICOID POTENCY	FORM/STRENGTH	DOSAGE RANGE
Betamethasone (Celestone)	0.6 mg	0	**Syr:** 0.6 mg/5 ml	**Initial:** 0.6-7.2 mg/d PO.
Betamethasone Sodium Phosphate & Betamethasone Acetate (Celestone Soluspan)	0.6 mg	0	**Inj:** 3 mg-3 mg/ml	**Initial:** 0.5-9 mg/d IM.
Cortisone Acetate	25 mg	2	**Tab:** 25 mg	**Initial:** 25-300 mg/d PO.
Dexamethasone (Decadron)	0.5 mg	0	**Sol:** 0.5 mg/5 ml **Tab:** 0.5 mg, 0.75 mg, 1 mg, 1.5 mg, 2 mg, 4 mg, 6 mg	**Initial:** 0.75-9 mg/d PO.
Dexamethasone Sodium Phosphate (Decadron Phosphate)	0.5 mg	0	**Inj:** 4 mg/ml	**Initial:** 0.5-9 mg/d IM/IV.
Hydrocortisone (Cortef)	20 mg	2	**Tab:** 5 mg, 10 mg, 20 mg	**Initial:** 20-240 mg/d PO.
Hydrocortisone Cypionate (Cortef)	20 mg	2	**Susp:** 10 mg/5 ml	**Initial:** 20-240 mg/d PO.

CORTICOSTEROID	EQUIVALENT POTENCY	MINERALOCORTICOID POTENCY	FORM/STRENGTH	DOSAGE RANGE
Hydrocortisone Sodium Succinate (Solu-Cortef)	20 mg	2	**Inj:** 100 mg, 250 mg, 500 mg, 1000 mg	**Initial:** 100-500 mg IM/IV.
Methylprednisolone (Medrol)	4 mg	0	**Tab:** 2 mg, 4 mg, 8 mg, 16 mg, 24 mg, 32 mg	**Initial:** 4-48 mg/d PO.
Methylprednisolone Acetate (Depo-Medrol)	4 mg	0	**Inj:** 20 mg/ml, 40 mg/ml, 80 mg/ml	**Initial:** 40-120 mg/wk IM.
Methylprednisolone Sodium Succinate (Solu-Medrol)	4 mg	0	**Inj:** 40 mg, 125 mg, 500 mg, 1 gm, 2 gm	**Initial:** 10-40 mg IV.
Prednisolone (Prelone)	5 mg	1	**Syr:** 5 mg/5 ml, 15 mg/5 ml	**Initial:** 5-60 mg/d PO.
Prednisolone Sodium Phosphate (Pediapred)	5 mg	1	**Sol:** 5 mg/5 ml	**Initial:** 5-60 mg/d PO.
Prednisone (Deltasone)	5 mg	1	**Sol:** 5 mg/ml, 5 mg/5 ml; **Tab:** 1 mg, 2.5 mg, 5 mg, 10 mg, 20 mg, 50 mg	**Initial:** 5-60 mg/d PO.
Triamcinolone (Aristocort)	4 mg	0	**Tab:** 4 mg	**Initial:** 4-60 mg/d PO.
Triamcinolone Acetonide (Kenalog-10)	4 mg	0	**Inj:** 10 mg/ml	**Intra-articular/ Intrabursal:** 2.5-20 mg/d.

Triamcinolone Acetonide (Kenalog-40)	4 mg	0	**Inj:** 40 mg/ml	**Initial:** 2.5-60 mg/d IM or intra-articular.
Triamcinolone Hexacetonide (Aristospan Intra-lesional, Aristospan Intra-articular)	4 mg	0	**Inj:** 5 mg/ml (intralesional), 20 mg/ml (intra-articular)	**Intra-articular:** 2-48 mg. **Intra-lesional:** Up to 0.5 mg/in^2 of area affected.

NAME	FORM/STRENGTH	DOSAGE	COMMENTS

Gout

URICOSURICS

Probenecid	**Tab:** 500 mg	**Adults:** 250 mg bid x 1 wk. **Titrate:** Increase by 500 mg q4wks. **Maint:** 500 mg bid. **Max:** 2 gm/d.	◙N ❋> R
Sulfinpyrazone	**Tab:** 100 mg	**Initial:** 100-200 mg bid w/ meals or milk x 1 wk. **Maint:** 200 mg bid, increase to 300 mg/d if needed. **Max:** 800 mg/d.	◙N ❋>

XANTHINE OXIDASE INHIBITORS

Allopurinol (Zyloprim)	**Tab:** 100 mg, 300 mg	**Adults: Usual:** 200-300 mg/d. **Prevention of Uric Acid Nephropathy w/ Chemotherapy: Usual:** 600-800 mg/d for 2-3d w/ high fluid intake.	◙C ❋> R

NAME	FORM/STRENGTH	DOSAGE	COMMENTS
MISCELLANEOUS			
Colchicine	**Inj:** 0.5 mg/ml; **Tab:** 0.5 mg, 0.6 mg	**Adults: Acute Gouty Arthritis:** 1-1.2 mg, then 0.5-0.6 mg/h or 1-1.2 mg q2h until pain relieved or diarrhea ensues up to 4-8 mg; wait 3d between courses to avoid toxicity. **Prophylaxis:** (<1 attack/yr) 0.5-0.6 mg/d 3-4x/wk; (>1 attack/wk) 0.5-0.6 mg/d, severe cases may need 2-3 tabs/d.	C > **H R**
Probenecid/Colchicine	**Tab:** 500-0.5 mg	**Adults: Initial:** 1 tab qd x 1 wk, then 1 tab bid. **Titrate:** May increase by 1 tab/d q4wks. **Max:** 4 tabs/d. Not for acute gouty attacks. May reduce dose by 1 tab q6mths if acute attacks have been absent ≥6 mths.	N > **R** CI in pregnancy.

Growth Hormone

NAME	FORM/STRENGTH	DOSAGE	COMMENTS
Somatropin (rDNA origin) (Saizen, Zorbtive)	**Inj:** (Saizen) 8.8 mg, 5 mg, (Zorbtive) 8.8 mg	**Saizen: Adults: Initial:** ≤0.005 mg/kg/d. **Maint:** After 4 wks, may increase to ≤0.01 mg/kg/d depending on patient tolerance. **Peds:** Individualize dose. **Usual:** 0.06 mg/kg IM/SQ TIW. If epiphyses are fused, d/c therapy. **Zorbtive: Adults:** 0.1 mg/kg SC qd x 4 wks. **Max:** 8 mg qd. Rotate injection site.	B >

Hypoglycemia

NAME	FORM/STRENGTH	DOSAGE	COMMENTS
Glucagon (GlucaGen)	**Inj:** 1 mg	**Severe Hypoglycemia: Adults & Peds: ≥25 kg:** 1 mg IM/IV/SC. **<25 kg or <6-8 yo:** 0.5 mg IM/IV/SC. May repeat x 1 dose after 15 min if no response while waiting for emergency assistance.	B >

Obesity

CENTRALLY ACTING ADRENERGIC AGENTS

Benzphetamine HCl CIII (Didrex)	**Tab:** 50 mg	**Adults & Peds: ≥12 yo: Initial:** 25-50 mg qd. **Maint:** 25-50 mg qd-tid.	X v
Diethylpropion HCl CIV (Tenuate)	**Tab:** 25 mg; **Tab,ER:** 75 mg	**Adults & Peds: ≥16 yo:** (Tab) 25 mg tab tid 1h ac & mid-evening prn. (Tab,ER) 75 mg qd mid-morning.	B >
Methamphetamine HCl CII (Desoxyn)	**Tab:** 5 mg	**Adults & Peds: ≥12 yo:** 5 mg 1/2 hr before each meal.	C v High potential for abuse.
Phendimetrazine CIII (Prelu-2, Bontril)	**Cap,ER:** 105 mg; **Tab:** 35 mg	**Adults & Peds: ≥12 yo:** (Tab) 35 mg tab bid-tid 1h ac. May decrease to 17.5 mg/dose. (Cap,ER) 105 mg qam 30-60 min ac.	N >
Phentermine HCl CIV (Adipex-P, Phentercot)	**Cap:** 15 mg, 18.75 mg, 30 mg, 37.5 mg; **Tab:** 8 mg, 37.5 mg	**Adults & Peds: ≥16 yo:** 30 mg 2h before breakfast, 37.5 mg before, or 1-2h after, breakfast, or 18.75 mg qd-bid.	N >
Phentermine Resin CIV (Ionamin)	**Cap:** 15 mg, 30 mg	**Adults & Peds: ≥16 yo:** 15-30 mg before breakfast or 10-14h before retiring.	N >

CENTRALLY ACTING SEROTONIN/NE AGENTS

Sibutramine (Meridia)	**Cap:** 5 mg, 10 mg, 15 mg	**Adults & Peds: ≥16 yo: Initial:** 10 mg qd. **Titrate:** May increase after 4 wks to 15 mg qd. **Max:** 15 mg/d. May continue for up to 2 yrs.	C v Do not give if severe renal/hepatic impairment.

NAME	FORM/STRENGTH	DOSAGE	COMMENTS
LIPASE INHIBITOR			
Orlistat (Xenical)	**Cap:** 120 mg	**Adults & Peds: ≥12yo:** 120 mg tid w/ meals containing fat. Take during or up to 1h after meals. Omit dose if miss meal. Take a MVI w/ fat-soluble vitamins at least 2h before or after dose.	◉B ❋v

Osteoporosis

BISPHOSPHONATES AND COMBINATIONS

NAME	FORM/STRENGTH	DOSAGE	COMMENTS
Alendronate Sodium (Fosamax)	**Sol:** 70 mg/75 ml; **Tab:** 5 mg, 10 mg, 35 mg, 40 mg, 70 mg	**Adults: Treatment in Females/Bone Mass Increase in Men:** 10 mg qd or 70 mg qwk. **Prevention: Females:** 5 mg qd or 35 mg qwk. **Glucocorticoid-Induced: Men/Women:** 5 mg qd. **Postmenopausal Women Not Receiving Estrogen:** 10 mg qd. Take at least 30 min before 1st food, beverage, or medication of the day. Take tab w/ 6-8 oz of water, followed by 2 oz of water. Do not lie down x 30 min after dose & until after 1st food of the day.	◉C ❋> **R**
Alendronate Sodium/Cholecalciferol (Fosamax Plus D)	**Tab:** 70 mg/2800 IU	**Adults: Treatment in Females/Bone Mass Increase in Men:** 1 tab q wk. Take at least 30 min before 1st food, beverage, or medication of the day. Take tab w/ 6-8 oz of water, followed by 2 oz of water. Do not lie down x 30 min after dose & until after 1st food of day.	◉C ❋> **R**

Ibandronate Sodium (Boniva)	**Tab:** 2.5 mg, 150 mg	**Treatment/Prevention: Female:** 2.5 mg qd or 150 mg once monthly. Take at least 60 min before 1st food, beverage, or medication. Do not lie down x 60 min after dose.	◙C ❁> **R**
Risedronate (Actonel)	**Tab:** 5 mg, 30 mg, 35 mg	**Adults: Treatment/Prevention: Postmenopausal:** 5 mg qd or 35 mg qwk. **Glucocorticoid-Induced:** 5 mg qd. Take at least 30 min before 1st food or drink of day other than water. Swallow in upright position w/ 6-8 oz of water. Do not lie down x 30 min after dose.	◙C ❁v **R**
Risedronate Sodium/Calcium Carbonate (Actonel with Calcium)	**Tab:** (Risedronate) 35 mg; **Tab:** (Calcium): 1250 mg	**Adults: Treatment/Prevention: Postmenopausal: Actonel:** 35 mg qwk on Day 1 of 7-day treatment cycle. Take at least 30 min before 1st food or drink of day other than water. Swallow in upright position w/ 6-8 oz of water. Do not lie down x 30 min after dose. **Calcium:** 1250 mg qd on Days 2-7 of 7-day treatment cycle.	◙C ❁v **R**

CALCITONIN

Calcitonin-Salmon (Fortical, Miacalcin)	**Inj:** 200 IU/ml (Miacalcin); **Nasal Spr:** 200 IU/spr (Fortical, Miacalcin)	**Treatment: Adults: Female: Intranasal:** 200 IU/day (1 spr), alternate nostrils, daily. **IM/SC:** 100 IU qod.	◙C ❁v

NAME	FORM/STRENGTH	DOSAGE	COMMENTS
ESTROGEN/PROGESTIN COMBINATION			
Estradiol/Levonorgestrel (Climara Pro)	**Patch:** 0.045 -0.015 mg/d	**Prevention: Adults:** Apply 1 patch qwk to lower abdomen (avoid breasts/waistline). Rotate application site; allow 1 wk between same site.	◉X ✿> 4, 10, 28
Estradiol/Norethindrone (Activella)	**Tab:** 1-0.5 mg	**Prevention: Adults: Female:** 1 tab qd.	◉X ✿> 28
Estradiol/Norgestimate (Prefest)	**Tab:** 1 mg-none, 1 mg-0.09 mg	**Prevention: Adults: Female:** 1 mg estradiol x 3d; alternate w/ 1 mg-0.09 mg tab x 3d on continuous schedule.	◉X ✿v 28
Estrogens, Conjugated/Medroxyprogesterone Acetate (Premphase, Prempro)	**Tab:** (Premphase) 0.625 mg conjugated estrogens & 0.625-5 mg, (Prempro) 0.3-1.5 mg, 0.45-1.5 mg, 0.625-2.5 mg, 0.625-5 mg	**Prevention: Adults: Female:** Treat w/ lowest effective dose. Adjust dose based on response.	◉X ✿> 10, 28
Ethinyl Estradiol/Norethindrone (Femhrt)	**Tab:** 2.5 mcg-0.5 mg, 5 mcg-1 mg	**Prevention: Female: Usual:** 1 tab qd.	◉X ✿> 4

Estradiol (Alora, Climara, Vivelle, Vivelle-Dot)	**Patch:** (Alora) 0.025 mg/d, 0.05 mg/d, 0.075 mg/d, 0.1 mg/d, (Climara) 0.025 mg/d, 0.0375 mg/d, 0.05 mg/d, 0.06 mg/d, 0.075 mg/d, 0.1 mg/d, (Vivelle, Vivelle-Dot) 0.025 mg/d, 0.0375 mg/d, 0.05 mg/d, 0.075 mg/d, 0.1 mg/d	**Prevention: Adults: Female:** (Climara) Apply 0.025 mg/d patch qwk. (Vivelle, Vivelle-Dot) 0.025 mg/d patch BIW is minimum effective dose. (Alora) Apply 0.025 mg/d patch BIW. **Titrate:** May increase depending on bone mineral density & adverse events.	◙X ❁> [4]
Estradiol (Estrace, Gynodiol)	**Tab:** (Estrace) 0.5 mg, 1 mg, 2 mg, (Gynodiol) 0.5 mg, 1 mg, 1.5 mg, 2 mg	**Prevention: Adults: Female:** 0.5 mg qd (23 days on & 5 days off)	◙X ❁v [4, 10, 28]
Estradiol (Menostar)	**Patch:** 14 mcg/d	**Prevention: Adults: Female:** Apply 1 patch (14 mcg/d) qwk.	◙X ❁> [4, 28]
Estrogens, Conjugated (Premarin)	**Tab:** 0.3 mg, 0.45 mg, 0.625 mg, 0.9 mg, 1.25 mg, 2.5 mg	**Prevention: Adults: Female:** 0.3 mg qd given continuously or cyclically (eg, 25d on, 5d off).	◙X ❁> [4, 28]

4 Contraindicated in pregnancy. Increased risk of endometrial carcinoma.

10 Attempt to taper or d/c at 3-6 mth intervals.

28 Not for prevention of CV disease or dementia. The WHI reported increased risks of MI, stroke, invasive breast cancer, pulmonary emboli, DVT, and probable dementia in postmenopausal women. Prescribe at lowest effective doses for shortest duration.

NAME	FORM/STRENGTH	DOSAGE	COMMENTS
Estropipate (Ogen, Ortho-Est)	**Tab:** (Ogen, Ortho-Est) 0.625 mg (0.75 mg estropipate), 1.25 mg (1.5 mg estropipate); (Ogen) 2.5 mg (3 mg estropipate)	**Prevention: Adults: Female:** 0.625 mg (0.75 mg estropipate) qd x 25d of a 31d cycle per mth.	■X ❀> [4, 10, 28]
PARATHYROID HORMONE			
Teriparatide [rDNA origin] (Forteo)	**Inj:** 250 mcg/ml	**Treatment in Females/Bone Mass Increase in Men: Adults:** 20 mcg qd SC into thigh or abdominal wall. Discard pen after 28d. Use for >2 yrs is not recommended. Administer initially under circumstances where patient can sit or lie down.	■C ❀v Avoid if risk of osteosarcoma.
SERM (SELECTIVE ESTROGEN RECEPTOR MODULATOR)			
Raloxifene HCl (Evista)	**Tab:** 60 mg	**Treatment/Prevention: Adults: Female:** 60 mg qd.	■X ❀v

Thyroid Agents

THYROID HORMONES

Levothyroxine Sodium, T4 (Levothroid, Levoxyl, Synthroid)	**Tab:** 0.025 mg, 0.05 mg, 0.075 mg, 0.088 mg, 0.1 mg, 0.112 mg, 0.125 mg, 0.137 mg, 0.15 mg, 0.175 mg, 0.2 mg, 0.3 mg	**Hypothyroidism: Adults <50 yo or >50 yo & Recently Treated for Hyperthyroidism or Hypothyroid for Short Time & Peds >12 yo where Growth/Puberty Complete:** 1.7 mcg/kg/d. >200 mcg/d seldom required. **>50 yo or <50 yo w/ Underlying Cardiac Disease: Initial:** 25-50 mcg/d until TSH normalized. **Peds: >12 yo where Growth/Puberty Incomplete:** 2-3 mcg/kg/d. **6-12 yo:** 4-5 mcg/kg/d. **1-5 yo:** 5-6 mcg/kg/d. **6-12 mths:** 6-8 mcg/kg/d. **3-6 mths:** 8-10 mcg/kg/d. **0-3 mths:** 10-15 mcg/kg/d. **Adults: Pituitary TSH Suppression: Thyroid Cancer, Well-Differentiated: Adjunct:** TSH suppression to <0.1 mU/L usually requires >2 mcg/kg/d. **High-Risk Tumors:** Target TSH supression may be <0.01 mU/L. **Benign Nodules/Nontoxic Multinodular Goiter:** Target TSH suppression of 0.1-1 mU/L.	◙A ❋>
Liothyronine, T3 (Cytomel)	**Tab:** 0.005 mg, 0.025 mg, 0.05 mg	**Adults: Initial:** 25 mcg qd. **Titrate:** Increase up to 25 mcg q1-2wks. **Maint:** 25-75 mcg qd. **Peds: Initial:** 5 mcg qd. **Titrate:** Increase by 5 mcg qd q3-4d until desired response. **Maint: >3 yo:** 25-75 mcg/d. **1-3 yo:** 50 mcg qd. **<1 yo:** 20 mcg qd.	◙A ❋>

4 Contraindicated in pregnancy. Increased risk of endometrial carcinoma.

10 Attempt to taper or d/c at 3-6 mth intervals.

28 Not for prevention of CV disease or dementia. The WHI reported increased risks of MI, stroke, invasive breast cancer, pulmonary emboli, DVT, and probable dementia in postmenopausal women. Prescribe at lowest effective doses for shortest duration.

NAME	FORM/STRENGTH	DOSAGE	COMMENTS
Liotrix (Thyrolar)	**Tab:** (1/4) 3.1-12.5 mcg, (1/2) 6.25-25 mcg, (1) 12.5-50 mcg, (2) 25-100 mcg, (3) 37.5-150 mcg	**Adults: Initial:** 6.25-25 mcg qd. **Titrate:** Increase by 3.1-12.5 mcg q2-3wks. **Usual:** 12.5-50 mcg to 25-100 mcg/d. **Peds: >12 yo:** 18.75-75 mcg qd. **6-12 yo:** 12.5-50 mcg to 18.75-75 mcg qd. **1-5 yo:** 9.35-37.5 mcg to 12.5-50 mcg qd. **6-12 mths:** 6.25-25 mcg to 9.35-37.5 mcg qd. **0-6 mths:** 3.1-12.5 mcg to 6.25-25 mcg qd.	◙A ❋>
Thyroid, Desiccated (Armour Thyroid)	**Tab:** 15 mg, 30 mg, 60 mg, 90 mg, 120 mg, 180 mg, 240 mg, 300 mg	**Adults: Initial:** 30 mg qd. **Titrate:** Increase by 15 mg q2-3wks. **Maint:** 60-120 mg/d. **Peds: >12 yo:** 1.2-1.8 mg/kg/d. **6-12 yo:** 2.4-3 mg/kg/d. **1-5 yo:** 3-3.6 mg/kg/d. **6-12 mths:** 3.6-4.8 mg/kg/d. **0-6 mths:** 4.8-6 mg/kg/d.	◙A ❋>
Thyrotropin alfa (Thyrogen)	**Inj:** 1.1 mg	**Thyroglobulin Testing: Adults & Peds: ≥16 yo:** 0.9 mg IM q24h x 2 doses or q72h x 3 doses into buttock.	◙C ❋>

Miscellaneous

BONE RESORPTION INHIBITOR

NAME	FORM/STRENGTH	DOSAGE	COMMENTS
Pamidronate Disodium (Aredia)	**Inj:** 30 mg, 90 mg	**Adults: Moderate Hypercalcemia:** 60-90 mg IV single dose over 4-24h. **Severe Hypercalcemia:** 90 mg IV single dose over 24h. **Retreatment:** May repeat after 7d. **Paget's Disease:** 30 mg IV over 4h x 3d. **Osteolytic Bone Lesions of Multiple Myeloma:** 90 mg IV over 4h once mthly. **Osteolytic Bone Metastases of Breast Cancer:** 90 mg IV over 2h q3-4wks. **Max:** 90 mg/single dose for all indications.	◙D ❋> **R**

Zoledronic Acid (Zometa)	**Inj:** 4 mg/5 ml	**Adults: Hypercalcemia of Malignancy: Max:** 4 mg IV over no less than 15 min. **Retreatment (if necessary):** Wait at least 7d from initial dose. **Multiple Myeloma/Bone Metastases:** 4 mg IV over 15 min q 3-4wks. Take w/ oral calcium 500 mg/d & vitamin D 400 IU/d.	◉D ✽v **R**

CALCIUM REGULATOR

Gallium Nitrate (Ganite)	**Inj:** 500 mg	**Adults: Cancer-related Hypercalcemia:** 200 mg/m² IV daily x 5d. **Mild hypercalcemia:** 100 mg/m²/d x 5d. If calcium levels are within normal range in <5d, may d/c treatment. Daily infusion must be given over 24 h.	◉C ✽v **R** Avoid concurrent use with nephrotoxic drugs.

URIC ACID AGENTS

Allopurinol Sodium (Aloprim)	**Inj:** 500 mg	**Elevated Serum/Urinary Uric Acid Levels: Adults: Initial:** 200-400 mg/m²/d IV as qd or in divided doses every 6, 8, or 12h. **Max:** 600 mg/d. **Peds: Initial:** 200 mg/m²/d IV as qd or in divided doses every 6, 8, or 12h.	◉C ✽> **R**
Rasburicase (Elitek)	**Inj:** 1.5 mg	**Peds: 1 mth-17 yo:** 0.15 or 0.2 mg/kg IV as single daily dose x 5d. Administer over 30 min, not as bolus infusion. Dosing >5d or >1 course not recommended. Initiate chemo 4-24h after 1st dose.	◉C ✽v [39]

[39] May cause severe hypersensitivity reactions including anaphylaxis. May cause severe hemolysis w/ G6PD deficiency. Use associated w/ methemoglobinemia. May interfere w/ uric acid measurements.

GASTROINTESTINAL AGENTS

Antidiarrheal Agents

NAME	FORM/STRENGTH	DOSAGE	COMMENTS
Atropine Sulfate/ Diphenoxylate HCl CV (Lomotil)	**Liq:** 0.025-2.5 mg/5 ml; **Tab:** 0.025-2.5 mg	**Adults: Initial:** 2 tabs or 10 ml qid. **Maint:** 2 tabs or 10 ml tid. **Max:** 20 mg diphenoxylate/d. **13-16 yo: Initial:** 2 tabs or 10 ml qd. **2-12 yo: Initial:** 0.3-0.4 mg/kg/d given qid. **Maint:** 1/4 of initial daily dose.	◙C ✽>
Attapulgite (Kaopectate)	**Liq:** 750 mg/15 ml; **Tab:** 750 mg	**Adults & Peds: ≥12 yo:** 1500 mg after loose BM. **6-12 yo:** 750 mg after loose BM. **Max:** 6 doses/d.	◙N ✽>
Bismuth Subsalicylate (Pepto-Bismol)	**Chewtab:** 262 mg; **Susp:** 262 mg/15 ml, 525 mg/15 ml; **Tab:** 262 mg	**Adults:** 2 tabs or 30 ml q0.5-1h. **Peds: 9-12 yo:** 1 tab q0.5-1h or 15 ml q1h. **6-9 yo:** 2/3 tab q0.5-1h or 10 ml q1h. **3-6 yo:** 1/3 tab q0.5-1h or 5 ml q1h. **Max:** 8 doses/d (reg str.), 4 doses/d (max str.).	◙N ✽>
Loperamide (Imodium A-D)	**Liq:** 1 mg/5 ml; **Tab:** 2 mg	**Adults & Peds: ≥12 yo:** 4 mg after 1st loose BM, then 2 mg after loose BM. **Max:** 8 mg/d. **9-11 yo (60-95 lbs):** 2 mg after 1st loose BM, then 1 mg after loose BM. **Max:** 6 mg/d. **6-8 yo (48-59 lbs):** 2 mg after 1st loose BM, then 1 mg after loose BM. **Max:** 4 mg/d. **2-5 yo (24-47 lbs):** 1 mg after 1st loose BM, then 1 mg after loose BM. **Max:** 3 mg/d.	◙N ✽>
Nitazoxanide (Alinia)	**Susp:** 100 mg/5 ml; **Tab:** 500 mg	***G. lamblia* Diarhhea: Adults & Peds: ≥12 yo:** 500 mg q12h x 3d. Take w/ food. ***C. parvum/G. lamblia* Diarrhea: Peds: 1-3 yrs:** 100 mg (5 ml) q12h x 3d. **4-11 yrs:** 200 mg (10 ml) q12h x 3d.	◙B ✽>

Antiemetics

5-HT$_3$ ANTAGONISTS

Dolasetron Mesylate (Anzemet)	**Inj:** 20 mg/ml; **Tab:** 50 mg, 100 mg	**Prevent Chemo N/V: Adults:** 1.8 mg/kg IV or 100 mg IV/PO. **Peds: 2-16 yo:** 1.8 mg/kg IV/PO, up to 100 mg IV/PO. Give IV 30 min before or PO within 1h before chemo. **Prevent Post-Op N/V: Adults:** 12.5 mg IV or 100 mg PO. **Peds: 2-16 yo:** 0.35 mg/kg IV, up to 12.5 mg IV; or 1.2 mg/kg PO, up to 100 mg PO. Give PO within 2h pre-op, IV 15 min before anesthesia cessation or at start of n/v. **Treat Post-op N/V: Adults:** 12.5 mg IV. **Peds: 2-16 yo:** 0.35 mg/kg IV up to 12.5 mg IV.	B >
Granisetron HCl (Kytril)	**Inj:** 1 mg/ml; **Sol:** 2 mg/10 ml; **Tab:** 1 mg	**Prevent Chemo N/V: Adults & Peds: 2-16 yo: IV:** 10 mcg/kg within 30 min before chemo. **Adults: PO:** 2 mg qd up to 1h before chemo or 1 mg bid (up to 1h before chemo & 12h later). **Prevent Radiation N/V: Adults: PO:** 2 mg qd within 1h of radiation. **Prevent Post-Op N/V: Adults: IV:** 1 mg over 30 sec before anesthesia induction or immediately before anesthesia reversal. **Treat Post-Op N/V: Adults: IV:** 1 mg over 30 sec.	B >

NAME	FORM/STRENGTH	DOSAGE	COMMENTS
Ondansetron HCl (Zofran)	**Inj:** 2 mg/ml, 32 mg/50 ml; **Sol:** 4 mg/5 ml; **Tab:** 4 mg, 8 mg, 24 mg; **Tab,Dissolve:** 4 mg, 8 mg	**Prevent Chemo-Induced N/V: Adults (>18 yo):** Single 32 mg dose IV over 15 min, 30 min before chemo or three 0.15 mg/kg doses IV over15 min, 1st dose 30 min before chemo w/ subsequent doses given 4 & 8h after 1st dose. **Peds: 6 mths-18 yo:** Three 0.15 mg/kg doses IV over 15 min, 1st dose 30 min before chemo with subsequent doses given 4 & 8h after 1st dose. **Prevent Highly Emetogenic Chemo N/V: Adults:** 24 mg tab PO 30 min before chemo. **Prevent Moderately Emetogenic Chemo N/V: Adults & Peds: ≥12 yo:** 8 mg PO 30 min before chemo, then 8h after 1st dose, then 8 mg bid x 1-2d. **4-11 yo:** 4 mg PO 30 min before chemo, then 4 & 8h after1st dose, then 4 mg tid x 1-2d. **Prevent Post-Op N/V: Adults:** 16 mg PO 1h before anesthesia. **Peds: >12 yo:** 4 mg IV/IM immediately before anesthesia or post-op. **1mth-12 yo: ≤40 kg:** 0.1 mg/kg IV single dose; **>40 kg:** 4 mg IV single dose. **Prevent Radiation N/V: Adults: Usual:** 8 mg PO tid. **Total Body Irradiation:** 8 mg PO 1-2h before therapy daily. **Single High-Dose Therapy To Abdomen:** 8 mg PO 1-2h before therapy then q8h after 1st dose x 1-2d after complete therapy. **Daily Fractionated Therapy To Abdomen:** 8 mg PO 1-2h before therapy then q8h after 1st dose. **Severe Hepatic Dysfunction: Max:** 8 mg/d IV single dose 30 min before chemo or 8 mg/d PO.	●B ❉> **H**

Palonosetron HCl (Aloxi)	**Inj:** 0.25 mg/5 ml	**Adults:** 0.25 mg IV single dose 30 min before chemo. Repeated dosing within a 7d interval is not recommended.	⦿B ✽v

ANTICHOLINERGICS

Scopolamine (Transderm Scop)	**Patch:** 0.33 mg/24h	**Adults: Motion Sickness:** 1 patch behind ear 4h prior to event. Replace after 3d. **Prevent Post-Op N/V:** 1 patch x 24h post-op.	⦿C ✽>
Trimethobenzamide (Tigan)	**Cap:** 300 mg; **Inj:** 100 mg/ml; **Sup:** 100 mg, 200 mg	**Nausea in Gastroenteritis/Post-op N/V: Adults: Cap:** 300 mg tid-qid. **Inj:** 200 mg IM tid-qid. **Sup:** 200 mg tid-qid. **Peds: Sup: 30-90 lbs:** 100-200 mg tid-qid. **<30 lbs:** 100 mg tid-qid.	⦿N ✽>

ANTIHISTAMINES

Dimenhydrinate (Dramamine)	**Chewtab:** 50 mg; **Tab:** 50 mg	**Motion Sickness: Adults:** 1-2 tabs q4-6h. **Max:** 400 mg/24h. **6-12 yo:** 1/2-1 tab q6-8h. **Max:** 150 mg/24h. **2-6 yo:** 1/4-1/2 tab q6-8h. **Max:** 75 mg/24h.	⦿N ✽>
Hydroxyzine HCl	**Inj:** 25 mg/ml, 50 mg/ml	**N/V: Adults:** 25-100 mg IM. **Peds:** 0.5 mg/lb IM.	⦿N ✽v CI in early pregnancy.
Meclizine HCl (Antivert)	**Tab:** 12.5 mg, 25 mg, 50 mg	**Adults & Peds: ≥12 yo: Vertigo: Usual:** 25-100 mg/d in divided doses. **Motion Sickness:** 25-50 mg 1h before trip/departure; repeat q24h prn.	⦿B ✽>

NAME	FORM/STRENGTH	DOSAGE	COMMENTS
Prochlorperazine (Compazine)	**Cap,ER:** 10 mg, 15 mg; **Inj:** 5 mg/ml; **Sup:** 2.5 mg, 5 mg, 25 mg; **Syr:** 5 mg/5 ml; **Tab:** 5 mg, 10 mg	**Severe N/V: Adults: PO:** 5-10 mg tab tid-qid; 10 mg cap q12h; 15 mg cap on arising. **PR:** 25 mg sup bid. **IM:** 5-10 mg 3-4h prn. **IV:** 2.5-10 mg (slow push). **Max:** 10 mg/IV single dose; 40 mg/d PO/IM/IV. **Peds: >2 yo & >20lbs: PO/PR: 20-29 lbs:** 2.5 mg qd-bid. **Max:** 7.5 mg/d. **30-39 lbs:** 2.5 mg bid-tid. **Max:** 10 mg/d. **40-85 lbs:** 2.5 mg tid or 5 mg bid. **Max:** 15 mg/d. **IM:** 0.06 mg/lb. **N/V w/ Surgery: Adults: IM/IV:** 5-10 mg IM 1-2h or 5-10 mg IV 15-30 min before anesthesia, or during or after surgery; repeat once if needed.	◙N ❊>
Promethazine (Phenergan)	(Generic) **Inj:** 25 mg/ml, 50 mg/ml; **Sup:** 12.5 mg, 25 mg, 50 mg; **Syr:** 6.25 mg/5 ml; **Tab:** 12.5 mg, 25 mg, 50 mg; (Phenergan) **Inj:** 25 mg/ml, 50 mg/ml; **Sup:** 12.5 mg, 25 mg, 50 mg; **Tab:** 12.5 mg, 25 mg, 50 mg	**Prevent N/V & Post-Op N/V: Adults:** 12.5-25 mg IM/IV q4h; 25 mg PO/PR initially, then 12.5-25 mg q4-6h prn. **Peds: ≥2 yo:** 0.5 mg/lb PO/PR/IM/IV q4-6h prn.	◙C ❊v

DOPAMINE ANTAGONIST/PROKINETIC

NAME	FORM/STRENGTH	DOSAGE	COMMENTS
Metoclopramide (Reglan)	(Generic) **Inj:** 5 mg/ml; **Syr:** 5 mg/5 ml; **Tab:** 5 mg, 10 mg; (Reglan) **Inj:** 5 mg/ml; **Tab:** 5 mg, 10 mg	**Adults: Prevent Chemo N/V:** 1-2 mg/kg 30 min before chemo, then q2h x 2 doses, then q3h x 3 doses. **Prevent Post-Op N/V:** 10-20 mg IM near end of surgery.	◙B ❊> **R**

SUBSTANCE P/NEUROKININ 1 RECEPTOR ANTAGONIST

Aprepitant (Emend)	**Tab:** 80 mg, 125 mg	**Adults: Day 1:** 125 mg 1h prior to chemotherapy. **Days 2 & 3:** 80 mg qam. Regimen should include a corticosteroid & a 5-HT_3 antagonist. **Concomitant Corticosteroid:** Reduce dexamethasone PO or methylprednisolone PO by 50% & methylprednisolone IV by 25%.	B >

MISCELLANEOUS

Dronabinol CIII (Marinol)	**Cap:** 2.5 mg, 5 mg, 10 mg	**Adults & Peds: Prevent Chemo N/V:** 5 mg/m² 1-3h before chemo, then 2-4h after chemo, up to 4-6 doses/d. **Titrate:** May increase by 2.5 mg/m² increments. **Max:** 15 mg/m²/dose.	C v
Droperidol (Inapsine)	**Inj:** 2.5 mg/ml	**Premed for Surgery/Diagnostic Procedures: Adults: Initial (Max):** 2.5 mg IM/IV. May give additional 1.25 mg cautiously for desired effect. **Peds: 2-12 yo: Initial (Max):** 0.1 mg/kg IM/IV. May give additional dose cautiously.	C > QT prolongation. Torsade de pointes. Arrhythmias.
Nabilone CII (Cesamet)	**Cap:** 1 mg	**Adults: Initial:** 1 or 2 mg bid; given 1-3 hrs before chemotherapy. A dose of 1 or 2 mg the night before may be useful. **Max:** 6 mg/d given in divided doses tid.	C v

Antispasmodics

Atropine Sulfate/ Hyoscyamine Sulfate/ Phenobarbital/Scopolamine (Donnatal)	**Tab/Eli (per 5 ml):** 0.0194-0.1037-16.2-0.0065 mg	**Adults:** 1-2 tabs or 5-10 ml tid-qid. **Peds: 100 lbs:** 5 ml q4h or 7.5 ml q6h. **75 lbs:** 3.75 ml q4h or 5 ml q6h. **50 lbs:** 2.5 ml q4h or 3.75 ml q6h. **30 lbs:** 1.5 ml q4h or 2 ml q6h. **20 lbs:** 1 ml q4h or 1.5 ml q6h. **10 lbs:** 0.5 ml q4h or 0.75 ml q6h.	C > **H**

NAME	FORM/STRENGTH	DOSAGE	COMMENTS
Atropine Sulfate/ Hyoscyamine Sulfate/ Phenobarbital/Scopolamine (Donnatal Extentabs)	**Tab:** 0.0582-0.3111-48.6-0.0195 mg	**Adults:** 1 tab q8-12h.	◙C ❁> H
Chlordiazepoxide HCl/Clidinium (Librax)	**Cap:** 5-2.5 mg	**Adults: Usual:** 1-2 caps tid-qid ac & qhs.	◙N ❁>
Dicyclomine HCl (Bentyl)	**Cap:** 10 mg; **Inj:** 10 mg/ml; **Syr:** 10 mg/ 5 ml; **Tab:** 20 mg	**Adults: Initial: PO:** 20 mg qid. **Maint:** 40 mg qid if tolerated. **IM:** 20 mg qid x 1-2d, followed by PO dose.	◙B ❁v
Hyoscyamine Sulfate (Cystospaz)	**Tab:** 0.15 mg	**Adults:** 0.15-0.3 mg qid prn.	◙C ❁>
Hyoscyamine Sulfate (Levbid, Levsin, Levsinex, NuLev)	(Levbid) **Tab,ER:** 0.375 mg. (Levsin) **Drops:** 0.125 mg/ml; **Eli:** 0.125 mg/5 ml; **Inj:** 0.5 mg/ml; **Tab:** 0.125 mg; **Tab,SL:** 0.125 mg. (Levsinex) **Cap,ER:** 0.375 mg. (NuLev) **Tab,Dissolve (ODT):** 0.125 mg.	**Adults & Peds: ≥12 yo: Drops/Eli/ODT/Tab/Tab,SL:** 0.125-0.25 mg q4h or prn. **Max:** 1.5 mg/24h. **Cap, Tab,ER:** 0.375-0.75 mg q12h; or 1 cap q8h. **Max:** 1.5 mg/24h. **2 to <12 yo: ODT/Tab/Tab,SL:** 0.0625-0.125 mg q4h or prn. **Max:** 0.75 mg/24h. **Eli:** Give q4h or prn. **10 kg:** 1.25 ml. **20 kg:** 2.5 ml. **40 kg:** 3.75 ml. **50 kg:** 5 ml. **Max:** 30 ml/24h. **Drops:** 0.25-1 ml q4h or prn. **Max:** 6 ml/24h. **<2 yo: Drops:** Give q4h or prn. **3.4 kg:** 4 gtts. **Max:** 24 gtts/24h. **5 kg:** 5 gtts. **Max:** 30 gtts/24h. **7 kg:** 6 gtts. **Max:** 36 gtts/24h. **10 kg:** 8 gtts. **Max:** 48 gtts/24h.	◙C ❁>
Propantheline Bromide	**Tab:** 15 mg	**Adults:** 15 mg (tid 30 min ac), & 30 mg qhs (total 75 mg/d).	◙C ❁>

Helicobacter pylori TREATMENT REGIMENS*

MEDICATION/DOSE	FREQUENCY
PPI**+ 1 gm amoxicillin bid + 500 mg clarithromycin bid	10-14d (7d with rabeprazole, pantoprazole, esomeprazole)
PPI+ 500 mg metronidazole + 500 mg clarithromycin	bid x 2 wks
RBC (400 mg ranitidine bismuth citrate) + 500 mg clarithromycin +1 gm amoxicillin OR 500 mg metronidazole OR 500 mg tetracycline	bid x 2 wks
BSS*** qid + 500 mg metronidazole tid + 500 mg tetracycline qid + PPI qd	as indicated x 2 wks
BSS + 250 mg metronidazole qid + 500 mg tetracycline qid + H_2 receptor antagonist qd	as indicated x 2 wks, & continue H_2R antagonist x 2 wks

*Suggested regimens for the treatment of *H. pylori* infection. Not all of the above regimens are FDA-approved. *Am J Gastroenterol* 1998; 93: 2330-2338.

**PPI= esomeprazole 40 mg qd, lansoprazole 30 mg bid, omeprazole 20 mg bid, rabeprazole 20 mg bid, or pantoprazole 40 mg bid

***BSS=bismuth subsalicylate 525 mg

NAME	FORM/STRENGTH	DOSAGE	COMMENTS
DUODENAL ULCER ADHERENT COMPLEX			
Sucralfate (Carafate)	**Susp:** 1 gm/10 ml; **Tab:** 1 gm	**Active Ulcer: Adults: Susp/Tab:** 1 gm qid x 4-8 wks. **Maint: Tab:** 1 gm bid.	■B ❁>

NAME	FORM/STRENGTH	DOSAGE	COMMENTS
H_2 ANTAGONISTS			
Cimetidine (Tagamet)	(Generic) **Cap:** 150 mg, 300 mg; **Inj:** 150 mg/ml, 300 mg/50 ml; **Sol:** 300 mg/5 ml; **Tab:** 200 mg, 300 mg, 400 mg, 800 mg; (Tagamet) **Tab:** 200 mg, 300 mg, 400 mg	**Adults & Peds: ≥16 yo: PO: Active DU:** 800 mg qhs or 300 mg qid or 400 mg bid x 4-8 wks. **Maint:** 400 mg qhs. **Active Benign GU:** 800 mg qhs or 300 mg qid x 6 wks. **IM/IV:** 300 mg q6-8h. **Max:** 2400 mg/d.	B v **R**
Famotidine (Pepcid, Pepcid RPD)	**Inj:** 0.4 mg/ml, 10 mg/ml; **Susp:** 40 mg/5 ml; **Tab:** 20 mg, 40 mg; **Tab,Dissolve:** 20 mg, 40 mg	**Adults: DU: PO:** 20 mg bid or 40 mg qhs x 4-8 wks. **Maint:** 20 mg qhs. **IV:** 20 mg q12h. **GU: PO:** 20 mg bid up to 6 wks. **Peds 1-16 yo: DU/GU:** 0.25 mg/kg IV/PO q12h or 0.5 mg/kg/d PO qhs. **Max:** 40 mg/d.	B v **R**
Nizatidine (Axid, Axid Oral Solution)	**Cap:** 150 mg, 300 mg; **Sol:** 15 mg/ml	**Adults:** 150 mg bid or 300 mg qhs up to 8 wks. **Maint:** 150 mg qhs up to 1 yr.	B v **R**
Ranitidine HCl (Zantac)	**Inj:** 1 mg/ml, 25 mg/ml; **Syr:** 15 mg/ml; **Tab:** 75mg, 150 mg, 300 mg; **Tab,Eff:** 25 mg, 150 mg	**Adults: GU/DU: PO:** 150 mg bid, or (DU) 300 mg after evening meal or qhs. **Maint:** 150 mg qhs. **IV/IM:** 50 mg q6-8h. **Continuous IV:** 6.25 mg/h. **Max:** 400 mg/d. **1 mth-16 yo: GU/DU: PO:** 2-4 mg/kg bid. **Max:** 300 mg/d. **Maint:** 2-4 mg/kg qd. **Max:** 150 mg/d. **DU: IV:** 2-4 mg/kg/d given q6-8h. **Max:** 50 mg q6-8h.	B > **R**
PROSTAGLANDIN E_1 ANALOG			
Misoprostol (Cytotec)	**Tab:** 100 mcg, 200 mcg	**NSAID Ulcer Prevention: Adults:** 200 mcg qid w/ food. May use 100 mcg dose if 200 mcg not tolerated.	X v Abortifacient.

Esomeprazole Magnesium (Nexium)	**Cap,Delay:** 20 mg, 40 mg	**Risk Reduction of NSAID-Associated Gastric Ulcer: Adults:** 20-40 mg qd x up to 6 mths.	B v **H**
Lansoprazole (Prevacid)	**Cap,Delay:** 15 mg, 30 mg; **Pkt,Delay:** 15 mg, 30 mg (granules/pkt); **Tab,Delay,Dissolve (SoluTab):** 15 mg, 30 mg	**Adults: DU:** 15 mg qd x 4 wks. **Maint:** 15 mg qd. **Benign GU:** 30 mg qd up to 8 wks. **NSAID-Associated GU: Healing:** 30 mg qd x 8 wks. **Risk Reduction:** 15 mg qd up to 12 wks.	B v **H**
Lansoprazole-Naproxen (Prevacid NapraPAC)	**Cap,Delay**: 15-500 mg	**NSAID-Associated GU: Risk Reduction: Adults:** 1 tab Naproxen + 1 cap Lansoprazole qam, before eating + 1 tab Naproxen qpm. **Max:** 1000 mg Naproxen/day. Take naproxen w/ full glass of water. Swallow lansoprazole whole.	B v **H R**
Omeprazole (Prilosec)	**Cap,Delay:** 10 mg, 20 mg, 40 mg	**Adults: DU:** 20 mg qd x 4-8 wks. **GU:** 40 mg qd x 4-8 wks.	C v
Omeprazole/Sodium Bicarbonate (Zegerid)	**Cap:** 20-1100 mg, 40-1100 mg; **Pow:** 20-1680 mg/pkt, 40-1680 mg/pkt	**Adults: Cap/Pow: DU:** 20 mg qd x 4-8 wks. **GU:** 40 mg qd x 4-8 wks. **Pow (40-1680 mg): Risk Reduction of Upper GI Bleeding in Critically Ill Patients: Initial:** 40 mg, followed by 40 mg 6-8 h later. **Maint:** 40 mg qd x 14d.	C v
Rabeprazole Sodium (Aciphex)	**Tab,Delay:** 20 mg	**DU Treatment: Adults:** 20 mg qd up to 4 wks.	B v

NAME	FORM/STRENGTH	DOSAGE	COMMENTS

GERD

DOPAMINE ANTAGONIST/PROKINETIC

NAME	FORM/STRENGTH	DOSAGE	COMMENTS
Metoclopramide (Reglan)	(Generic) **Syr:** 5 mg/5 ml; **Tab:** 5 mg, 10 mg; (Reglan) **Tab:** 5 mg, 10 mg	**Adults:** 10-15 mg qid 30 min ac & qhs. **Max:** 12 wks of therapy. **Intermittent Symptoms:** Up to 20 mg single dose prior to provoking situation.	◉B ❋> **R**

H_2 ANTAGONISTS

NAME	FORM/STRENGTH	DOSAGE	COMMENTS
Cimetidine (Tagamet)	(Generic) **Sol:** 300 mg/5 ml; **Tab:** 200 mg, 300 mg, 400 mg, 800 mg; (Tagamet) **Tab:** 200 mg, 300 mg, 400 mg	**Adults & Peds: ≥16 yo: PO:** 400 mg qid or 800 mg bid x 12 wks.	◉B ❋v **R**
Famotidine (Pepcid)	**Inj:** 0.4 mg/ml, 10 mg/ml; **Susp:** 40 mg/5 ml; **Tab:** 20 mg, 40 mg; **Tab,Dissolve:** 20 mg, 40 mg.	**Adults: PO:** 20 mg bid up to 6 wks. **Peds: 1-16 yo: IV/PO:** 0.25 mg/kg IV q12h (up to 40 mg/d) or 0.5 mg/kg PO bid (up to 40 mg bid). **3 mths-1 yo: PO:** 0.5 mg/kg bid x up to 8 wks. **<3 mths: PO:** 0.5 mg/kg qd x up to 8 wks. **Esophagitis: Adults: PO:** 20-40 mg bid x up to 12 wks.	◉B ❋v **R**
Nizatidine (Axid, Axid Oral Solution)	**Cap:** 150 mg, 300 mg; **Sol:** 15 mg/ml	**Adults:** 150 mg bid up to 12 wks. **Peds: ≥12 yo: Erosive Esophagitis/GERD: Sol:** 150 mg bid up to 8 wks. **Max:** 300 mg/d.	◉B ❋v **R**

Ranitidine HCl (Zantac)	**Inj:** 1 mg/ml, 25 mg/ml; **Syr:** 15 mg/ml; **Tab:** 75 mg, 150 mg, 300 mg; **Tab,Eff:** 25 mg, 150 mg	**Adults: PO: Symptomatic:** 150 mg bid. **Erosive Esophagitis:** 150 mg qid. **Maint:** 150 mg bid. **IV/IM:** 50 mg q6-8h. **Continuous IV:** 6.25 mg/h. **Max:** 400 mg/d. **1 mth-16 yo: Symptomatic/ Erosive Esophagitis:** 2.5-5 mg/kg PO bid.	B > R

PROTON PUMP INHIBITORS AND COMBINATIONS

Esomeprazole (Nexium, Nexium I.V.)	**Cap,Delay:** (Mg salt) 20 mg, 40 mg; **Inj:** (Na salt) 20 mg, 40 mg	**Adults: PO: Symptomatic GERD:** 20 mg qd x 4 wks; additional 4 wks w/ continued symptoms. **Erosive Esophagitis: Healing:** 20-40 mg qd x 4-8 wks; additional 4-8 wks if not healed. **Maint:** 20 mg qd x up to 6 mths. **IV:** 20-40 mg qd x up to 10 days. Change to PO ASAP. **Peds: 12-17 yo: PO: Symptomatic GERD:** 20-40 mg qd x up to 8 wks.	B v H
Lansoprazole (Prevacid, Prevacid I.V.)	**Cap,Delay:** 15 mg, 30 mg; **Inj:** 30 mg; **Pkt,Delay:** 15 mg, 30 mg (granules/pkt); **Tab,Delay, Dissolve (SoluTab):** 15 mg, 30 mg.	**Adults: PO: Symptomatic GERD:** 15 mg qd x up to 8 wks. **Erosive Esophagitis:** 30 mg qd x up to 8 wks. May repeat x 8 wks, if needed. If recurrence, may consider additional 8 wks. **Maint:** 15 mg qd. **IV: Erosive Esophagitis:** 30 mg/d x up to 7d. Switch to PO when possible. **Peds: PO: 12-17 yo: Symptomatic GERD/Nonerosive:** 15 mg qd x up to 8 wks. **Symptomatic GERD/Erosive Esophagitis:** 30 mg qd x up to 8 wks. **1-11 yo: Symptomatic GERD/Erosive Esophagitis: ≤30 kg:** 15 mg qd x up to 12 wks. **>30 kg:** 30 mg qd x up to 12 wks. **Titrate:** May increase up to 30 mg bid after 2 wks if symptomatic.	B v H

NAME	FORM/STRENGTH	DOSAGE	COMMENTS
Omeprazole (Prilosec)	**Cap,Delay:** 10 mg, 20 mg, 40 mg	**Adults: Symptomatic GERD:** 20 mg qd x up to 4 wks. **Erosive Esophagitis:** 20 mg qd x 4-8 wks. **Maint:** 20 mg qd. **Peds: ≥2 yo: >20 kg: GERD/ Erosive Esophagitis:** 20 mg qd. **<20 kg:** 10 mg qd.	●C ❉v
Omeprazole/Sodium Bicarbonate (Zegerid)	**Cap:** 20-1100 mg, 40-1100 mg; **Pow:** 20-1680 mg/pkt, 40-1680 mg/pkt	**Adults: Cap/Pow: Symptomatic GERD:** 20 mg qd x up to 4 wks. **Erosive Esophagitis:** 20 mg qd x 4-8 wks. **Maint:** 20 mg qd.	●C ❉v
Pantoprazole Sodium (Protonix, Protonix I.V.)	**Inj:** 40 mg; **Tab,Delay:** 20 mg, 40 mg	**Adults: Erosive Esophagitis: PO:** 40 mg qd x up to 8 wks. May repeat course. **Maint:** 40 mg qd. **GERD: IV:** 40 mg qd x 7-10d.	●B ❉v
Rabeprazole Sodium (Aciphex)	**Tab,Delay:** 20 mg	**Adults: Erosive/Ulcerative GERD: Healing:** 20 mg qd x 4-8 wks. May repeat x 8 wks if needed. **Maint:** 20 mg qd. **Symptomatic GERD:** 20 mg qd x 4 wks. May repeat x 4 wks if needed.	●B ❉v

Laxatives

BOWEL EVACUANTS

Bisacodyl/Polyethylene Glycol with Electrolytes (Halflytely Bowel Prep Kit)	**Kit (Tab,Delay-Sol):** 5 mg-2000 ml	**Adults:** Swallow all 4 bisacodyl tabs at noon (do not chew or crush). After first bowel movement (or max of 6 h) begin drinking solution, 240 ml every 10 min (approx. 8 glasses). Drink ALL solution.	●C ❉>
Polyethylene Glycol with Electrolytes (Colyte)	**Pow for Sol:** 3754 ml, 4000 ml	**Adults: GI Exam Prep: PO** 240 ml q10min until fecal discharge is clear. **NG Tube:** 20-30 ml/min (1.2-1.8 L/h).	●C ❉>

BULK-FORMING AGENTS

Calcium Polycarbophil (FiberCon)	**Tab:** 625 mg	**Adults & Peds: ≥12 yo:** 2 tabs qd. **Max:** 2 tabs qid. **6-12 yo:** 1 tab qd. **Max:** 1 tab qid.	N ❃>
Methylcellulose (Citrucel)	**Pow:** 2 gm/heaping tbs; **Tab:** 500 mg	**Adults & Peds: ≥12 yo:** 1 heaping tbs up to tid, or 2 tabs up to 6x/d. **6-12 yo:** 1/2 tbs qd or 1 tab up to 6x/d. Dissolve pow in 8 oz of cold water & follow pow/tabs w/ additional glass of water.	N ❃>
Psyllium (Metamucil)	**Pow:** 3.4 gm psyllium husk/dose	**Adults & Peds: ≥12 yo:** 1 tsp, 1 tbs, or 1 pkt (depending on product). **6-12 yo:** 1/2 adult dose. May take qd-tid. Mix w/ 8 oz of liquid.	N ❃>

COLONIC ACIDIFIER

Lactulose (Constulose, Enulose)	**Sol:** 10 gm/15 ml	**Adults:** 15-30 ml qd. **Max:** 60 ml/d.	B ❃>

OSMOTIC AGENT

Polyethylene Glycol (MiraLax)	**Pow:** 17 gm/tbs	**Adults:** Dissolve 17 gm in 8 oz of water, juice, soda, coffee, or tea & drink qd up to 2 wks.	C ❃>

SALINE LAXATIVES

Magnesium Citrate (Citrate of Magnesia)	**Liq:** 10 oz bottle	**Adults:** Drink 240 ml prn. **Peds:** Drink 120 ml; repeat if necessary.	N ❃>
Magnesium Hydroxide (Milk of Magnesia)	**Liq:** 400 mg/5 ml	**Adults & Peds: ≥12 yo:** 30-60 ml qhs or qam. **6-11 yo:** 15-30 ml. **2-5 yo:** 5-15 ml.	N ❃>

NAME	FORM/STRENGTH	DOSAGE	COMMENTS
Sodium Biphosphate (Fleet Phospho-Soda, Fleet Enema)	**Sol:** (Phospho-Soda) 1.5 oz, 3 oz; **Enema:** (Adult) 4.5 oz, (Ped) 2.25 oz	**Phospho-Soda: Adults & Peds: ≥12 yo:** 20-45 ml. **10-11 yo:** 10-20 ml. **5-9 yo:** 5-10 ml. Dilute dose w/ 4 oz clear liquid, then follow w/ 8 oz clear liquid. Take on empty stomach in am at least 30 min before a meal or hs. **Enema: ≥12 yo:** (Adult Enema) 1 bottle PR. **5-11 yo:** (Ped Enema) 1 bottle PR. **2 to <5 yo:** (Ped Enema) Use 1/2 bottle PR.	◙N ❀>
STIMULANT/STOOL SOFTENERS			
Docusate Sodium/Sennosides (Peri-Colace)	**Tab:** 50-8.6 mg	**Adults:** 2-4 tabs daily. **Peds: ≥12 yo:** 2-4 tabs daily. **6-<12 yo:** 1-2 tabs daily. **2-<6 yo: Max:** 1 tab daily.	◙N ❀>
STIMULANTS			
Bisacodyl (Dulcolax)	**Sup:** 10 mg; **Tab,Delay:** 5 mg	**Adults & Peds: ≥12 yo:** 2-3 tabs or 1 sup qd as single dose. **6-12 yo:** 1 tab or 1/2 sup qd.	◙N ❀>
Cascara Sagrada	**Liq:** 120 ml; **Tab:** 325 mg	**Adults:** 1 tab or 5 ml qhs.	◙N ❀>
Castor Oil (Purge)	**Liq:** (Purge) 95%	**Adults: Usual:** 15-60 ml. **Peds 2-12 yo:** 5-15 ml.	◙N ❀>
Senna (Senokot, SenokotXTRA)	**Granules:** 15 mg/tsp; **Tab:** 8.6 mg, 17 mg	**Adults & Peds: ≥12 yo:** 2 tabs or 1 tsp qd. **Max**: 4 tabs or 2 tsp bid. **6-12 yo:** 1 tab or 1/2 tsp qd. **Max:** 2 tabs or 1 tsp bid. **2-6 yo:** 1/2 tab or 1/4 tsp qd. **Max:** 1 tab or 1/2 tsp bid. SenokotXTRA dose is 1/2 of reg str tab.	◙N ❀>
STOOL SOFTENERS			
Docusate Calcium (Surfak)	**Cap:** 240 mg	**Adults & Peds: ≥12 yo:** 240 mg qd until bowel movement.	◙N ❀>

Docusate Sodium (Colace)	**Cap:** 50 mg, 100 mg; **Liq:** 10 mg/ml; **Syr:** 20 mg/5 ml	**Adults & Peds: ≥12 yo:** 50-200 mg qd. **6-12 yo:** 40-120 mg/d liq. **3-6 yo:** 2 ml liq tid. Mix liq/ syr w/ 6-8 oz of milk, juice or formula. **Retention/Flushing Enemas:** Add 5-10 ml liq to enema fluid.	◙N ✽ >
Glycerin (Fleet Glycerin Suppositories, Fleet Babylax, Fleet Liquid Glycerin Suppository)	**Enema:** (Babylax) 2.3 gm; **Sup:** (Child) 1 gm, (Adult) 2 gm, (Adult Max Strength) 3 gm; **Liquid Glycerin Sup:** 5.6 gm	**Adults & Peds: ≥6 yo:** 1 Liq Sup (5.6 gm) or 1 sup (2 or 3 gm) PR. **2-6 yo:** 1 Babylax (2.3 gm) or 1 sup (1 gm) PR.	◙N ✽>

Ulcerative Colitis

ANTI-INFLAMMATORY/IMMUNOMODULATORY AGENTS

Sulfasalazine (Azulfidine, Azulfidine EN-tabs)	**Tab:** 500 mg; **Tab,Delay:** 500 mg	**Adults: Initial:** 1-4 gm/d in divided doses. **Maint:** 2 gm/d. **Peds: ≥2 yo:** 40-60 mg/kg/24h divided in 3-6 doses. **Maint:** 7.5 mg/kg qid.	◙B ✽>

SALICYLATES

Balsalazide Disodium (Colazal)	**Cap:** 750 mg	**Adults:** 2250 mg tid x 8 wks (up to 12 wks if needed).	◙B ✽>
Mesalamine (Asacol, Canasa, Pentasa, Rowasa)	**Cap,ER:** (Pentasa) 250 mg, 500mg; **Enema:** (Rowasa) 4 gm/60 ml; **Sup:** (Canasa) 500 mg, 1000 mg; **Tab,Delay:** (Asacol) 400 mg	**Adults: Asacol: Active Ulcerative Colitis:** 800 mg PO tid x 6 wks. **Remission Maint:** 1.6 gm/d in divided doses. **Canasa: Initial:** 500 mg PR bid or 1000 mg PR qhs. **Titrate:** May increase 500 mg bid to tid after 2 wks if inadequate response. Retain x 1-3h. **Rowasa:** 4 gm enema qhs x 3-6 wks; retain x 8h. **Pentasa:** 1 gm PO qid up to 8 wks.	◙B ✽>

NAME	FORM/STRENGTH	DOSAGE	COMMENTS
Olsalazine Sodium (Dipentum)	**Cap:** 250 mg	**Adults:** 500 mg bid.	◙C ❁>

Zollinger-Ellison Agents

H_2 ANTAGONISTS

NAME	FORM/STRENGTH	DOSAGE	COMMENTS
Cimetidine (Tagamet)	(Generic) **Inj:** 150 mg/ml, 300 mg/50 ml; **Sol:** 300 mg/5 ml; **Tab:** 200 mg, 300 mg, 400 mg, 800 mg; (Tagamet) **Tab:** 200 mg, 300 mg, 400 mg	**Adults: PO:** 300 mg qid. **Max:** 2400 mg/d. **IM/IV:** 300 mg q6-8h. **Max:** 2400 mg/d.	◙B ❁v **R**
Famotidine (Pepcid)	**Inj:** 0.4 mg/ml, 10 mg/ml; **Susp:** 40 mg/5 ml; **Tab:** 20 mg, 40 mg; **Tab,Dissolve:** 20 mg, 40 mg	**Adults: PO: Initial:** 20 mg q6h. **Max:** 160 mg q6h. **IV:** 20 mg q12h or greater if required.	◙B ❁v **R**
Ranitidine HCl (Zantac)	**Inj:** 1 mg/ml, 25 mg/ml; **Syr:** 15 mg/ml; **Tab:** 75 mg, 150 mg, 300 mg; **Tab,Eff:** 25 mg, 150 mg	**Adults: PO:** 150 mg bid. May give up to 6 gm/d w/ severe disease. **IM/IV (Intermittent):** 50 mg q6-8h. **IV (Continuous):** 1 mg/kg/h IV. **Titrate:** May increase after 4 h by 0.5 mg/kg/h increments. **Max:** 2.5 mg/kg/h or 220 mg/h.	◙B ❁> **R**

Lansoprazole (Prevacid)	**Cap,Delay:** 15 mg, 30 mg; **Pkt,Delay:** 15 mg,30 mg (granules/pkt); **Tab,Delay,Dissolve (SoluTab):** 15 mg, 30 mg.	**Adults:** 60 mg qd. **Max:** 90 mg bid. Divide dose if >120 mg/d.	B v **H**
Omeprazole (Prilosec)	**Cap,Delay:** 10 mg, 20 mg, 40 mg	**Adults:** 60 mg qd, then adjust as needed. Divide dose if >80 mg/d. Doses up to 120 mg tid have been given.	C v
Pantoprazole Sodium (Protonix, Protonix I.V.)	**Inj:** 40 mg; **Tab,Delay:** 20 mg, 40 mg	**Adults: PO:** 40 mg bid. **Max:** 240 mg/d. **IV:** 80 mg q12h, adjust based on acid output. **Max:** 240 mg/d.	B v

Miscellaneous

Alosetron HCl (Lotronex)	**Tab:** 0.5 mg, 1 mg	**Diarrhea-Predominant Irritable Bowel Syndrome (Women): Adults: Initial:** 1 mg qd x 4 wks. **Titrate:** May increase to 1 mg bid. D/C after 4 wks if symptoms uncontrolled on 1 mg bid.	B > [43]
Infliximab (Remicade)	**Inj:** 100 mg	**Adults: Crohn's Disease/Fistulizing Crohn's Disease/Ulcerative Colitis: Induction:** 5 mg/kg IV at 0, 2, & 6 wks. **Maint:** 5 mg/kg q8wks. **Peds: Crohn's Disease: Induction:** 5 mg/kg IV at 0, 2, & 6 wks. **Maint:** 5 mg/kg q8wks.	B v TB, fungal, & other opportunistic infections reported.
Lubiprostone (Amitiza)	**Cap:** 24 mcg	**Chronic Idiopathic Constipation: Adults:** 24 mcg bid w/ food.	C v

[43] Serious GI adverse events reported; D/C if constipation or symptoms of ischemic colitis develop.

NAME	FORM/STRENGTH	DOSAGE	COMMENTS
Tegaserod Maleate (Zelnorm)	**Tab:** 2 mg, 6 mg	**Irritable Bowel Syndrome w/ Constipation: Adults (Women):** 6 mg bid x 4-6 wks. If respond, may repeat course. **Chronic Idiopathic Constipation: Adults: <65 yo:** 6 mg bid before meals.	B v
Ursodiol (Actigall)	**Cap:** 300 mg	**Gallstone Dissolution:** 8-10 mg/kg/d in 2-3 divided doses. **Prevention:** 300 mg bid.	B >

GYNECOLOGY

Anti-Infective Agents

ANTIBACTERIALS

NAME	FORM/STRENGTH	DOSAGE	COMMENTS
Clindamycin Phosphate (Cleocin Vaginal, Cleocin Vaginal Ovules, Clindamax Vaginal, Clindesse)	**Cre:** 2%; **Sup:** (Ovules) 100 mg	**Bacterial Vaginosis: Post-menarchal Females: Ovules:** 1 sup intravaginally qhs x 3d. **Adults: Cre:** (Cleocin Vaginal/Clindamax Vaginal) 1 applicatorful intravaginally qhs x 3-7d (non-pregnant) or x 7d (pregnant). (Clindesse) 1 applicatorful intravaginally any time of day (non-pregnant).	B >
Metronidazole (Flagyl, Flagyl ER)	**Cap:** 375 mg; **Tab:** 250 mg, 500 mg; **Tab,ER:** 750 mg	**Adults: Flagyl: Trichomoniasis:** 375 mg (cap) bid or 250 mg (tab) tid x 7d. **Alternate Regimen:** If non-pregnant, 2 gm (tab) single or divided dose. **Bacterial Vaginosis:** (Flagyl ER) 750 mg qd x 7d on empty stomach.	B v **H** CI in 1st trimester.
Metronidazole (MetroGel-Vaginal)	**Gel:** 0.75%	**Bacterial Vaginosis: Adults:** 1 applicatorful intravaginally qd-bid x 5d.	B v
Sulfanilamide (AVC)	**Cre:** 15%	**Vulvovaginal Candidiasis: Adults:** 1 applicatorful intravaginally qd-bid. Continue x 30d.	B v

Tinidazole (Tindamax)	**Tab:** 250 mg, 500 mg	**Trichomoniasis: Adults:** 2 gm single dose w/ food. Treat sexual partner w/ same dose.	◙X (1st trimester) ◙C (2nd/3rd trimester) ✽v **R** Avoid unnecessary use.

ANTIFUNGALS

Butoconazole Nitrate (Gynazole-1, Mycelex-3)	**Cre:** 2%	**Vulvovaginal Candidiasis: Adults:** (Gynazole-1) 1 applicatorful intravaginally once. (Mycelex-3) 1 applicatorful intravaginally qhs x 3d.	◙C ✽>
Clotrimazole (Gyne-Lotrimin Combination, Gyne-Lotrimin 3)	**Cre-Sup:** (Gyne-Lotrimin Combination) 1%-100 mg, (Gyne-Lotrimin 3) 2%-200 mg	**Vulvovaginal Candidiasis: Adults & Peds: ≥12 yo:** (Gyne-Lotrimin 3) 1 applicatorful or 1 insert intravaginally qhs x 3d. (Gyne-Lotrimin Combination) 1 sup intravaginally qhs for 7d. Apply cre prn.	◙N ✽>
Clotrimazole (Mycelex 7)	**Cre:** 1%	**Vulvovaginal Candidiasis: Adults & Peds: ≥12 yo:** 1 applicatorful intravaginally qhs x 7d.	◙N ✽>
Fluconazole (Diflucan)	**Tab:** 150 mg	**Vaginal Candidiasis: Adults:** 150 mg single dose.	◙C ✽v
Miconazole Nitrate (Monistat 3, Monistat 7, Monistat Dual-Pak)	**Cre-Sup:** (Monistat 3) 4%-200 mg; (Monistat 7)2%-100 mg; (Dual-Pak) 2%-1200 mg	**Vulvovaginal Candidiasis: Adults & Peds: ≥12 yo:** (Monistat 3) 200 mg sup or 4% intravaginally qhs x 3d. (Monistat 7) 100 mg sup or 2% intravaginally qhs x 7d. (Monistat Dual-Pak) 1200 mg intravaginally qhs. Apply 2% cream bid up to 7d for external itching.	◙C ✽>
Terconazole (Terazol 3, Terazol 7)	**Cre-Sup:** (Terazol 3) 0.8%-80 mg; **Cre:** (Terazol 7) 0.4%	**Vulvovaginal Candidiasis: Adults:** (Terazol 3) 1 applicatorful of 0.8% or 80 mg sup intravaginally qhs x 3d. (Terazol 7) 1 applicatorful of 0.4% intravaginally qhs x 7d.	◙C ✽>

NAME	FORM/STRENGTH	DOSAGE	COMMENTS
Tioconazole (Monistat 1, Vagistat 1)	**Oint:** 6.5%	**Vulvovaginal Candidiasis: Adults & Peds: ≥12 yo:** Insert contents of applicator intravaginally once hs.	N >

Contraceptives

NAME	FORM/STRENGTH	DOSAGE	COMMENTS
Copper (ParaGard)	**IUD:** 68.7 mg	**Adults:** Insert intrauterine device any time during cycle. Replace q10yrs.	N v CI in pregnancy.
Estradiol Cypionate/ Medroxyprogesterone Acetate (Lunelle)	**Susp:** 5-25 mg/0.5 ml	**Adults:** 0.5 ml IM monthly.	X v
Ethinyl Estradiol/ Levonorgestrel (Seasonale)	**Tab:** 0.03-0.15 mg	**Adults:** 1 tab qd x 91d, then repeat. Start 1st Sunday after menses begin.	X v
Levonorgestrel (Mirena)	**IUD:** 52 mg	**Adults:** Insert intravaginally initially within 7d of menses onset. May replace any time in the cycle. May insert 6 wks postpartum or until involution of uterus is complete, & immediately after 1st trimester abortion. Replace q5yrs.	X v
Levonorgestrel (Norplant)	**Implant:** 36 mg	**Adults:** Implant 216 mg (6 implants) during 1st 7d of menses onset. Replace by end of 5th year.	X >
Medroxyprogesterone Acetate (Depo-Provera)	**Inj:** 150 mg/ml	**Adults:** 150 mg IM q3mths. Give 1st inj during 1st 5d of menses; within 1st 5d postpartum if not nursing; or 6 wks postpartum if nursing.	X >
Mifepristone (Mifeprex)	**Tab:** 200 mg	**Day 1:** 600 mg single dose. **Day 3:** If treatment fails, 400 mcg misoprostol. **Day 14:** Confirm complete termination.	X v [46]

[46] Serious and sometimes fatal infections and bleeding occur very rarely

ORAL CONTRACEPTIVES

DRUG	ESTROGEN	PROGESTIN	STRENGTH (ESTROGEN-PROGESTIN)
MONOPHASIC			
Alesse, Aviane, Lessina, Levlite	Ethinyl Estradiol	Levonorgestrel	20 mcg-0.1 mg
Apri, Desogen, Ortho-Cept	Ethinyl Estradiol	Desogestrel	30 mcg-0.15 mg
Brevicon, Necon 0.5/35, Nortrel 0.5/35	Ethinyl Estradiol	Norethindrone	35 mcg-0.5 mg
Demulen 1/35, Zovia 1/35E	Ethinyl Estradiol	Ethynodiol Diacetate	35 mcg-1 mg
Demulen 1/50, Zovia 1/50E	Ethinyl Estradiol	Ethynodiol Diacetate	50 mcg-1 mg
Levlen, Levora, Nordette, Portia	Ethinyl Estradiol	Levonorgestrel	30 mcg-0.15 mg
Loestrin 1/20, Loestrin Fe 1/20 Microgestin Fe 1/20, Junel 1/20	Ethinyl Estradiol	Norethindrone Acetate	20 mcg-1 mg
Loestrin 21 1.5/30, Loestrin Fe 1.5/30, Microgestin 1.5/30, Junel 1.5/30	Ethinyl Estradiol	Norethindrone Acetate	30 mcg-1.5 mg
Lo/Ovral, Low-Ogestrol, Cryselle	Ethinyl Estradiol	Norgestrel	30 mcg-0.3 mg
Necon 1/35, Norinyl 1/35, Ortho-Novum 1/35, Norcept-E 1/35, Nortrel 1/35, Norethin 1/35E	Ethinyl Estradiol	Norethindrone	35 mcg-1 mg

DRUG	ESTROGEN	PROGESTIN	STRENGTH (ESTROGEN-PROGESTIN)
Necon 1/50, Norinyl 1/50, Ortho-Novum 1/50, Norethin 1/50M	Mestranol	Norethindrone	50 mcg-1 mg
Ortho-Cyclen, Previfem, Sprintec, Mononessa	Ethinyl Estradiol	Norgestimate	35 mcg-0.25 mg
Balziva, Ovcon 35	Ethinyl Estradiol	Norethindrone	35 mcg-0.4 mg
Ovcon 50	Ethinyl Estradiol	Norethindrone	50 mcg-1 mg
Ogestrel-28	Ethinyl Estradiol	Norgestrel	50 mcg-0.5 mg
Seasonale	Ethinyl Estradiol	Levonorgestrel	30 mcg-0.15 mg
Yasmin	Ethinyl Estradiol	Drospirenone	30 mcg-3 mg
Yaz	Ethinyl Estradiol	Drospirenone	20 mcg-3 mg
BIPHASIC			
Aranelle, Gencept 10/11, Necon 10/11, Ortho-Novum 10/11	Ethinyl Estradiol	Norethindrone	**Phase 1:** 35 mcg-0.5 mg **Phase 2:** 35 mcg-1 mg
Mircette, Kariva	Ethinyl Estradiol	Desogestrel	**Phase 1:** 20 mcg-0.15 mg **Phase 2:** 10 mcg-NONE
TRIPHASIC			
Cyclessa, Velivet	Ethinyl Estradiol	Desogestrel	**Phase 1:** 25 mcg-0.1 mg **Phase 2:** 25 mcg-0.125 mg **Phase 3:** 25 mcg-0.15 mg

Estrostep	Ethinyl Estradiol	Norethindrone	**Phase 1:** 20 mcg-1 mg **Phase 2:** 30 mcg-1 mg **Phase 3:** 35 mcg-1 mg
Ortho-Novum 7/7/7, Necon 7/7/7, Nortrel 7/7/7	Ethinyl Estradiol	Norethindrone	**Phase 1:** 35 mcg-0.5 mg **Phase 2:** 35 mcg-0.75 mg **Phase 3:** 35 mcg-1 mg
Ortho Tri-Cyclen Tri-Sprintec, Tri-Previfem	Ethinyl Estradiol	Norgestimate	**Phase 1:** 35 mcg-0.18 mg **Phase 2:** 35 mcg-0.215 mg **Phase 3:** 35 mcg-0.25 mg
Ortho Tri-Cyclen Lo	Ethinyl Estradiol	Norgestimate	**Phase 1:** 25 mcg-0.18 mg **Phase 2:** 25 mcg-0.215 mg **Phase 3:** 25 mcg-0.25 mg
Expresse, Tri-Levlen, Triphasil, Trivora	Ethinyl Estradiol	Levonorgestrel	**Phase 1:** 30 mcg-0.05 mg **Phase 2:** 40 mcg-0.075 mg **Phase 3:** 30 mcg-0.125 mg
Tri-Norinyl	Ethinyl Estradiol	Norethindrone	**Phase 1:** 35 mcg-0.5 mg **Phase 2:** 35 mcg-1 mg **Phase 3:** 35 mcg-0.5 mg
PROGESTIN ONLY			
Ortho-Micronor, Nor-Q.D, Camila, Errin		Norethindrone	0.35 mg
EMERGENCY			
Plan B		Levonorgestrel	0.75 mg

Dysmenorrhea

NSAIDS

NAME	FORM/STRENGTH	DOSAGE	COMMENTS
Celecoxib (Celebrex)	**Cap:** 100 mg, 200 mg, 400 mg	**Adults: Day 1:** 400 mg, then 200 mg if needed. **Maint:** 200 mg bid prn.	C v **H** [66, 67]
Diclofenac Potassium (Cataflam)	**Tab:** 50 mg	**Adults:** 50 mg tid or 100 mg x 1 dose, then 50 mg tid. **Max:** 150 mg/d (200 mg/d on Day 1).	B v [66, 67]
Ibuprofen (Motrin)	**Susp:** 100 mg/5 ml; **Tab:** 400 mg, 600 mg, 800 mg	**Adults:** 400 mg q4h prn.	C v **R** [66, 67]
Ketoprofen	**Cap:** 50 mg, 75 mg	**Adults:** 25-50 mg q6-8h prn. **Max:** 300 mg/d.	C v **H R** [66, 67]
Mefenamic Acid (Ponstel)	**Cap:** 250 mg	**Adults & Peds ≥14 yo:** 500 mg, then 250 mg q6h, up to 3d.	C v [66, 67]
Naproxen (Naprosyn)	**Susp:** 25 mg/ml; **Tab:** 250 mg, 375 mg, 500 mg	**Adults: Initial:** 500 mg, then 250 mg q6-8h prn.	C v [66, 67]
Naproxen Sodium (Anaprox, Anaprox DS, Naprelan)	**Tab:** (Anaprox) 275 mg, (Anaprox DS) 550 mg; **Tab,ER:** (Naprelan) 375 mg, 500 mg	**Adults: Tab: Initial:** 550 mg, then 550 mg q12h or 275 mg q6-8h prn. **Max:** 1100 mg/d for maint. **Tab,ER: Intial:** 1000-1500 mg qd. **Max:** 1000 mg/d for maint.	C v [66, 67]

Endometriosis

ANDROGEN

Danazol (Danocrine)	**Cap:** 50 mg, 100 mg, 200 mg	**Adults: Mild:** 100-200 mg bid. **Moderate-Severe:** 400 mg bid. Start during menstruation & continue x 3-6 mths; may extend to 9 mths.	◙X ❃v

GONADOTROPINS

Goserelin Acetate (Zoladex)	**Implant:** 3.6 mg	**Adults:** 3.6 mg SC in upper abdominal wall q28d x up to 6 mths.	◙X ❃v
Leuprolide Acetate (Lupron Depot)	**Inj:** (Depot) 3.75 mg, (Depot-3 Month) 11.25 mg	**Adults:** 11.25 mg IM q3mths or 3.75 mg IM monthly, alone or w/ norethindrone acetate 5 mg/d. **Max:** 6 mths of therapy. May retreat with the combo up to 6 mths if symptoms recur.	◙X ❃v
Nafarelin Acetate (Synarel)	**Spr:** 200 mcg/inh	**Adults:** **≥18 yo:** 1 spr into one nostril qam & 1 spr into other nostril qpm. Initiate b/w Days 2-4 of menstrual cycle. Increase to 1 spr/nostril qam & qpm after 2 mths if amenorrhea has not occurred. Treat x 6 mths.	◙X ❃v

PROGESTOGEN

Norethindrone Acetate (Aygestin)	**Tab:** 5 mg	**Adults:** Assume interval between menses is 28d. **Initial:** 5 mg qd x 2 wks. **Titrate:** Increase by 2.5 mg/d q2wks until 15 mg/d. Continue x 6-9 mths or until breakthrough bleeding demands temporary termination.	◙X ❃> **H**

66 NSAIDs may cause an increased risk of serious CV thrombotic events, MI, stroke and serious GI adverse events including bleeding, ulceration, and perforation of the stomach or intestines.

67 Contraindicated for treatment of peri-operative pain in CABG surgery.

Hormone Replacement Therapy

NAME	FORM/STRENGTH	DOSAGE	COMMENTS
Estradiol Acetate (Femring, Femtrace)	**Vaginal Ring:** (Femring) 0.05 mg/d, 0.1 mg/d **Tab:** (Femtrace) 0.45 mg, 0.9 mg, 1.8 mg	**Adults: Femring: Initial:** Use lowest effective dose. Insert ring vaginally. Replace q3mths. Re-evaluate periodically. **Femtrace:** 1 tab qd. Use lowest effective dose. Re-evaluate periodically.	X > 4, 28
Estradiol (Alora, Climara, Vivelle, Vivelle-Dot)	**Patch:** (Alora) 0.025 mg/d, 0.05 mg/d, 0.075 mg/d, 0.1 mg/d, (Climara) 0.025 mg/d, 0.0375 mg/d, 0.05 mg/d, 0.06 mg/d, 0.075 mg/d, 0.1 mg/d, (Vivelle, Vivelle-Dot) 0.025 mg/d, 0.0375 mg/d, 0.05 mg/d, 0.075 mg/d, 0.1 mg/d	**Vasomotor Symptoms, Vulval/Vaginal Atrophy, Hypoestrogenism: Adults: Alora: Initial:** Apply 0.05 mg/d 2x/wk. **Vivelle, Vivelle-Dot: Initial:** 0.0375 mg/d 2x/wk. **Alora, Vivelle, Vivelle-Dot:** Use continuously without intact uterus. **Climara: Initial:** 0.025 mg/d qwk. **Titrate:** Adjust dose. Use cyclic schedule (3 wks on, 1 wk off) w/ intact uterus.	X > 4, 10, 28
Estradiol (Estrace, Gynodiol)	**Tab:** (Estrace) 0.5 mg, 1 mg, 2 mg, (Gynodiol) 0.5 mg, 1 mg, 1.5 mg, 2 mg; **Cre:** (Estrace) 0.01 mg/gm	**Adults: Vulval/Vaginal Atrophy: Cre:** (Estrace) 2-4 gm/d x 1-2 wks, then 1-2 gm/d x 1-2 wks. **Maint:** 1 gm 1-3 times/wk. **Menopause/Vulval/Vaginal Atrophy: Tab:** (Estrace, Gynodiol) 1-2 mg/d (3 wks on, 1 wk off). **Maint:** Minimum effective dose. **Hypoestrogenism:** 1-2 mg/d. **Maint:** Minimum effective dose.	X v 4, 10, 28
Estradiol (Estrasorb)	**Emul:** 2.5 mg/gm	**Vasomotor Symptoms: Adults:** 2 pouches (0.05 mg/d) qam. Apply 1 pouch to each leg from the upper thigh to the calf. Rub in for 3 min.	X > 4, 10, 28

Estradiol (EstroGel)	**Gel:** 0.06%	**Vasomotor Symptoms, Vulvar/Vaginal Atrophy: Adults:** Apply 1 compression (1.25 g) to one arm from wrist to shoulder qd.	X > [4, 28]
Estradiol/Levonorgestrel (Climara Pro)	**Patch:** 0.045-0.015 mg/d	**Vasomotor Symptoms: Adults:** Apply 1 patch qwk to lower abdomen (avoid breasts/waistline). Rotate application site; allow 1 wk between same site.	X > [4, 10, 28]
Estradiol/Norethindrone Acetate (CombiPatch)	**Patch:** 0.05-0.14 mg/d, 0.05-0.25 mg/d	**Adults: Menopause, Vulval/Vaginal atrophy, Hypoestrogenism: Intact Uterus: Continuous Combined Regimen:** 0.05-0.14 mg 2x/wk. **Continuous Sequential Regimen:** Wear estradiol-only patch for 1st 14d of 28d cycle, replace 2x/wk. 0.05-0.14 mg 2x/wk for remaining 14d.	X v [10, 28]
Estradiol/Norethindrone (Activella)	**Tab:** 1-0.5 mg	**Vulval/Vaginal atrophy, Vasomotor Symptoms: Adults: Intact Uterus:** 1-0.5 mg qd.	X > [28]
Estradiol/Norgestimate (Prefest)	**Tab:** 1 mg-none, 1 mg-0.09 mg	**Vasomotor symptoms, Vulvar/Vaginal Atrophy: Adults: Intact Uterus:** 1 mg estradiol x3d alternating w/ 1-0.09 mg x3d on continuous schedule.	X v [28]
Estrogens, Conjugated (Cenestin)	**Tab:** 0.3 mg, 0.45 mg, 0.625 mg, 0.9 mg, 1.25 mg	**Adults: Vasomotor Symptoms: Initial:** 0.45 mg qd. Adjust dose based on response. **Vulvar/Vaginal Atrophy:** 0.3 mg qd.	N > CI in pregnancy. [4, 10, 28]

[4] Contraindicated in pregnancy. Increased risk of endometrial carcinoma.

[10] Attempt to taper or d/c at 3-6 mth intervals.

[28] Not for prevention of CV disease or dementia. The WHI reported increased risks of MI, stroke, invasive breast cancer, pulmonary emboli, DVT, and probable dementia in postmenopausal women. Prescribe at lowest effective doses for shortest duration.

NAME	FORM/STRENGTH	DOSAGE	COMMENTS
Estrogens, Conjugated (Premarin)	**Tab:** 0.3 mg, 0.45 mg, 0.625 mg, 0.9 mg, 1.25 mg, 2.5 mg; **Vag Cre:** 0.625 mg/gm	**Adults: Tab: Vasomotor Symptoms/Vulvar/Vaginal Atrophy:** 0.3 mg continuous or cyclically (eg, 25d on, 5d off). **Female Hypogonadism:** 0.3-0.625 mg qd cyclically. **Female Castration/Primary Ovarian Failure:** 1.25 mg qd cyclically. **Cre: Atrophic Vaginitis/Kraurosis Vulvae:** 1/2-2 gm intravaginally qd cyclically (3 wks on, 1 wk off).	X > 4, 10, 28
Estrogens, Conjugated/ Medroxyprogesterone Acetate (Premphase, Prempro)	**Tab:** (Premphase) 0.625 mg conjugated estrogens & 0.625-5 mg, (Prempro) 0.3-1.5 mg, 0.45-1.5 mg, 0.625-2.5 mg, 0.625-5 mg	**Menopause/Atrophy: Adults:** Treat w/ lowest effective dose. Adjust dose based on response.	X > 10, 28
Estrogens, Esterified (Menest)	**Tab:** 0.3 mg, 0.625 mg, 1.25 mg, 2.5 mg	**Adults: Vasomotor Symptoms:** 1.25 mg qd cyclically (3 wks on, 1 wk off). **Atrophic Vaginitis/Kraurosis Vulvae:** 0.3-1.25 mg qd cyclically. **Female Hypogonadism:** 2.5-7.5 mg/d in divided doses for 20d, then 10d off therapy; repeat until menses occurs. **Female Castration/Primary Ovarian Failure:** 1.25 mg qd cyclically. **Maint:** Lowest effective dose.	X v 4, 10, 28
Estrogens, Esterified/ Methyltestosterone (Estratest, Estratest H.S.)	**Tab:** 1.25-2.5 mg, (H.S.) 0.625-1.25 mg	**Vasomotor Symptoms: Adults:** 0.625-1.25 mg or 1.25-2.5 mg qd cyclically (3 wks on, 1 wk off).	X v 4, 10, 28

Estropipate (Ogen, Ortho-Est)	**Tab:** (Ogen, Ortho-Est) 0.625 mg (0.75 mg estropipate), 1.25 mg (1.5 mg estropipate), (Ogen) 2.5 mg (3 mg estropipate)	**Adults: Vasomotor Symptoms:** 0.75-6 mg/d (as estropipate). **Vulval/Vaginal Atrophy:** 0.75-6 mg/d (as estropipate), cyclically. **Female Hypogonadism/Female Castration/Primary Ovarian Failure:** 1.5-9 mg/d (as estropipate) for 1st 3 wks of cycle, then 8-10d off.	X > [4, 10, 28]
Ethinyl Estradiol/Norethindrone Acetate (femhrt)	**Tab:** 2.5 mcg-0.5 mg, 5 mcg-1 mg	**Vasomotor Symptoms: Adults:** 1 tab qd.	X > [10, 28]

Premenstrual Dysphoric Disorder

SSRIS

Fluoxetine (Sarafem)	**Cap:** 10 mg, 20 mg	**Adults: Continuous: Initial:** 20 mg qd. **Maint:** 20 mg/d up to 6 mths. **Max:** 60 mg/d. **Intermittent: Initial:** 20 mg qd; start 14d before menses onset through 1st full day of menses. **Maint:** 20 mg/d up to 3 mths. **Max:** 60 mg/d.	C v **H** [29]
Paroxetine HCl (Paxil CR)	**Tab,CR:** 12.5 mg, 25 mg, 37.5 mg	**Adults: Initial:** 12.5 mg qd continuous or limited to luteal phase. **Titrate:** Wait at least 1 wk between dose changes.	D > **H R** [29]

[4] Contraindicated in pregnancy. Increased risk of endometrial carcinoma.

[10] Attempt to taper or d/c at 3-6 mth intervals.

[28] Not for prevention of CV disease or dementia. The WHI reported increased risks of MI, stroke, invasive breast cancer, pulmonary emboli, DVT, and probable dementia in postmenopausal women. Prescribe at lowest effective doses for shortest duration.

[29] Antidepressants may increase the risk of suicidality in children and adolescents.

NAME	FORM/STRENGTH	DOSAGE	COMMENTS
Sertraline (Zoloft)	**Tab:** 25 mg, 50 mg, 100 mg; **Sol:** 20 mg/ml	**Initial:** 50 mg qd continuous or limit to luteal cycle phase. **Titrate:** Increase by 50 mg/cycle up to 150 mg/d for continuous or 100 mg/d for luteal phase dosing. If 100 mg/d is established for luteal phase dosing, then titrate by 50 mg/d x 3d at beginning of each luteal phase dosing period.	C > H [29]

Miscellaneous

NAME	FORM/STRENGTH	DOSAGE	COMMENTS
Danazol (Danocrine)	**Cap:** 50 mg, 100 mg, 200 mg	**Fibrocystic Breast Disease: Adults:** 50-200 mg bid. Start during menstruation.	X v
Estradiol (Estring)	**Vag Ring:** 2 mg/ring	**Postmenopausal Urogenital Symptoms: Adults:** Insert ring into upper 1/3 of the vaginal vault, remove & replace after 90d.	X v [4, 10]

Hematopoietic Agents

Darbepoetin Alfa (Aranesp)	**Inj:** (Syr) 0.025 mg/ 0.42 ml, 0.04 mg/0.4 ml, 0.06 mg/0.3 ml, 0.1 mg/ 0.5 ml, 0.15 mg/0.3 ml, 0.2 mg/0.4 ml, 0.3 mg/0.6 ml, 0.5 mg/ml; **SDV:** 0.025 mg/ml, 0.04 mg/ ml, 0.06 mg/ml, 0.1 mg/ ml, 0.15 mg/0.75 ml, 0.2 mg/ml, 0.3 mg/ml	**Adults: CRF: Initial:** 0.45 mcg/kg IV/SC wkly. **Titrate:** Adjust to target Hgb <12 gm/dL. If Hgb increases >1 gm/dL in a 2-wk period or is approaching 12 gm/dL, decrease dose by 25%. If Hgb continues to increase, hold dose until Hgb begins to decrease, & reinitiate at 25% below previous dose. Do not increase more than once monthly. **Malignancy: Initial:** 2.25 mcg/kg SC wkly. **Titrate:** Increase to 4.5 mcg/kg if Hgb increase is <1 gm/dL after 6 wks of therapy. If Hgb increases >1 gm/dL in a 2-wk period or if Hgb >12 gm/dL, decrease dose by 25%. If Hgb >13 gm/dL, hold dose until Hgb falls to 12 gm/dL & reinitiate at 25% below previous dose.	◙C ❊>
Epoetin Alfa (Epogen, Procrit)	**Inj:** 2000 U/ml, 3000 U/ml, 4000 U/ml, 10,000 U/ml, 20,000 U/ml, 40,000 U/ml	**Adults: CRF: Initial:** 50-100 U/kg IV/SC TIW. **Maint:** Adjust based on Hgb. **AZT Therapy:** 100 U/kg IV/SC TIW x 8 wks. **Titrate:** Increase by 50-100 U/kg TIW up to 300 U/kg TIW. **Maint:** Adjust based on AZT & Hgb. **Chemotherapy: Initial:** 150 U/kg SC TIW x 8 wks. **Titrate:** May increase to 300 U/kg TIW after 8 wks of therapy. **Maint:** Adjust based on Hgb. **Surgery:** 300 U/kg/d SC x10d prior to surgery, on day of, & 4d after surgery; or 600 U/kg SC wkly on Days 21,14, & 7 prior to surgery, & a 4th dose on day of surgery. **Peds: CRF: Initial:** 50 U/kg TIW IV/SC. **Maint:** Adjust based on Hgb.	◙C ❊>

4 Contraindicated in pregnancy. Increased risk of endometrial carcinoma.
10 Attempt to taper or d/c at 3-6 mth intervals.
29 Antidepressants may increase the risk of suicidality in children and adolescents.

NAME	FORM/STRENGTH	DOSAGE	COMMENTS
Filgrastim (Neupogen)	**Inj:** 300 mcg/0.5 ml, 300 mcg/ml, 480 mcg/0.8 ml, 480 mcg/1.6 ml	**Adults: Myelosuppressive Chemotherapy: Initial:** 5 mcg/kg/d IV/SC. **BMT Cancer: Initial:** 10 mcg/kg/d IV/SC. **Congenital Neutropenia: Initial:** 6 mcg/kg SC bid. **Idiopathic/Cyclic Neutropenia: Initial:** 5 mcg/kg SC qd. **Maint:** Adjust dose for above based on neutrophil count. **Peripheral Blood Progenitor Cell Collection: Initial:** 10 mcg/kg/d SC 4d before & x 6-7d w/ leukapheresis on Days 5, 6 & 7.	C >
Oprelvekin (Neumega)	**Inj:** 5 mg	**Severe Thrombocytopenia Prevention: Adults:** 50 mcg/kg SC qd. Initiate 6-24h after chemo completion. Continue therapy until post-nadir platelets ≥50,000 cells/mcL. D/C at least 2d before next chemo cycle. **Max:** 21d of therapy.	C v
Pegfilgrastim (Neulasta)	**Inj:** 6 mg/0.6 ml	**Infection/Febrile Neutropenia w/ Non-Myeloid Malignancies: Adults:** 6 mg SC, once per chemotherapy cycle. Do not administer in the period 14d before & 24h after chemotherapy.	C >
Sargramostim (Leukine)	**Inj:** 250 mcg, 500 mcg/ml	**Adults: BMT Myeloid Reconstitution:** 250 mcg/m²/d IV post bone marrow infusion, continue until ANC >1500 cells/mm³ x 3d. **BMT Failure/Engraftment Delay:** 250 mcg/m²/d IV x 14d, repeat after 7d if needed; 500 mcg m²/d IV x 14d after another 7d off therapy, if needed. **Post Peripheral Blood Progenitor Cell (PBPC) Transplant:** 250 mcg m²/d SC until ANC >1500 cells/mm³ x 3d. **PBPC Mobilization:** 250 mcg/m²/d IV/SC, continue through PBPC collection period. **Post-Chemo in AML:** 250 mcg /m²/d IV until ANC >1500 cells/mm³ x 3d or max of 42d.	C >

Vaccines/Toxoids/Immunoglobulins

Anthrax Vaccine Adsorbed (Biothrax)	**Inj:** 5 ml	**Pre-exposure Prophylaxis: Adults: 18-65 yo:** 0.5 ml SC at 0, 2, 4 wks, then 0.5 ml at 6, 12, 18 mths. **Booster:** 0.5 ml yearly.	D ❋>
Diphtheria Toxoid/Tetanus Toxoid/Acellular Pertussis Vaccine Adsorbed (Adacel, Daptacel, Infanrix, Tripedia)	**Inj:** (Adacel) 2 LFU-5 LFU-2.5 mcg/0.5 ml. (Daptacel) 15 LFU-5 LFU-23 mcg/0.5 ml; (Infanrix) 25 LFU-10 LFU-58 mcg/0.5 ml; (Tripedia) 6.7 LFU-5 LFU-46.8 mcg/0.5 ml	**Adults & Peds: 11-63 yo: Adacel:** 0.5 ml IM. **Peds: ≥6 wks up to 7 yo: Infanrix, Tripedia:** 3 doses of 0.5 ml IM at 4-8 wk intervals. **Booster:** Give at 15-20 mths, at least 6 mths after 3rd dose. **Daptacel:** 4 doses of 0.5 ml IM w/ 1st 3 doses at 6-8 wk intervals. The interval between 3rd & 4th dose should be at least 6 mths.	C ❋>
Diphtheria/Tetanus Toxoids Adsorbed	**Inj:** 2-5 LFU/0.5 ml, 6.6-5 LFU/0.5 ml, 10-5 LFU/0.5 ml	**>7 yo:** 0.5 ml IM in the vastus lateralis or deltoid. Repeat 4-8 wks later. Give 3rd dose 6-12 mths after 2nd dose. **Booster:** 0.5 ml IM every 10 yrs. **6 wks-12 mths:** 0.5 ml IM x 3 doses 4-8 wks apart. 4th dose 6-12 mths after 3rd dose. **1-6 yo:** 0.5 ml IM x 2 doses 4-8 wks apart. 3rd dose 6-12 mths after 2nd dose. **Booster: If received 4 doses:** 0.5 ml IM before entering school.	C ❋>
Haemophilus b Conjugate & Hepatitis B Vaccine Recombinant (Comvax)	**Inj:** 7.5-5-125 mcg/0.5 ml	**Peds: ≥6 wks:** 0.5 ml IM at 2, 4, & 12-15 mths of age. If cannot follow schedule, wait at least 6 wks between 1st 2 doses. 2nd & 3rd dose should be close to 8-11 mths apart.	C ❋>

NAME	FORM/STRENGTH	DOSAGE	COMMENTS
Haemophilus b Conjugate Vaccine (ActHIB)	**Inj:** 10 mcg	**Peds: Reconstituted w/ DTP or Saline:** 0.5 ml IM at 2, 4, & 6 mths old; 4th dose at 15-18 mths; 5th dose at 4-6 yo. **Reconstituted w/ Tripedia (as 4th dose in series):** 0.5 ml IM at 15-18 mths; 5th dose at 4-6 yo. **Unvaccinated: 7-11 mths:** 2 doses at 8 wk intervals w/ a booster at 15-18 mths. **12-14 mths:** 1 dose followed by a booster 2 mths later.	C ❁>
Hepatitis A Inactivated, Hepatitis B Recombinant (Twinrix)	**Inj:** 720 U-20 mcg	**Adults:** 1 ml IM at 0-, 1- & 6-mth schedule.	C ❁>
Hepatitis A Vaccine, Inactivated (Havrix, Vaqta)	**Inj:** (Havrix) 720 EL.U/0.5 ml, 1440 EL.U/ml; (Vaqta) 25 U/0.5 ml, 50 U/ml	**Havrix: Adults:** 1440 EL.U. IM. **Peds: 1-18 yo:** 720 EL.U. IM. All ages require booster dose at 6-12 mths following primary dose. **Vaqta: Adults:** 50 U IM, repeat 6-18 mths later. **Peds: 1-18 yo:** 25 U IM, repeat 6-18 mths later.	C ❁>
Hepatitis B Immune Globulin (BayHep, Nabi-HB)	**Inj:** 0.5 ml, 1 ml, 5 ml	**Percutaneous or Permucosal Exposure, HBsAg-Positive or High Risk Source: Vaccinated:** 0.06 ml/kg IM x 1 dose immediately plus either HB vaccine booster or second dose of HBIG 1 mth later. **Unvaccinated:** Initiate HB vaccine series.	C ❁>
Hepatitis B Vaccine, Recombinant (Engerix-B, Recombivax HB)	**Inj:** (Engerix-ped) 10 mcg/0.5 ml, (Recombivax HB-ped) 5 mcg/0.5 ml, (Engerix-adult) 20 mcg/ml, (Recombivax HB adult) 10 mcg/ml	**Engerix: Adults: >19 yo:** 20 mcg/ml IM at 0, 1, 6 mths. **Peds: ≤19 yo:** 10 mcg/0.5 ml IM at 0, 1, 6 mths. **Booster: Adults & Peds: ≥11 yo:** 20 mcg IM. **≤10 yo:** 10 mcg IM. **Recombivax: Adults: ≥20 yo:** 10 mcg IM at 0, 1, 6 mths. **Peds: 0-19 yo:** 5 mcg IM at 0, 1, 6 mths.	C ❁>

Human Papillomavirus Recombinant Vaccine (Gardasil)	**Inj:** 0.5 ml	**Adults & Peds: ≥9 yo:** Give 3 separate 0.5 ml IM doses in the deltoid region of upper arm or higher anterolateral area of the thigh. **1st dose:** At elected date; **2nd dose:** 2 mths after first dose; **3rd dose:** 6 mths after first dose.	◙B ❁>
Influenza Virus Vaccine Live, Intranasal (FluMist)	**Nasal Spr:** 0.5 ml/spr	**Adults & Peds: ≥9 yo:** 0.25 ml per nostril. **5-8 yo: Not Previously Vaccinated w/ FluMist:** 0.25 ml per nostril x 2 doses 60d (+/- 14d) apart. **Previously Vaccinated w/ FluMist:** 0.25 ml per nostril.	◙C ❁>
Influenza Virus Vaccine, Subvirion (FluShield, Fluzone)	**Inj:** 45 mcg/0.5 ml	**Adults & Peds: ≥3 yrs:** 0.5 ml IM. **6-35 mths:** 0.25 ml IM. **<9 yo (Not Previously Vaccinated):** Repeat dose min 1 mth apart. Administer in deltoid muscle to older children & thigh muscle in infants & young children.	◙C ❁>
Influenza Virus Vaccine, Subvirion (Fluvirin)	**Inj:** 45 mcg/0.5 ml	**Adults & Peds: ≥4 yo:** 0.5 ml IM. **Peds: <9 yo (Not Previously Vaccinated):** Repeat dose min 1 mth apart. Administer in deltoid muscle to older children & thigh muscle in young children.	◙C ❁>
Measles Virus Vaccine Live (Attenuvax)	**Inj:** 1000 $TCID_{50}$	**Peds: 12-15 mths:** 0.5 ml SC in upper arm. If vaccinated <12 mths old, revaccinate at 12-15 mths old. Revaccinate prior to school entry.	◙C ❁>
Measles/Mumps/Rubella Virus Vaccine Live (M-M-R II)	**Inj:** 0.5 ml/dose	**Adults & Peds: >12 mths:** 0.5 ml SC in upper arm. Recommended primary vaccination is at 12-15 mths; repeat before elementary school entry. If vaccinated at 6-12 mths due to outbreak, give another dose at 12-15 mths & before elementary school entry.	◙C ❁>
Meningitis Vaccine (Menomune-A/c/y/w-135)	**Inj:** 0.05 mg	**Adults & Peds: ≥2 yo:** 0.05 ml SC.	◙C ❁>

NAME	FORM/STRENGTH	DOSAGE	COMMENTS
Mumps Virus Vaccine (Mumpsvax)	**Inj:** 20,000 $TCID_{50}$	**Adults & Peds: ≥12 mths:** 0.5 ml SC in outer aspect of upper arm. Give primary vaccine at 12-15 mths. Revaccinate prior to elementary school.	◙C ❀>
Pneumococcal Vaccine, Diphtheria Protein (Prevnar)	**Inj:** 16 mcg/0.5 ml	**Peds: *S. pneumoniae*/Otitis Media:** 0.5 ml IM. 1st dose at 6 wks-2 mths old, then q2mths x 2 more doses. 4th dose given at 12-15 mths. **Unvaccinated: ≥24 mths-9 yo:** 0.5 ml IM single dose. **12-23 mths:** 0.5 ml IM x 2 doses given at least 2 mths apart. **7-11 mths:** 0.5 ml IM. 1st 2 doses at least 4 wks apart, then 3rd dose after 1 yo birthday at least 2 mths after 2nd dose.	◙C ❀v
Pneumococcal Vaccine (Pneumovax 23, Pnu-Imune 23)	**Inj:** 0.5 ml/dose	**Adults & Peds: ≥2 yo:** Usual: 0.5 ml SC/IM in deltoid muscle or lateral mid-thigh.	◙C ❀>
Rabies Immune Globulin, Human (BayRab, Imogam)	**Inj:** 150 IU/ml	**Adults:** 20 IU/kg infiltrated in the area around the wound & the rest IM in gluteal area.	◙C ❀>
Rabies Vaccine (Imovax, RabAvert)	**Inj:** 2.5 IU	**Adults: Pre-exposure:** 1 ml IM on Days 0, 7 & either 21 or 28 (3 total doses), booster shots as needed based on titers. **Post-exposure:** (Imovax) 1 ml IM on Days 0, 3, 7, 14 & 30 (ACIP recommendations). (Rabavert) 1 ml IM on Days 0, 3, 7, 14 & 28.	◙C ❀>
Rotavirus Vaccine, Live, Oral, Pentavalent (RotaTeq)	**Susp:** 2 ml	**Rotavirus Gastroenteritis Prevention: Peds:** Administer series of 3 doses orally starting at 6-12 wks of age, w/ subsequent doses administered at 4-10 wk intervals. Third dose should not be given after 32 wks of age. Do not mix w/ any other vaccines or solutions. Do not reconstitute or dilute.	◙N ❀>

Rubella Virus Vaccine Live (Meruvax)	**Inj:** 1000 $TCID_{50}$	**Peds: 12-15 mths:** 0.5 mlSC in outer aspect of upper arm. Revaccinate w/ MMR II prior to elementary school entry.	C > CI in pregnancy.
Tetanus & Diphtheria Toxoids Adsorbed (Td)	**Inj:** 5 LFU-2 LFU/0.5 ml	**Adults & Peds: >7 yo:** 0.5 ml IM in the vastus lateralis or deltoid. Repeat 4-8 wks later. Give 3rd dose 6-12 mths after 2nd dose. **Booster:** 0.5 ml IM q10yrs.	C >
Tetanus Immunoglobulin (BayTet)	**Inj:** 250 U	**Prophylactic: Adults & Peds: ≥7 yo:** 750 U IM. **Peds: <7 yo:** 4 U/kg or 250 U. **Active Case:** Adjust dose to severity of infection.	C >
Tetanus Toxoid (Tetanus Toxoid Adsorbed Purogenated)	**Inj:** 0.5 ml/dose	**Adults & Peds: ≥1 yo:** 0.5 ml IM. Repeat at 4-8 wks then 6-12 mths after 2nd dose. **Booster:** 0.5 ml IM q10yrs. **<1 yo:** 3 doses of 0.5 ml IM 4-8 wks apart, then 4th dose (0.5 ml) 6-12 mths after 3rd dose. Last dose before 4 yo. **Booster:** 0.5 ml at 4-6 yo.	C >
Varicella Virus Vaccine Live (Varivax)	**Inj:** 1350 PFU/vial	**Adults & Peds: ≥13 yo:** 0.5 ml SC, repeat in 4-8 wks. **1-12 yo:** 0.5 ml SC x 1 dose.	C > CI in pregnancy.
Varicella-Zoster Immune Globulin	**Inj:** 125 U/vial, 625 U/vial	**Adults & Peds: IM (gluteal): >40 kg:** 625 U. **30.1-40 kg:** 500 U. **20.1-30 kg:** 375 U. **10.1-20 kg:** 250 U. **0-10 kg:** 125 U.	C >
Zoster Vaccine Live (Zostavax)	**Inj:** 19,400 PFU/0.65 ml	**Adults: ≥60 yo:** Inject SC immediately after reconstitution w/ supplied diluent.	C >

IMMUNIZATIONS

RECOMMENDED CHILDHOOD AND ADOLESCENT IMMUNIZATION SCHEDULE UNITED STATES • 2006

Vaccine ▼ / Age ▶	Birth	1 month	2 months	4 months	6 months	12 months	15 months	18 months	24 months	4–6 years	11–12 years	13–14 years	15 years	16–18 years
Hepatitis B[1]	HepB	HepB		*HepB*[1]			HepB				HepB Series			
Diphtheria, Tetanus, Pertussis[2]			DTaP	DTaP	DTaP		DTaP			DTaP	Tdap		Tdap	
Haemophilus influenzae type b[3]			Hib	Hib	*Hib*[3]	Hib								
Inactivated Poliovirus			IPV	IPV			IPV			IPV				
Measles, Mumps, Rubella[4]						MMR				MMR		MMR		
Varicella[5]							Varicella				Varicella			
Meningococcal[6]							Vaccines within broken line are for selected populations		MPSV4		MCV4		MCV4 / MCV4	
Pneumococcal[7]			PCV	PCV	PCV	PCV			PCV		PPV			
Influenza[8]						Influenza (Yearly)					Influenza (Yearly)			
Hepatitis A[9]										HepA Series				

Range of recommended ages | Catch-up immunization | 11–12 year old assessment

This schedule indicates the recommended ages for routine administration of currently licensed childhood vaccines, as of December 1, 2005, for children through age 18 yrs. Any dose not administered at the recommended age should be administered at any subsequent visit when indicated and feasible. Indicates age groups that warrant special effort to administer those vaccines not previously administered. Additional vaccines may be licensed and recommended during the year. Licensed combination vaccines may be used whenever any components of the combination are indicated and other components of the vaccine are not contraindicated and if approved by the Food and Drug Administration for that dose of the series. Providers should consult the respective ACIP statement for detailed recommendations. Clinically significant adverse events that follow immunization should be reported to the Vaccine Adverse Event Reporting System (VAERS). Guidance about how to obtain and complete a VAERS form is available at **www.vaers.hhs.gov** or by telephone, 800-822-7967.

1. **Hepatitis B vaccine (HepB).** ***AT BIRTH:*** **All newborns** should receive monovalent HepB soon after birth and before hospital discharge. **Infants born to mothers who are HBsAg-positive** should receive HepB and 0.5 mL of hepatitis B immune globulin (HBIG) within 12 hrs of birth. **Infants born to mothers whose HBsAg status is unknown** should receive HepB within 12 hrs of birth. The mother should have blood drawn as soon as possible to determine her HBsAg status; if HBsAg-positive, the infant should receive HBIG as soon as possible (no later than age 1 week). **For infants born to HBsAg-negative mothers,** the birth dose can be delayed in rare circumstances but only if a physician's order to withhold the vaccine and a copy of the mother's original HBsAg-negative laboratory report are documented in the infant's medical record. **FOLLOWING THE BIRTHDOSE:** The HepB series should be completed with either monovalent HepB or a combination vaccine containing HepB. The second dose should be administered at age 1–2 mths. The final dose should be administered at age ≥24 wks. It is permissible to administer 4 doses of HepB (e.g., when combination vaccines are given after the birth dose); however, if monovalent HepB is used, a dose at age 4 mths is not needed. **Infants born to HBsAg-positive mothers** should be tested for HBsAg and antibody to HBsAg after completion of the HepB series, at age 9–18 mths (generally at the next well-child visit after completion of the vaccine series).
2. **Diphtheria and tetanus toxoids and acellular pertussis vaccine (DTaP).** The fourth dose of DTaP may be administered as early as age 12 mths, provided 6 mths have elapsed since the third dose and the child is unlikely to return at age 15–18 mths. The final dose in the series should be given at age ≥4 yrs. **Tetanus and diphtheria toxoids and acellular pertussis vaccine (Tdap – adolescent preparation)** is recommended at age 11–12 yrs for those who have completed the recommended childhood DTP/DTaP vaccination series and have not received a Td booster dose. Adolescents 13–18 yrs who missed the 11–12-year Td/Tdap booster dose should also receive a single dose of Tdap if they have completed the recommended childhood DTP/DTaP vaccination series. Subsequent **tetanus and diphtheria toxoids (Td)** are recommended every 10 yrs.
3. ***Haemophilus influenzae*** **type b conjugate vaccine (Hib).** Three Hib conjugate vaccines are licensed for infant use. If PRP-OMP (PedvaxHIB® or ComVax® [Merck]) is administered at ages 2 and 4 mths, a dose at age 6 mths is not required. DTaP/Hib combination products should not be used for primary immunization in infants at ages 2, 4 or 6 mths but can be used as boosters after any Hib vaccine. The final dose in the series should be administered at age ≥12 mths.

4. **Measles, mumps, and rubella vaccine (MMR).** The second dose of MMR is recommended routinely at age 4–6 yrs but may be administered during any visit, provided at least 4 wks have elapsed since the first dose and both doses are administered beginning at or after age 12 mths. Those who have not previously received the second dose should complete the schedule by age 11–12 yrs.
5. **Varicella vaccine.** Varicella vaccine is recommended at any visit at or after age 12 mths for susceptible children (i.e., those who lack a reliable history of chickenpox). Susceptible persons aged ≥13 yrs should receive 2 doses administered at least 4 wks apart.
6. **Meningococcal vaccine (MCV4).** Meningococcal conjugate vaccine (MCV4) should be given to all children at the 11–12 yr old visit as well as to unvaccinated adolescents at high school entry (15 yrs of age). Other adolescents who wish to decrease their risk for meningococcal disease may also be vaccinated. All college freshmen living in dormitories should also be vaccinated, preferably with MCV4, although **meningococcal polysaccharide vaccine (MPSV4)** is an acceptable alternative. Vaccination against invasive meningococcal disease is recommended for children and adolescents aged ≥2 yrs with terminal complement deficiencies or anatomic or functional asplenia and certain other high risk groups (see *MMWR* 2005;54 [RR-7]:1-21); use MPSV4 for children aged 2–10 yrs and MCV4 for older children, although MPSV4 is an acceptable alternative.
7. **Pneumococcal vaccine.** The heptavalent **pneumococcal conjugate vaccine (PCV)** is recommended for all children aged 2–23 mths and for certain children aged 24–59 mths. The final dose in the series should be given at age ≥12 mths. **Pneumococcal polysaccharide vaccine (PPV)** is recommended in addition to PCV for certain high-risk groups. See *MMWR* 2000; 49(RR-9):1-35.
8. **Influenza vaccine.** Influenza vaccine is recommended annually for children aged ≥6 mths with certain risk factors (including, but not limited to, asthma, cardiac disease, sickle cell disease, human immunodeficiency virus [HIV], diabetes, and conditions that can compromise respiratory function or handling of respiratory secretions or that can increase the risk for aspiration), healthcare workers, and other persons (including household members) in close contact with persons in groups at high risk (see *MMWR* 2005;54[RR-8]:1-55). In addition, healthy children aged 6–23 mths and close contacts of healthy children aged 0–5 mths are recommended to receive influenza vaccine because children in this age group are at substantially increased risk for influenza-related hospitalizations. For healthy persons aged 5–49 yrs, the intranasally administered, live, attenuated influenza vaccine (LAIV) is an acceptable alternative to the intramuscular trivalent inactivated influenza vaccine (TIV). See *MMWR* 2005;54(RR-8):1-55. Children receiving TIV should be administered a dosage appropriate for their age (0.25 mL if aged 6–35 mths or 0.5 mL if aged ≥3 yrs). Children aged ≤8 yrs who are receiving influenza vaccine for the first time should receive 2 doses (separated by at least 4 wks for TIV and at least 6 wks for LAIV).
9. **Hepatitis A vaccine (HepA).** HepA is recommended for all children at 1 yr of age (i.e.,12–23 mths). The 2 doses in the series should be administered at least 6 mths apart. States, counties, and communities with existing HepA vaccination programs for children 2–18 yrs of age are encouraged to maintain these programs. In these areas, new efforts focused on routine vaccination of 1-year-old children should enhance, not replace, ongoing programs directed at a broader population of children. HepA is also recommended for certain high risk groups (see *MMWR* 1999; 48[RR-12]1-37).

ADHD/Narcolepsy Agents

NOREPINEPHRINE REUPTAKE INHIBITOR

Atomoxetine HCl (Strattera)	**Cap:** 10 mg, 18 mg, 25 mg, 40 mg, 60 mg	**ADHD: Adults & Peds: ≥6 yo & >70 kg: Initial:** 40 mg/d given qam or evenly divided doses in am & late afternoon/ early pm. **Titrate:** Increase after minimum of 3d to target dose of about 80 mg/d. After 2-4 wks, may increase to max of 100 mg/d. **Max:** 100 mg/d. **≥6 yo & ≤70 kg: Initial:** 0.5 mg/kg/d given qam or evenly divided doses in am & late afternoon/early pm. **Titrate:** Increase after minimum of 3d to target dose of about 1.2 mg/kg/d. **Max:** 1.4 mg/kg/d or 100 mg, whichever is less. Adjust w/ CYP450 2D6 inhibitors.	◙C ❁> **H** Increased risk of suicidal ideation in children or adolescents.

SYMPATHOMIMETICS

Amphetamine & Dextroamphetamine Mixture CII (Adderall, Adderall XR)	**Cap,ER:** 5 mg, 10 mg, 15 mg, 20 mg, 25 mg, 30 mg; **Tab:** 5 mg, 7.5 mg, 10 mg, 12.5 mg, 15 mg, 20 mg, 30 mg	**ADHD: Adderall: Peds: ≥6 yo:** 5 mg qd-bid. **Titrate:** May increase qwk by 5 mg. **Max:** 40 mg/d. **3-5 yo:** 2.5 mg qd. **Titrate:** May increase qwk by 2.5 mg until optimal response. **Adderall XR: Adults: Initial:** 20 mg qam. **Peds: ≥6 yo: Initial:** 10 mg qam. **Titrate:** May increase qwk by 5-10 mg/d. **Max:** 30 mg/d. **Peds: 13-17 yo: Initial:** 10 mg/d. **Titrate:** May increase to 20 mg/d after 1 wk. May switch from Adderall to Adderall XR at same total daily dose taken qd. **Narcolepsy: Adderall: Adults & Peds: ≥12 yo: Initial:** 10 mg/d. **Titrate:** May increase by 10 mg qwk. **Usual:** 5-60 mg/d. **6-12 yo: Initial:** 5 mg/d. **Titrate:** May increase by 5 mg qwk.	◙C ❁v [49]

[49] High potential for abuse; avoid prolonged use.

NAME	FORM/STRENGTH	DOSAGE	COMMENTS
Dexmethylphenidate HCl CII (Focalin, Focalin XR)	**Tab:** (Focalin) 2.5 mg, 5 mg, 10 mg; **Tab,ER:** (Focalin XR) 5 mg, 10 mg, 20 mg	**ADHD: Methylphenidate Naive: Focalin: Initial: Adults & Peds: ≥6 yo:** 2.5 mg bid at least 4 h apart. **Titrate:** May adjust wkly by 2.5-5 mg/d. **Max:** 20 mg/d. **Focalin XR: Initial: Adults:** 10 mg/d. **Titrate:** May adjust wkly by 10 mg/d. **Max:** 20 mg/d. **Peds: ≥6 yo:** 5 mg/d. **Titrate:** May adjust wkly by 5 mg/d. **Max:** 20 mg/d. **Currently on Methylphenidate: Focalin/Focalin XR: Initial:** Take 1/2 methylphenidate dose. **Max:** 20 mg/d. D/C if no improvement after 1 mth.	◙C ❀>
Dextroamphetamine CII (Dexedrine, Dexedrine Spansules, DextroStat)	**Cap,ER:** (Spansules) 5 mg, 10 mg, 15 mg; **Tab:** (Dexedrine) 5 mg, (DextroStat) 5 mg, 10 mg	**ADHD: Peds: ≥6 yo: Initial:** 5 mg qd-bid. **Titrate:** Increase qwk by 5 mg. **Max:** 40 mg/d. **3-5 yo: Initial:** 2.5 mg qd. **Titrate:** Increase qwk by 2.5 mg. **Narcolepsy: Adults & Peds: ≥12 yo: Initial:** 10 mg qd. **Titrate:** Increase qwk by 10 mg/d. **Usual:** 5-60 mg/d. **6-12 yo: Initial:** 5 mg/d. **Titrate:** Increase qwk by 5 mg. Give Cap,ER qd or tab q4-6h.	◙C ❀v High potential for abuse.
Methamphetamine HCl CII (Desoxyn)	**Tab:** 5 mg	**ADHD: Peds: ≥6 yo: Initial:** 5 mg qd-bid. **Titrate:** Increase by 5 mg qwk until optimum response. **Usual:** 20-25 mg/d given bid.	◙C ❀v High potential for abuse.
Methylphenidate CII (Concerta, Metadate CD, Metadate ER, Methylin, Methylin ER, Ritalin, Ritalin LA, Ritalin-SR)	**Cap,ER:** (Metadate CD) 10 mg, 20 mg, 30 mg, (Ritalin LA) 10 mg, 20 mg, 30 mg, 40 mg; **Sol:** (Methylin) 5 mg/5 ml, 10 mg/5 ml; **Tab:** (Methylin, Ritalin)	**ADHD: Adults: Ritalin/Methylin:** 10-60 mg/d divided bid-tid 30-45 min ac. **Peds: ≥6 yo: Ritalin/Methylin:** 5 mg bid. **Titrate:** May increase by 5-10 mg qwk. **Max:** 60 mg/d. **Ritalin LA: Initial:** 10-20 mg qam. **Titrate:** May adjust wkly by 10 mg increments. **Max:** 60 mg/d. **Concerta: Adults/Peds: ≥6 yo: Methylphenidate-Naive or Receiving Other Stimulant:**	◙C ❀> Caution with history of drug dependence or alcoholism.

	5 mg, 10 mg, 20 mg; **Chewtab:** (Methylin) 2.5 mg, 5 mg, 10 mg; **Tab,ER:** (Concerta) 18 mg, 27 mg, 36 mg, 54 mg, (Metadate ER, Methylin ER) 10 mg, 20 mg, (Ritalin-SR) 20 mg	**Initial:** 18 mg qam. **Titrate:** May adjust dose at weekly intervals. **Max: 6-12 yo:** 54 mg/d; **13-17 yo:** 72 mg/d not to exceed 2 mg/kg/d. **Previous Methylphenidate Use: Initial:** 18 mg qam if previous dose 10-15 mg/d; 36 mg qam if previous dose 20-30 mg/d; 54 mg qam if previous dose 30-45 mg/d. Initial conversion should not exceed 54 mg/day. **Titrate:** May adjust dose at wkly intervals. **Max:** 72 mg/day. **Metadate CD:** 20 mg qd. **Titrate:** May adjust by 10-20 mg increments wkly. **Max:** 60 mg/d. May use Ritalin-SR, Methylin ER, or Metadate ER when 8h extended-release dose corresponds to titrated 8h immediate-release dose.	
Methylphenidate CII (Daytrana)	**Patch:** 10 mg/9 h, 15 mg/9 h, 20 mg/9 h, 30 mg/9 h	**ADHD: Adults & Peds ≥6 yo:** Individualize dose. Apply to hip area 2 h before effect is needed and remove 9 h after application. **Recommended Titation Schedule: Week 1:** 10 mg/9 h. **Week 2:** 15 mg/9 h. **Week 3:** 20 mg/9 h. **Week 4:** 30 mg/9 h.	C > Caution with history of drug dependence or alcoholism.

MISCELLANEOUS

Modafinil CIV (Provigil)	**Tab:** 100 mg, 200 mg	**Adults & Peds: ≥ 16 yo:** 200 mg qd. **Narcolepsy/OSAHS:** Take in AM. **SWSD:** Take 1h prior to start of work shift.	C > **H**

Alzheimer's Therapy

CHOLINESTERASE INHIBITORS

Donepezil (Aricept, Aricept ODT)	**Sol:** 1 mg/ml; **Tab:** 5 mg, 10 mg; **Tab,Dissolve:** 5 mg, 10 mg	**Adults: Initial:** 5 mg qhs x 4-6 wks. **Maint:** 10 mg qd.	C v

NAME	FORM/STRENGTH	DOSAGE	COMMENTS
Galantamine HBr (Razadyne, Razadyne ER)	**Sol:** 4 mg/ml; **Tab:** 4 mg, 8 mg, 12 mg; **Tab,ER:** 8 mg, 16 mg, 24 mg	**Adults: Sol/Tab: Initial:** 4 mg bid with am & pm meals. **Titrate:** Increase to 8 mg bid after 4 wks if tolerated, then increase to 12 mg bid after 4 wks if tolerated. **Usual:** 16-24 mg/d. **Max:** 24 mg/d. **Tab,ER: Initial:** 8 mg qd w/ am meal. **Titrate:** Increase to 16 mg qd after 4 wks, then increase to 24 mg/d after 4 wks if tolerated. **Usual:** 16-24 mg/d. **Max:** 24 mg/d.	●B ❉v **H R**
Rivastigmine (Exelon)	**Cap:** 1.5 mg, 3 mg, 4.5 mg, 6 mg; **Sol:** 2 mg/ml	**Adults: Initial:** 1.5 mg bid. **Titrate:** May increase by 1.5 mg bid q2wks. **Max:** 12 mg/d. Suspend therapy if not tolerated. If interrupt longer than several days, reinitiate w/ lowest daily dose.	●B ❉v
Tacrine (Cognex)	**Cap:** 10 mg, 20 mg, 30 mg, 40 mg	**Adults: Initial:** 10 mg qid. **Titrate:** Increase to 20 mg qid after 4 wks, then increase at 4-wk intervals to 30 mg qid then to 40 mg qid if no significant transaminase elevations.	●C ❉> **H**
NMDA-RECEPTOR ANTAGONIST			
Memantine HCl (Namenda)	**Sol:** 2 mg/ml; **Tab:** 5 mg, 10 mg	**Adults: Initial:** 5 mg qd. **Maint:** 10 mg bid. **Titrate:** Increase at intervals no less than 1 wk to 10 mg/d (5 mg bid), 15 mg/d (5 mg & 10 mg as separate doses), then 20 mg/d (10 mg bid).	●B ❉> **R**

Antianxiety/Hypnotic Agents

BARBITURATES

NAME	FORM/STRENGTH	DOSAGE	COMMENTS
Pentobarbital CII (Nembutal Sodium)	**Inj:** 50 mg/ml	**Adults:** 150-200 mg IM. **Peds: Usual:** 2-6 mg/kg/24h IM. **Max:** 100 mg IM. Avoid IV use if possible.	●D ❉> **H R**

Phenobarbital CIV	**Eli:** 20 mg/5 ml; **Inj:** 30 mg/ml, 60 mg/ml, 65 mg/ml, 130 mg/ml; **Tab:** 15 mg, 30 mg, 32.4 mg, 60 mg, 64.8 mg, 97.2 mg, 100 mg	**Adults: Daytime Sedation:** 30-120 mg/d PO given in 2-3 doses, or IM/IV given in 2-9 doses. **Peds: Pre-op Sedation:** 1-3 mg/kg IM/IV.	D >
Secobarbital CII (Seconal)	**Cap:** 100 mg	**Adults: Hypnotic:** 100 mg qhs. **Peds: Pre-op:** 2-6 mg/kg. **Max:** 100 mg.	D > **H R**

BENZODIAZEPINES

Alprazolam CIV (Niravam, Xanax, Xanax XR)	**Tab,Dissolve (ODT):** (Niravam) 0.25 mg, 0.5 mg, 1 mg, 2 mg; **Tab:** (Xanax) 0.25 mg, 0.5 mg, 1 mg, 2 mg; **Tab,ER:** (Xanax XR) 0.5 mg, 1 mg, 2 mg, 3 mg	**Adults: Niravam/Xanax: Anxiety: Initial:** 0.25-0.5 mg tid. **Titrate:** May increase q3-4d. **Max:** 4 mg/d. **Panic Disorder: Initial:** 0.5 mg tid. **Titrate:** Increase by 1 mg/d q3-4d. **Usual:** 1-10 mg/d. **Xanax XR: Panic Disorder: Initial:** 0.5-1 mg qd, preferably in am. **Titrate:** Increase by 1 mg/d q3-4d. **Maint:** 1-10 mg/d. **Usual:** 3-6 mg/d.	D v **H**
Chlordiazepoxide CIV (Librium)	**Cap:** 5 mg, 10 mg, 25 mg; **Inj:** 100 mg	**Adults: Mild-Moderate Anxiety:** 5-10 mg PO tid-qid. **Severe Anxiety: Initial:** 20-25 mg PO tid-qid or 50-100 mg IM/IV. **Maint:** 5-25 mg PO tid-qid or 25-50 mg IM/IV tid-qid. **Peds: ≥6 yo: Initial:** 5 mg PO bid-qid. **Max:** 10 mg PO bid-tid. **≥12 yo: Acute/Severe Anxiety:** 25-50 mg PO, then 12.5-50 mg tid-qid prn.	N >

NAME	FORM/STRENGTH	DOSAGE	COMMENTS
Clorazepate CIV (Tranxene T-Tab, Tranxene-SD)	**Tab:** (T-Tab) 3.75 mg, 7.5 mg, 15 mg; **Tab,ER:** (SD) 11.25 mg, 22.5 mg	**Anxiety: Adults & Peds: >9 yo: Tab: Initial:** 15 mg qhs. **Usual:** 30 mg/d in divided doses. **Max:** 60 mg/d. **Tab,ER:** 22.5 mg qd if controlled on 7.5 mg tid or 11.25 mg qd if controlled on 3.75 mg tid.	N v
Diazepam CIV (Valium)	**Inj:** 5 mg/ml; **Tab:** 2 mg, 5 mg, 10 mg	**Anxiety: Adults: PO:** 2-10 mg bid-qid. **IM/IV:** (moderate) 2-5 mg or (severe) 5-10 mg, repeat in 3-4h if needed. **Peds: ≥6 mths: Initial:** 1-2.5 mg PO tid-qid.	N >
Estazolam CIV (ProSom)	**Tab:** 1 mg, 2 mg	**Insomnia: Adults: >18 yo: Initial:** 1 mg qhs. **Maint:** 1-2 mg qhs.	X v
Lorazepam CIV (Ativan)	**Tab:** 0.5 mg, 1 mg, 2 mg	**Adults & Peds: >12 yo: Anxiety: Initial:** 2-3 mg/d given bid-tid. **Usual:** 2-6 mg/d. **Insomnia:** 2-4 mg qhs.	N v
Midazolam CIV (Versed)	**Inj:** 1 mg/ml, 5 mg/ml; **Syr:** 2 mg/ml	**Sedation & Anxiolysis: Pre-op: Adults: <60 yo: IM:** 0.07-0.08 mg/kg (approx. 5 mg) IM. **IV:** Individualize dose. Up to 2.5 mg over 2 min, titrate as needed. **Max:** 5 mg. **Peds: PO:** 0.25-1 mg/kg single dose. **Max:** 20 mg/dose. **IM:** 0.1-0.15 mg/kg, up to 0.5 mg/kg. **Max:** 10 mg/dose. **IV: 12-16 yo:** Adult dose. **6-12 yo:** 0.025-0.05 mg/kg, up to 0.4 mg/kg. **Max:** 10 mg/dose. **6 mths-5 yo:** 0.05-0.1 mg/kg, up to 0.6 mg/kg. **Max:** 6 mg/dose.	D > Associated with respiratory depression & respiratory arrest.
Temazepam CIV (Restoril)	**Cap:** 7.5 mg, 15 mg, 22.5 mg, 30 mg	**Adults: ≥18 yo: Insomnia:** 7.5-30 mg qhs. **Transient Insomnia:** 7.5 mg qhs.	X >
Triazolam CIV (Halcion)	**Tab:** 0.125 mg, 0.25 mg	**Insomnia: Adults: ≥18 yo: Usual:** 0.25 mg qhs. **Max:** 0.25 mg qhs. **Low-weight Patients:** 0.125 mg qhs. **Max:** 0.25 mg qhs.	X v

SEROTONIN/NE REUPTAKE INHIBITORS

Venlafaxine (Effexor XR)	**Cap,ER:** 37.5 mg, 75 mg, 150 mg	**Generalized Anxiety Disorder/Social Anxiety Disorder: Adults: Initial:** 75 mg/d, or 37.5 mg/d increase to 75 mg/d after 4-7d. **Titrate:** Increase by 75 mg/d at intervals of no less than 4 d. **Max:** 225 mg/d. **Panic Disorder: Initial:** 37.5 mg/d x 7d. **Titrate:** Increase by 75 mg/d at intervals of no less than 7d. **Max:** 225 mg/d.	C v H R [29]

SSRIS

Escitalopram Oxalate (Lexapro)	**Sol:** 5 mg/5 ml; **Tab:** 5 mg, 10 mg, 20 mg	**Generalized Anxiety Disorder: Adults: Initial:** 10 mg qd, in am or pm. **Titrate:** May increase to 20 mg after at least 1 wk. **Elderly:** 10 mg qd.	C v H [29]
Fluoxetine (Prozac)	**Cap:** 10 mg, 20 mg, 40 mg; **Sol:** 20 mg/5ml; **Tab:** 10 mg	**Panic Disorder: Adults: Initial:** 10 mg/d. May increase to 20 mg/d after 1 wk. May increase further after several wks if needed. **Max:** 60 mg/d.	C v H [29]
Paroxetine HCl (Paxil, Paxil CR)	**Susp:** 10 mg/5 ml; **Tab:** 10 mg, 20 mg, 30 mg, 40 mg; **Tab,CR:** 12.5 mg, 25 mg, 37.5 mg	**Adults: Panic Disorder: Susp/Tab: Initial:** 10 mg qam. **Usual:** 40 mg/d. **Max:** 60 mg/d. **Social Anxiety Disorder: Susp/Tab: Initial/Usual:** 20 mg qam. **Tab,CR: Initial:** 12.5 mg/d. May increase wkly by 12.5 mg/d. **Max:** 37.5 mg/d. **GAD/PTSD: Initial:** 20 mg qam. **Usual:** 20-50 mg qam. May increase wkly by 10 mg/d. **Tab,CR: Panic Disorder: Initial:** 12.5 mg qam. May increase wkly by 12.5 mg/d. **Max:** 75 mg qam.	D > H R [29]
Paroxetine Mesylate (Pexeva)	**Tab:** 10 mg, 20 mg, 30 mg, 40 mg	**Panic Disorder: Adults: Initial:** 10 mg/d. **Titrate:** 10 mg/d wkly. **Max:** 40 mg/d.	C > H R [29]

29 Antidepressants may increase the risk of suicidality in children and adolescents.

NAME	FORM/STRENGTH	DOSAGE	COMMENTS
Sertraline (Zoloft)	**Tab:** 25 mg, 50 mg, 100 mg; **Sol:** 20 mg/ml	**Panic Disorder/Social Anxiety Disorder/PTSD: Adults: Initial:** 25 mg qd. **Titrate:** Increase to 50 mg qd after 1 wk. Adjust wkly. **Max:** 200 mg/d.	◙C ❁> H[29]
MISCELLANEOUS			
Buspirone (BuSpar, Vanspar)	**Tab:** (Buspar) 5 mg, 10 mg, 15 mg, 30 mg; (Vanspar) 7.5 mg	**Anxiety: Adults: ≥18 yo: Initial:** 7.5 mg bid. **Titrate:** Increase by 5 mg/d q2-3d. **Usual:** 20-30 mg/d. **Max:** 60 mg/d.	◙B ❁v
Chloral Hydrate CIV	**Cap:** 500 mg; **Sup:** 325 mg, 650 mg; **Syr:** 500 mg/5 ml	**Adults: Insomnia:** 500 mg-1 gm 15-30 min before retiring. **Sedative:** 250 mg tid. **Peds: Insomnia:** 50 mg/kg or 1.5 gm/m². **Max:** 1 gm. **Sedative:** 8 mg/kg or 250 mg/m² tid. **Max:** 500 mg tid.	◙C ❁>
Eszopiclone CIV (Lunesta)	**Tab:** 1 mg, 2 mg, 3 mg	**Insomnia: Adults 18-65 yo: Initial:** 2 mg qhs **Max:** 3 mg qhs. **≥65 yo: Difficulty Falling Asleep: Initial:** 1 mg qhs. **Max:** 2 mg qhs. **Difficulty Staying Asleep: Intial/Max:** 2 mg qhs.	◙C ❁> H
Ethchlorvynol CIV (Placidyl)	**Cap:** 500 mg, 750 mg	**Insomnia: Adults: Initial:** 500-750 mg qhs. **Max:** 1000 mg qhs.	◙C ❁v
Hydroxyzine (Atarax, Vistaril)	(Atarax) **Syr:** 10 mg/5 ml; (Generic) **Inj:** 25 mg/ml, 50 mg/ml; **Syr:** 10 mg /5 ml; **Tab:** 10 mg, 25 mg, 50 mg; (Vistaril) **Cap:** 25 mg, 50 mg;	**Anxiety: Adults: PO:** 50-100 mg qid. **Peds: PO: <6 yo:** 50 mg/d in divided doses. **>6 yo:** 50-100 mg/d in divided doses. **Psych/Emotional Emergency: Adults: IM:** 50-100 mg stat, then q4-6h prn.	◙N ❁v CI in early pregnancy.

	Susp: 25 mg/5 ml; (Generic) **Cap:** 25 mg, 50 mg, 100 mg; **Susp:** 25 mg/5 ml		
Meprobamate CIV (Miltown)	**Tab:** 200 mg, 400 mg	**Anxiety: Adults: Usual:** 1200-1600 mg/d given tid-qid. **Max:** 2400 mg/d. **6-12 yo:** 200-600 mg/d given bid-tid.	◙N ❁>
Ramelteon (Rozerem)	**Tab:** 8 mg	**Adults:** 8 mg within 30 min of bedtime. Do not take w/ or after high fat meal.	◙C ❁v **H**
Zaleplon CIV (Sonata)	**Cap:** 5 mg, 10 mg	**Insomnia: Adults:** 10 mg qhs. **Low-Wt Patients: Initial:** 5 mg qhs. **Max:** 20 mg qhs. **Debilitated Patients:** 5 mg qhs. **Max:** 10 mg qhs.	◙C ❁v **H**
Zolpidem Tartrate CIV (Ambien, Ambien CR)	**Tab:** 5 mg, 10 mg; **Tab,ER** 6.25 mg, 12.5 mg	**Insomnia: Adults: ≥18 yo:** 10 mg qhs. **Elderly/ Debilitated/Hepatic Insufficiency:** 5 mg qhs. Decrease dose w/ other CNS depressants. **Tab, ER:**12.5 mg qhs. **Elderly/Debilitated/Hepatic Insufficiency:** 6.25 mg qhs.	◙B (Ambien) ◙C (Ambien CR) ❁v **H**

Anticonvulsants

BENZODIAZEPINES

Clonazepam CIV (Klonopin)	**Tab:** 0.5 mg, 1 mg, 2 mg	**Seizure Disorder: Adults: Initial:** Up to 0.5 mg tid. **Titrate:** Increase by 0.5-1 mg q3d. **Max:** 20 mg/d. **Peds: Up to 10 yo or 30 kg: Initial:** 0.01-0.03 mg/kg/d (up to 0.05 mg/kg/d) given bid-tid. **Titrate:** Increase by 0.25-0.5 mg q3d. **Maint:** 0.1-0.2 mg/kg/d given tid.	◙D ❁v

29 Antidepressants may increase the risk of suicidality in children and adolescents.

NAME	FORM/STRENGTH	DOSAGE	COMMENTS
Diazepam CIV (Diastat, Valium)	(Diastat) **Rectal gel:** 2.5 mg, 5 mg, 10 mg, 15 mg, 20 mg; (Valium) **Inj:** 5 mg/ml; **Tab:** 2 mg, 5 mg, 10 mg	**Diastat:** 0.2-0.5 mg/kg rounded upward. **2-5 yo:** 0.5 mg/kg. **6-11 yo:** 0.3 mg/kg. **≥12 yo:** 0.2 mg/kg. May give 2nd dose 4-12h later. **Max:** 5 episodes/mth or 1 episode q5d. **Valium: PO: Adults:** 2-10 mg bid-qid. **Peds: ≥6 mths: Initial:** 1-2.5 mg tid-qid. **Status Epilepticus: IV: Adults: Initial:** 5-10 mg, may repeat q10-15min. **Max:** 30 mg. **Peds: 30 days-5 yo:** 0.2-0.5 mg, q2-5min. **Max:** 5 mg. **≥5 yo:** 1 mg q2-5min. **Max:** 10 mg.	◉D (Diastat) ◉N (Valium) ❋v (Diastat) ❋> (Valium)
Lorazepam CIV (Ativan)	**Inj:** 2 mg/ml, 4 mg/ml	**Status Epilepticus: Adults: ≥18 yo:** 2 mg/min IV x 2 min, may repeat x 1 dose after 10-15 min. **Max:** 8 mg.	◉D ❋v

HYDANTOIN DERIVATIVES

NAME	FORM/STRENGTH	DOSAGE	COMMENTS
Ethotoin (Peganone)	**Tab:** 250 mg	**Tonic-Clonic & Complex Partial Seizures: Adults:** Give q4-6h. **Initial:** 1 gm or less. **Titrate:** Increase over several days. **Maint:** 2-3 gm/d. **Peds:** Give q4-6h. **Initial:** Up to 750 mg/d. **Maint:** 500 mg-1 gm.	◉C ❋v
Fosphenytoin Sodium (Cerebyx)	**Inj:** 50 mg/ml	**Adults: LD:** 10-20 mg PE/kg IV/IM (≤150 mg PE/min). **Maint:** 4-6 mg PE/kg/d. **Status Epilepticus: LD:** 15-20 mg PE/kg; administer as 100-150 mg PE/min.	◉D ❋v **H R**
Phenytoin (Dilantin)	**Cap,ER:** 30 mg, 100 mg; **Chewtab:** 50 mg; **Susp:** 125 mg/5 ml	**Tonic-Clonic & Complex Partial Seizures/Seizure Treatment or Prevention w/ Neurosurgery: Adults: Cap,ER: Initial:** 100 mg tid-qid. **Titrate:** Increase q7-10d. **Max:** 200 mg tid. May give ER qd if controlled on 300 mg/d. **LD:** 400 mg PO, then 300 mg q2h	◉N ❋v

		x 2 doses (total 1 gm). Start maint 24h later. **Chewtab: Initial:** 100 mg tid. **Titrate:** Increase q7-10d. **Usual:** 300-400 mg/d. **Max:** 600 mg/d. **Susp: Initial:** 125 mg tid. **Titrate:** Increase q7-10d. **Max:** 625 mg/d. **Peds: Initial:** 5 mg/kg/d given bid-tid. **Titrate:** Increase q7-10d. **Maint:** 4-8 mg/kg/d. **Max:** 300 mg/d. **>6 yo:** May require min adult dose (300 mg/d).	

SUCCINIMIDES

Ethosuximide (Zarontin)	**Cap:** 250 mg; **Syr:** 250 mg/5 ml	**Absence Seizures: Adults & Peds: ≥6 yo:** 500 mg qd. **3-6 yo: Initial:** 250 mg qd. **Titrate:** Increase daily dose by 250 mg q4-7d. Usual optimal dose for peds is 20 mg/kg/d. **Max:** 1.5 gm/d.	◉N ❁>
Methsuximide (Celontin)	**Cap:** 150 mg, 300 mg	**Absence Seizures: Adults & Peds: Initial:** 300 mg qd x 7d. **Titrate:** Increase wkly by 300 mg/d wkly x 3 wks. **Max:** 1.2 gm/d.	◉N ❁>

SULFONAMIDE

Zonisamide (Zonegran)	**Cap:** 25 mg, 50 mg, 100 mg	**Partial Seizures: Adults & Peds: ≥16 yo: Initial:** 100 mg qd. **Titrate:** Increase by 100 mg q2wks, given qd-bid. **Max:** 400 mg/d.	◉C ❁v **H R**

NAME	FORM/STRENGTH	DOSAGE	COMMENTS
MISCELLANEOUS			
Carbamazepine (Carbatrol, Tegretol, Tegretol XR)	**Cap,ER:** (Carbatrol) 200 mg, 300 mg; **Chewtab:** 100 mg; **Susp:** 100 mg/5 ml; **Tab:** 200 mg; **Tab,ER:** (XR) 100 mg, 200 mg, 400 mg	**Partial/Tonic-Clonic/Mixed Seizures: Adults & Peds: ≥12 yo: Initial: Cap,ER/Chewtab/Tab/Tab,ER:** 200 mg bid. **Susp:** 100 mg qid. **Maint:** 800-1200 mg/d. **Max: >15 yo:** 1200 mg/d. **12-15 yo:** 1000 mg/d. **6 mths-12 yo: Cap,ER: Usual/Max:** ≤35 mg/kg/d. **6-12 yo: Chewtab/Tab/Tab,ER: Initial:** 100 mg bid. **Susp:** 50 mg qid. **Maint:** 400-800 mg/d. **Max:** 1000 mg/d. **6 mths-6 yo: Chewtab/Tab: Initial:** 10-20 mg/kg/d given bid-tid. **Susp:** 10-20 mg/kg/d given qid. **Max:** 35 mg/kg/d.	●D ✽v **H** Aplastic anemia. Agranulocytosis.
Divalproex Sodium (Depakote)	**Cap,Delay:** 125 mg; **Tab,Delay:** 125 mg, 250 mg, 500 mg	**Complex Partial Seizures: Adults & Peds: >10 yo: Initial:** 10-15 mg/kg/d. **Titrate:** Increase by 5-10 mg/kg/wk. **Max:** 60 mg/kg/d. **Absence Seizures: Adults: Initial:** 15 mg/kg/d. **Titrate:** Increase by 5-10 mg/kg/wk. **Max:** 60 mg/kg/d.	●D ✽v Hepatotoxic. Teratogenic. Pancreatitis.
Divalproex Sodium (Depakote ER)	**Tab,ER:** 250 mg, 500 mg	**Complex Partial Seizures: Adults & Peds: >10 yo: Initial:** 10-15 mg/kg qd. **Titrate:** Increase by 5-10 mg/kg/wk. **Usual:** <60 mg/kg/d. **Absence Seizures: Adults & Peds: >10 yo: Initial:** 15 mg/kg qd. **Titrate:** Increase by 5-10 mg/kg/wk. **Max:** 60 mg/kg/d.	●D ✽v Hepatotoxic. Teratogenic. Pancreatitis.
Felbamate (Felbatol)	**Susp:** 600 mg/5 ml; **Tab:** 400 mg, 600 mg	**Partial & Generalized Seizures: Adults & Peds: ≥14 yo: Initial:** 300 mg qid or 400 mg tid. **Max:** 3.6 gm/d. **Lennox-Gastaut Adjunct Therapy: Peds: 2-14 yo: Initial:** 15 mg/kg/d. **Titrate:** Increase wkly by 15 mg/kg/d to 45 mg/kg/d.	●C ✽> **H R** Hepatic failure. Aplastic anemia.

Gabapentin (Neurontin)	**Cap:** 100 mg, 300 mg, 400 mg; **Sol:** 250 mg/5 ml; **Tab:** 600 mg, 800 mg	**Partial Seizures: Adults & Peds: ≥12 yo: Initial:** 300 mg tid. **Titrate:** Increase up to 1.8 gm/d. **Max:** 3.6 gm/d. **3-12 yo: Initial:** 10-15 mg/kg/d given tid. **Titrate:** Increase over 3d. **Usual: ≥5 yo:** 25-35 mg/kg/d given tid. **3-4 yo:** 40 mg/kg/d given tid. **Max:** 50 mg/kg/d.	C > **R**
Lamotrigine (Lamictal, Lamictal CD)	**Chewtab:** (CD) 2 mg, 5 mg, 25 mg; **Tab:** 25 mg, 100 mg, 150 mg, 200 mg	**Lennox-Gastaut/Partial Seizures:** Special dosing requirements w/ VPA. **Adults & Peds: >12 yo: Concomitant EIAEDs w/ VPA:** 25 mg qod x 2 wks, then 25 mg qd x 2 wks. **Titrate:** Increase q1-2 wks by 25-50 mg/d. **Maint:** 100-400 mg/d, given qd or bid. **Concomitant EIAEDs w/o VPA:** 50 mg qd x 2 wks, then 50 mg bid x 2 wks. **Titrate:** Increase q1-2wks by 100 mg/d. **Maint:** 150-250 mg bid. **Conversion to Monotherapy from Single EIAED: ≥16 yrs:** 50 mg qd x 2 wks, then 50 mg bid x 2 wks. **Titrate:** Increase q1-2wks by 100 mg/d. **Maint:** 250 mg bid. Withdraw EIAED over 4 wks. **Conversion to Monotherapy from VPA: ≥16 yrs: Step 1:** Follow Concomitant AEDs w/ VPA dosing regimen to achieve Lamictal dose of 200 mg/d. Maintain previous VPA dose. **Step 2:** Maintain Lamictal 200 mg/d. Decrease VPA to 500 mg/d by decrements of ≤500 mg/d per wk. Maintain VPA 500 mg/d x 1 wk. **Step 3:** Increase to Lamictal 300 mg/d x 1 wk. Decrease VPA simultaneously to 250 mg/d x 1 wk. **Step 4:** D/C VPA. Increase Lamictal 100 mg/d every wk to maint dose of 500 mg/d. **Peds: 2-12 yo: ≥6.7 kg: Concomitant EIAEDs w/o VPA:** 0.3 mg/kg bid x 2 wks, then 0.6 mg/kg bid x 2 wks. **Titrate:** Increase q1-2wks by 1.2 mg/kg/d. **Maint:** 2.5-7.5 mg/kg bid. **Max:** 400 mg/d. Round dose down to nearest whole tab.	C v **H R** Serious rashes, Stevens-Johnson syndrome reported.

NAME	FORM/STRENGTH	DOSAGE	COMMENTS
Levetiracetam (Keppra)	**Sol:** 100 mg/ml; **Tab:** 250 mg, 500 mg, 750 mg	**Partial Onset Seizures: Adults & Peds: ≥16 yo: Initial:** 500 mg bid. **Titrate:** Increase q2wks by 1000 mg/d. **Max:** 3 gm/d. **Peds: ≥4-<16 yo: Initial:** 10 mg/kg bid. **Titrate:** Increase q2wks by 20 mg/kg/d. **Maint:** 30 mg/kg bid.	C > R
Magnesium Sulfate	**Inj:** 40 mg/ml, 80 mg/ml	**Nephritic Seizures: Peds:** 20-40 mg/kg IM to control seizures.	A >
Oxcarbazepine (Trileptal)	**Susp:** 300 mg/5 ml; **Tab:** 150 mg, 300 mg, 600 mg	**Partial Seizures: Monotherapy: Adults: Initial:** 300 mg bid. **Titrate:** Increase by 300 mg/d q3d. **Maint:** 1200 mg/d. **4-16 yo: Initial:** 4-5 mg/kg bid. **Titrate:** Increase by 5 mg/kg/d q3d. **Maint (mg/d): 20 kg: Initial:** 600 mg. **Max:** 900 mg. **25-30 kg: Initial:** 900 mg. **Max:** 1200 mg. **35-40 kg: Initial:** 900 mg. **Max:** 1500 mg. **45 kg: Initial:** 1200 mg. **Max:** 1500 mg. **50-55 kg: Initial:** 1200 mg. **Max:** 1800 mg. **60-65 kg: Initial:** 1200 mg. **Max:** 2100 mg. **70 kg: Initial:** 1500 mg. **Max:** 2100 mg. **Adjunct Therapy: Adults: Initial:** 300 mg bid. **Titrate:** Increase wkly by max of 600 mg/d. **Maint:** 600 mg bid. **4-16 yo: Initial:** 4-5 mg/kg bid. **Max:** 600 mg/d. **Titrate:** Increase over 2 wks. **Maint (mg/d): 20-29 kg:** 900 mg. **29.1-39 kg:** 1200 mg. **>39 kg:** 1800 mg. **Conversion to Monotherapy: Adults: Initial:** 300 mg bid while reducing other AEDs. **Titrate:** Increase wkly by 600 mg/d. **Maint:** 2400 mg/d. **4-16 yo: Initial:** 4-5 mg/kg bid while reducing other AEDs. **Titrate:** Increase wkly by max of 10 mg/kg/d to target dose. Withdraw other AEDs over 3-6 wks.	C v R

Pregabalin CV (Lyrica)	**Cap:** 25 mg, 50 mg, 75 mg, 100 mg, 150 mg, 200 mg, 225 mg, 300 mg	**Partial Seizures: Adults: Initial:** 150 mg/d divided bid-tid. **Max:** 600 mg/d.	C v R
Primidone (Mysoline)	**Tab:** 50 mg, 250 mg	**Grand Mal/Psychomotor/Focal Seizures: Adults & Peds: ≥8 yo: Initial/Titrate: Days 1-3:** 100-125 mg qhs. **Days 4-6:** 100-125 mg bid. **Days 7-9:** 100-125 mg tid. **Day 10-Maint:** 250 mg tid. **Max:** 500 mg qid. **<8 yo: Initial/Titrate: Days 1-3:** 50 mg qhs. **Days 4-6:** 50 mg bid. **Days 7-9:** 100 mg bid. **Day 10-Maint:** 125-250 mg tid or 10-25 mg/kg/d in divided doses.	N >
Tiagabine (Gabitril)	**Tab:** 2 mg, 4 mg, 6 mg, 8 mg, 10 mg, 12 mg, 16 mg	**Partial Seizures: Adjunctive Therapy: Adults: Initial:** 4 mg qd. **Titrate:** May increase weekly by 4-8 mg until clinical response. **Max:** 56 mg/d. Give in divided doses bid-qid. Take with food.**Peds: 12-18 yo: Initial:** 4 mg qd. **Titrate:** May increase to 8 mg qd at beginning of Week 2, then increase weekly by 4-8 mg until clinical response. **Max:** 32 mg/d. Give in divided doses bid-qid. Take with food.	C >
Topiramate (Topamax)	**Cap:** 15 mg, 25 mg; **Tab:** 25 mg, 50 mg, 100 mg, 200 mg	**Partial Onset/Tonic-Clonic Seizures: Monotherapy: Adults & Peds: ≥10 yo: Initial:** 25 mg qam & qpm for 1 wk. **Titrate:** Increase am & pm dose by 25 mg qwk until 200 mg qam & qpm. **Partial Onset/Tonic-Clonic/Lennox-Gastaut Seizures: Adjunctive Therapy: Adults & Peds: ≥17 yo: Initial:** 25-50 mg qd. **Titrate:** Increase qwk by 25-50 mg. **Usual:** 100-200 mg bid (partial seizures) or 200 mg bid (tonic-clonic seizures). **Max:** 1600 mg/d. **Peds: 2-16 yo: Initial:**61-3 mg/kg/d qpm x 1 wk. **Titrate:** Increase by 1-3 mg/kg/d q1-2wks. **Usual:** 5-9 mg/kg/d given as bid.	C > R

NAME	FORM/STRENGTH	DOSAGE	COMMENTS
Valproate Sodium (Depacon)	**Inj:** 100 mg/ml	**Complex Partial Seizure: Adults & Peds: ≥10 yo: IV: Initial:** 10-15 mg/kg/d. **Titrate:** Increase wkly by 5-10 mg/kg/d. **Max:** 60 mg/kg/d. **Simplex/Complex Absence Seizure: Adults: IV: Initial:** 15 mg/kg/d. **Titrate:** Increase wkly by 5-10 mg/kg/d. **Max:** 60 mg/kg/d.	D v **H** Hepatic failure. Teratogenic. Pancreatitis.
Valproic Acid (Depakene)	**Cap:** 250 mg; **Syr:** 250 mg/5 ml	**Complex Partial Seizure: Adults & Peds: ≥10 yo: Initial:** 10-15 mg/kg/d. **Titrate:** Increase wkly by 5-10 mg/kg/d. **Max:** 60 mg/kg/d. **Simplex/Complex Absence Seizure: Adults: Initial:** 15 mg/kg/d. **Titrate:** Increase wkly by 5-10 mg/kg/d. **Max:** 60 mg/kg/d.	D v **H** Hepatic failure. Teratogenic. Pancreatitis.

Antidepressant Agents

DOPAMINE/NOREPINEPHRINE REUPTAKE INHIBITOR

NAME	FORM/STRENGTH	DOSAGE	COMMENTS
Bupropion HCl (Wellbutrin XL)	**Tab,ER:** 150 mg, 300 mg	**Adults: ≥18 yo: Initial:** 150 mg qam, may increase to 300 mg qam after 3d. **Usual:** 300 mg qam. **Max:** 450 mg qam. Swallow whole.	B v **H R** 29
Bupropion (Wellbutrin, Wellbutrin SR)	**Tab:** 75 mg, 100 mg; **Tab,ER:** 100 mg, 150 mg, 200 mg	**Adults: ≥18 yo: Tab: Initial:** 100 mg bid. **Maint:** 100 mg tid. **Max:** 450 mg/d. **Tab,ER: Initial:** 150 mg qam. **Maint:** 150 mg bid. **Max:** 200 mg bid.	B v **H R** 29

MAOIS

NAME	FORM/STRENGTH	DOSAGE	COMMENTS
Phenelzine (Nardil)	**Tab:** 15 mg	**Adults & Peds: ≥16 yo: Initial:** 15 mg tid. **Titrate/Maint:** Increase to 60-90 mg/d until max benefit, then reduce dose to 15 mg qd or 15 mg qod.	N > 29

Selegiline (Emsam)	**Patch:** 6 mg/24 h, 9 mg/24 h, 12 mg/24 h	**Adults:** Apply to dry, intact skin on the upper torso, upper thigh, or outer surface of upper arm once every 24 h. **Initial/Target Dose:** 6 mg/24 h. **Titrate:** May increase in increments of 3 mg/24 h at intervals no less than 2 wks. **Max:** 12 mg/24 h. **Elderly:** 6 mg/24 h. Increase dose cautiously and monitor closely.	◙ C ❁> [29]
Tranylcypromine (Parnate)	**Tab:** 10 mg	**Adults: Initial:** 30 mg/d in divided doses. **Titrate:** Increase by 10 mg/d q1-3wks. **Max:** 60 mg/d.	◙N ❁> [29]
SEROTONIN/NOREPINEPHRINE REUPTAKE INHIBITORS			
Duloxetine (Cymbalta)	**Cap,Delay:** 20 mg, 30 mg, 60 mg	**Adults: Initial:** 40 mg/d (given as 20 mg bid) to 60 mg/d (given once daily or as 30 mg bid). Re-evaluate periodically. Do not chew or crush.	◙C ❁v **H R** [29]
Venlafaxine (Effexor, Effexor XR)	**Cap,ER:** 37.5 mg, 75 mg, 150 mg; **Tab:** 25 mg, 37.5 mg, 50 mg, 75 mg, 100 mg	**Adults: ≥18 yo: Tab: Initial:** 37.5 mg bid or 25 mg tid. **Titrate:** Increase by 75 mg/d q4d to 150-225 mg/d. **Max:** 375 mg/d. **Cap,ER: Initial:** 75 mg/d. **Titrate:** Increase by 75 mg/d at intervals not less than 4d. **Max:** 225 mg/d.	◙C ❁v **H R** [29]
SSRIS			
Citalopram (Celexa)	**Sol:** 10 mg/5 ml; **Tab:** 10 mg, 20 mg, 40 mg	**Adults: Initial:** 20 mg qd, in am or pm. **Titrate:** May increase by 20 mg at intervals ≥1 wk, to 40 mg/d. **Max:** 60 mg/d.	◙C ❁v **H** [29]

[29] Antidepressants may increase the risk of suicidality in children and adolescents.

NAME	FORM/STRENGTH	DOSAGE	COMMENTS
Escitalopram Oxalate (Lexapro)	**Sol:** 5 mg/5 ml; **Tab:** 5 mg, 10 mg, 20 mg	**Adults: Initial:** 10 mg qd, in am or pm. **Titrate:** May increase to 20 mg after at least 1 wk. **Elderly:** 10 mg qd.	◙C ❄v **H** 29
Fluoxetine (Prozac)	**Cap:** 10 mg, 20 mg, 40 mg; **Sol:** 20 mg/5 ml; **Tab:** 10 mg	**Adults: Daily Dosing: Initial:** 20 mg qam. **Titrate:** Increase dose if no improvement after several wks. Doses >20 mg/d, give qam or bid (am & noon). **Max:** 80 mg/d. **Peds: ≥8 yo: Higher Wt Peds: Initial:** 10 or 20 mg/d. After 1 wk at 10 mg/d, may increase to 20 mg/d. **Lower Wt Peds: Initial:** 10 mg/d. **Titrate:** May increase to 20 mg/d after several wks if clinical improvement not observed.	◙C ❄v **H** 29
Fluoxetine (Prozac Weekly)	**Cap,ER:** 90 mg	**Adults: Initial:** One 90 mg cap 7d after the last daily dose of Prozac 20 mg. Must be stabilized on 20 mg/d prior to initiation.	◙C ❄v **H** 29
Paroxetine HCl (Paxil, Paxil CR)	**Susp:** 10 mg/5 ml; **Tab:** 10 mg, 20 mg, 30 mg, 40 mg; **Tab,CR:** 12.5 mg, 25 mg, 37.5 mg	**Adults: Susp/Tab: Initial:** 20 mg qam. **Max:** 50 mg/d. **Tab,CR: Initial:** 25 mg/d. **Titrate:** May increase wkly by 12.5 mg/d. **Max:** 62.5 mg/d.	◙D ❄> **H R** 29
Paroxetine Mesylate (Pexeva)	**Tab:** 10 mg, 20 mg, 30 mg, 40 mg	**Adults: Initial:** 20 mg/d. **Max:** 50 mg/d.	◙C ❄> **H R** 29
Sertraline (Zoloft)	**Sol:** 20 mg/ml; **Tab:** 25 mg, 50 mg, 100 mg	**Adults: Initial:** 50 mg qd. **Titrate:** Adjust wkly. **Max:** 200 mg/d.	◙C ❄> **H** 29

TETRACYCLICS

Maprotiline	**Tab:** 25 mg, 50 mg, 75 mg	**Adults: Outpatients: Initial:** 25-75 mg qd x 2 wks. **Maint:** Increase by 25 mg. **Max:** 225 mg/d. **Adults: Hospitalized: Initial:** 100-150 mg qd. **Maint:** 150-225 mg/d. **Max:** 225 mg/d.	B > 29
Mirtazapine (Remeron, Remeron SolTab)	**Tab,Dissolve:** 15 mg, 30 mg, 45 mg; **Tab:** 15 mg, 30 mg, 45 mg	**Adults: Initial:** 15 mg qhs. **Titrate:** Increase q1-2wks. **Maint:** 15-45 mg qd. **Max:** 45 mg qd.	C > 29

TRICYCLIC ANTIDEPRESSANTS

Amitriptyline	**Inj:** 10 mg/ml; **Tab:** 10 mg, 25 mg, 50 mg, 75 mg, 100 mg, 150 mg	**Adults: PO: Initial:** (Outpatient) 75 mg/d in divided doses or 50-100 mg qhs. (Inpatient) 100 mg/d. **Titrate:** (Outpatient) Increase by 25-50 mg qhs. (Inpatient) Increase to 200 mg/d. **Maint:** 50-100 mg qhs. **Max:** (Outpatient) 150 mg/d. (Inpatient) 300 mg/d. **Peds: ≥12 yo & Elderly:** 10 mg tid or 20 mg qhs. **Adults & Peds: ≥12 yo: IM: Initial:** 20-30 mg qid.	C v 29
Amoxapine	**Tab:** 25 mg, 50 mg, 100 mg, 150 mg	**Adults & Peds: ≥16 yo: Initial:** 50 mg bid-tid. **Titrate:** Increase to 100 mg bid-tid. **Maint:** Effective dose given qhs. **Max:** 300 mg/d.	C > 29
Desipramine HCl (Norpramin)	**Tab:** 10 mg, 25 mg, 50 mg, 75 mg, 100 mg, 150 mg	**Adults: Usual:** 100-200 mg qd. **Max:** 300 mg/d. **Adolescents: Usual:** 25-100 mg qd. **Max:** 150 mg/d.	N > 29

29 Antidepressants may increase the risk of suicidality in children and adolescents.

NAME	FORM/STRENGTH	DOSAGE	COMMENTS
Doxepin (Sinequan)	(Generic) **Cap:** 10 mg, 25 mg, 50 mg, 75 mg, 100 mg, 150 mg; **Sol:** 10 mg/ml; (Sinequan) **Cap:** 10 mg, 25 mg, 50 mg, 75 mg	**Adults & Peds: ≥12 yo: Mild Illness: Usual:** 25-50 mg/d. **Mild-Moderate: Initial:** 75 mg/d. **Usual:** 75-150 mg/d. **Severely Ill:** Up to 300 mg/d.	●N ❀> 29
Imipramine HCl (Tofranil)	**Tab:** 10 mg, 25 mg, 50 mg	**Adults: Initial:** (Inpatients) 100 mg/d; may increase to 200 mg/d x 2 wks, then 250-300 mg/d if needed. (Outpatients) 75 mg/d; may increase to 150 mg/d, then to 200 mg/d if needed. **Maint:** 50-150 mg/d. **Adolescents: Initial:** 30-40 mg qhs. **Max:** 100 mg/d.	●N ❀v 29
Imipramine Pamoate (Tofranil-PM)	**Cap:** 75 mg, 100 mg, 125 mg, 150 mg	**Adults: Initial:** (Inpatients) 100-150 mg/d; may increase to 200 mg/d x 2 wks, then 250-300 mg/d if needed. (Outpatients) 75 mg/d; may increase to 150 mg/d, then to 200 mg/d if needed. **Maint:** 75-150 mg/d. **Adolescents:** May use if daily dose ≥75 mg.	●N ❀v 29
Nortriptyline HCl (Pamelor)	**Cap:** 10 mg, 25 mg, 50 mg, 75 mg; **Sol:** 10 mg/5 ml	**Adults: Usual:** 25 mg tid-qid. **Max:** 150 mg/d. **Adolescents:** 30-50 mg/d.	●N ❀> 29
Protriptyline HCl (Vivactil)	**Tab:** 5 mg, 10 mg	**Adults: Initial:** 15-40 mg/d given tid-qid. **Max:** 60 mg/d. **Adolescents: Initial:** 5 mg tid. **Maint:** Increase gradually if necessary.	●N ❀> 29

Trimipramine Maleate (Surmontil)	**Cap:** 25 mg, 50 mg, 100 mg	**Adults: Outpatients: Initial:** 75 mg/d in divided doses. **Maint:** 50-150 mg/d. **Max:** 200 mg/d. **Adults: Inpatients: Initial:** 100 mg/d in divided doses. **Titrate:** Increase gradually to 200 mg/d. **Max:** 250-300 mg/d. **Adolescents: Initial:** 50 mg/d. **Max:** 100 mg/d.	C ❋> [29]

MISCELLANEOUS

Trazodone (Desyrel)	**Tab:** 50 mg, 100 mg, 150 mg, 300 mg	**Adults: ≥18 yo: Initial:** 150 mg/d in divided doses. **Titrate:** Increase by 50 mg/d q3-4d. **Max:** (Outpatients) 400 mg/d, (Inpatients) 600 mg/d.	C ❋> [29]

Antiparkinson's Agents

ANTICHOLINERGIC AGENTS

Benztropine Mesylate	**Inj:** 1 mg/ml; **Tab:** 0.5 mg, 1 mg, 2 mg	**Adults: Initial:** 0.5-1 mg PO/IV/IM qhs. **Usual:** 1-2 mg/d. **Max:** 6 mg/d.	N ❋>
Trihexyphenidyl	**Eli:** 2 mg/5 ml; **Tab:** 2 mg, 5 mg	**Adults: Idiopathic:** 1 mg on Day 1. **Titrate:** Increase by 2 mg q3-5d. **Usual:** 6-10 mg/d. **Max:** 15 mg/d. **Drug-Induced: Initial:** 1 mg, increase until achieve control. **Usual:** 5-15 mg/d.	N ❋>

COMT INHIBITOR

Entacapone (Comtan)	**Tab:** 200 mg	**Adults:** 200 mg w/ each levodopa/carbidopa dose. **Max:** 1600 mg/d.	C ❋>

29 Antidepressants may increase the risk of suicidality in children and adolescents.

NAME	FORM/STRENGTH	DOSAGE	COMMENTS
Tolcapone (Tasmar)	**Tab:** 100 mg, 200 mg	**Adults: Initial:** 100 mg tid. Use 200 mg tid if clinical benefit justified. May need to decrease levodopa dose.	◙C ❋> Risk of acute fulminant liver failure.
DOPAMINE AGONISTS			
Apomorphine HCl (Apokyn)	**Inj:** 10 mg/ml	**Adults: Initial: Test Dose** 2 mg SC; closely monitor BP. **Titrate:** Increase by 1 mg q few days. **Max:** 6 mg/d. **Renal Impairment: Initial:** 1 mg SC.	◙C ❋v **R** CI with $5HT_3$ antagonists
Bromocriptine Mesylate (Parlodel)	**Cap:** 5 mg; **Tab:** 2.5 mg	**Adults: Initial:** 1.25 mg bid. **Titrate:** Increase by 2.5 mg/d q2-4wks. **Max:** 100 mg/d.	◙B ❋v
Pergolide Mesylate (Permax)	**Tab:** 0.05 mg, 0.25 mg, 1 mg	**Adults: Initial:** 0.05 mg/d for 1st 2d. **Titrate:** Increase by 0.1-0.15 mg/d q3d over next 12d, then increase by 0.25 mg/d q3d. **Max:** 5 mg/d. Give in 3 divided doses.	◙B ❋v
Pramipexole (Mirapex)	**Tab:** 0.125 mg, 0.25 mg, 0.5 mg, 1 mg, 1.5 mg	**Adults: Initial:** 0.125 mg tid. **Titrate:** Increase q5-7d according to titration table. **Maint:** 0.5-1.5 mg tid.	◙C ❋v **R**
Ropinirole HCl (Requip)	**Tab:** 0.25 mg, 0.5 mg, 1 mg, 2 mg, 3 mg, 4 mg, 5 mg	**Adults: Initial:** 0.25 mg tid. **Titrate/Maint:** Increase wkly by 0.25 mg tid x 4 wks. After wk 4, increase wkly by 1.5 mg/d up to 9 mg/d, then by 3 mg/d wkly to 24 mg/d.	◙C ❋v

DOPAMINE PRECURSOR/DOPA-DECARBOXYLASE INHIBITOR

Carbidopa/Levodopa (Parcopa, Sinemet, Sinemet CR)	**Tab:** (Sinemet) 10-100 mg, 25-100 mg, 25-250 mg; **Tab,Dissolve:** (Parcopa) 10-100 mg, 25-100 mg, 25-250 mg; **Tab,ER:** (Sinemet CR) 25-100 mg, 50-200 mg.	**Adults: ≥18 yo: Tab/Tab,Dissolve: Initial:** 10-100 mg tid-qid or 25-100 mg tid. **Titrate:** May increase by 1 tab qd or qod until 8 tabs/d. **Maint:** 70-100 mg/d carbidopa required. **Max:** 200 mg/d carbidopa. **Tab,ER: No Prior Levodopa Use: Initial:** 1 tab 50-200 mg bid at intervals ≥6 hrs. Do not chew or crush. **Titrate:** Increase/decrease dose or interval accordingly. Adjust dose q3d. **Usual:** 400-1600 mg/d levodopa, given in 4-8 hr intervals while awake. **Conversion to Extended-Release Tabs:** See labeling.	◙C ❃>

DOPAMINE PRECURSOR/DOPA-DECARBOXYLASE INHIBITOR/COMT INHIBITOR

Carbidopa/Levodopa/ Entacapone (Stalevo 50, Stalevo 100, Stalevo 150)	**Tab:** 12.5/50/200 mg, 25/100/200 mg, 37.5/150/200 mg	**Adults: Currently Taking Carbidopa/Levodopa & Entacapone:** May switch directly to corresponding strength of levodopa/carbidopa. **Currently Taking Carbidopa/Levodopa but not Entacapone:** First titrate individually w/ carbidopa/levodopa product & entacapone product then transfer to corresponding dose. **Max:** 8 tabs/d.	◙C ❃>

MAOIS

Rasagiline (Azilect)	**Tab:** 0.5 mg, 1 mg	**Adults: Monotherapy:** 1 mg qd. **Adjunctive Therapy: Initial:** 0.5 mg qd. **Titrate:** May increase to 1 mg qd. Adjust dose of levodopa with concomitant use. **Concomitant Ciprofloxacin or Other CYP1A2 Inhibitors/Hepatic Impairment:** 0.5 mg qd.	◙C ❃> H

NAME	FORM/STRENGTH	DOSAGE	COMMENTS
Selegeline HCl (Eldepryl)	**Cap:** 5 mg	**Adults:** 5 mg bid, at breakfast & lunch. **Max:** 10 mg/d.	◙C ❋v

Antipsychotic Agents

BENZISOXAZOLE DERIVATIVE

NAME	FORM/STRENGTH	DOSAGE	COMMENTS
Risperidone (Risperdal, Risperdal Consta, Risperdal M-Tab)	**Inj:** 25 mg, 37.5 mg, 50 mg; **Sol:** 1 mg/ml; **Tab:** 0.25 mg, 0.5 mg, 1 mg, 2 mg, 3 mg, 4 mg; **Tab,Dissolve:** 0.5 mg, 1 mg, 2 mg, 3 mg, 4 mg	**Schizophrenia: Adults: Inj:** 25 mg IM q2wks. **Max:** 50 mg/dose. Give 1st inj w/ oral dosage form or other oral antipsychotic. Continue x 3 wks, then d/c oral. **Titrate:** Increase at intervals of no more than q4wks. **PO: Initial:** 1 mg bid. **Maint:** 2-8 mg/d given qd-bid. **Max:** 16 mg/d.	◙C ❋v **H R** 30
Ziprasidone (Geodon)	**Cap:** 20 mg, 40 mg, 60 mg, 80 mg; **Inj:** 20 mg/ml	**Schizophrenia: Adults: Initial: PO:** 20 mg bid w/ food. **Max:** 80 mg bid. **Acute Agitation: IM:** 10 mg q2h or 20 mg q4h up to 40 mg/d x 3d.	◙C ❋v 30

BUTYROPHENONES

NAME	FORM/STRENGTH	DOSAGE	COMMENTS
Haloperidol (Haldol, Haldol Decanoate)	(Haldol) **Inj:** (decanoate) 50 mg/ml, 100 mg/ml, (lactate) 5 mg/ml; (Generic) **Cnt:** 2 mg/ml; **Inj:** (decanoate) 50 mg/ml, 100 mg/ml, (lactate) 5 mg/ml; **Tab:** 0.5 mg, 1 mg, 2 mg, 5 mg, 10 mg, 20 mg	**Adults: Usual: PO:** 0.5-5 mg bid-tid. **IM:** (Lactate) 2-5 mg q4-8h or q1h prn. **Max:** 100 mg/d. (Decanoate) Give q4wks. 10-20x daily PO dose up to 100 mg. Give remainder of dose 3-7d later if initial dose >100 mg. **Peds: 3-12 yo (15-40 kg): PO:** 0.05-0.15 mg/kg/d given bid-tid. **Max:** 6 mg/d.	◙C ❋v

Clozapine (Clozaril)	**Tab:** 12.5 mg, 25 mg, 100 mg	**Schizophrenia/Suicidal Behavior Risk Reduction: Adults: Initial:** 12.5 mg qd-bid. **Titrate:** Increase by 25-50 mg/d, up to 300-450 mg/d by end of 2nd wk, then increase wkly or bi-wkly by up to 100 mg. **Usual:** 100-900 mg/d given tid. **Max:** 900 mg/d. If at risk of suicial behavior then treat for at least 2 yrs then assess; reassess thereafter at regular intervals. To d/c, gradually reduce dose over 1-2 wks.	◙B ❁v [26, 30]
Clozapine (Fazaclo)	**Tab,Dissolve:** 25 mg, 100 mg	**Schizophrenia: Adults: Initial:** 12.5 mg qd-bid. **Titrate:** Increase by 25-50 mg/d, up to 300-450 mg/d by end of 2nd wk, then increase wkly or bi-wkly by up to 100 mg. **Ususal:** 100-900 mg/d given tid. **Max:** 900 mg/d. To d/c, gradually reduce dose over 1-2 wks.	◙B ❁v [26]
Loxapine (Loxitane)	**Cap:** 5 mg, 10 mg, 25 mg, 50 mg; **Cnt:** 25 mg/ml; **Inj:** 50 mg/ml	**Adults: PO: Initial:** 10 mg bid, up to 50 mg/d for severely disturbed. **Titrate:** Increase rapidly over 7-10d. **Maint:** 60-100 mg/d. **Max:** 250 mg/d. **IM:** 12.5-50 mg q4-6h. Individualize dose.	◙N ❁v
Olanzapine (Zyprexa, Zyprexa Zydis, Zyprexa IntraMuscular)	**Inj:** 10 mg; **Tab:** 2.5 mg, 5 mg, 7.5 mg, 10 mg, 15 mg, 20 mg; **Tab,Dissolve:** 5 mg, 10 mg, 15 mg, 20 mg	**Schizophrenia: Adults: PO: Initial/Usual:** 5-10 mg qd. **Titrate:** Adjust wkly by 5 mg/d. **Max:** 20 mg/d. **Agitation Associated w/ Schizophrenia: Inj: Initial:** 10 mg IM. **Range:** 2.5-10 mg IM. **Max:** 3 doses of 10 mg IM q2-4h. May initiate PO therapy when clinically appropriate.	◙C ❁v [30]

26 Risk of agranulocytosis, seizures, myocarditis, other cardiovascular/respiratory effects. Increased mortality in elderly patients with dementia-related psychosis.

30 Increased risk of death in elderly patients with dementia-related psychosis.

NAME	FORM/STRENGTH	DOSAGE	COMMENTS
Quetiapine Fumarate (Seroquel)	**Tab:** 25 mg, 50 mg, 100 mg, 200 mg, 300 mg, 400 mg	**Schizophrenia: Adults: Initial:** 25 mg bid. **Titrate:** Increase by 25-50 mg bid-tid daily on Day 2 & Day 3, up to target dose of 300-400 mg/d by Day 4. May adjust by 25-50 mg bid q2d thereafter. **Max:** 800 mg/d.	◙C ❀v H 30
DIHYDROINDOLONE DERIVATIVES			
Molindone (Moban)	**Tab:** 5 mg, 10 mg, 25 mg, 50 mg	**Adults & Peds: ≥12 yo: Initial:** 50-75 mg/d. **Titrate:** Increase to 100 mg/d in 3-4d, & adjust to patient response. **Maint:** (mild) 5-15 mg tid-qid, (moderate) 10-25 mg tid-qid, (severe) 225 mg/d.	◙N ❀>
PARTIAL D2/5HT1A AGONIST/5HT2A ANTAGONIST			
Aripiprazole (Abilify)	**Sol:** 1 mg/ml; **Tab:** 2 mg, 5 mg, 10 mg, 15 mg, 20 mg, 30 mg	**Schizophrenia: Adults: Initial/Target:** 10-15 mg qd. **Titrate:** Should not increase before 2 wks. **Maint:** Periodically reassess need for therapy. Oral solution can be given on a mg-per-mg basis up to 25 mg. Patients receiving 30 mg tablets should receive 25 mg of solution. Adjust dose w/ CYP3A4 inducers/inhibitors or w/ CYP2D6 inhibitors.	◙C ❀v 30
PHENOTHIAZINES			
Chlorpromazine	**Cap,ER:** 30 mg, 75 mg, 150 mg; **Inj:** 25 mg/ml; **Sup:** 25 mg, 100 mg; **Syr:** 10 mg/5 ml; **Tab:** 10 mg, 25 mg, 50 mg, 100 mg, 200 mg	**Adults: Inpatient: Acute State:** 25 mg IM, then 25-50 mg IM in 1h if needed. **Titrate:** Increase up to 400 mg q4-6h until controlled then switch to PO. **Max:** 1 gm/d PO. **Outpatient:** 10 mg PO tid-qid or 25 mg PO bid-tid. **Titrate:** After 1-2d, increase by 20-50 mg BIW.	◙N ❀v

Fluphenazine (Prolixin, Prolixin Decanoate)	(Generic) **Cnt:** 5 mg/ml; **Inj:** (Decanoate) 25 mg/ml, (HCl) 2.5 mg/ml; **Eli:** 2.5 mg/5 ml, **Tab:** 1 mg, 2.5 mg, 5 mg, 10 mg; (Prolixin) **Cnt:** 5 mg/ml; **Inj:** (Decanoate) 25 mg/ml; **Eli:** 2.5 mg/5 ml; **Tab:** 5 mg, 10 mg	**Adults: PO: Initial:** 2.5-10 mg/d given q6-8h. **Titrate:** Increase up to 40 mg/d. **Maint:** 1-5 mg qd. **Inj, HCl: Initial:** 1.25 mg IM q6-8h. **Max:** 10 mg/d. **Decanoate: Initial:** 12.5-25 mg IM/SC q4-6wks. **Max:** 100 mg/dose.	◙N ❋>
Mesoridazine Besylate (Serentil)	**Cnt:** 25 mg/ml; **Inj:** 25 mg/ml; **Tab:** 10 mg, 25 mg, 100 mg	**Schizophrenia: Adults: PO: Initial:** 50 mg tid. **Maint:** 100-400 mg/d. **IM: Initial:** 25 mg. **Maint:** 25-200 mg/d.	◙N ❋> QTc prolongation.
Perphenazine (Trilafon)	**Inj:** 5 mg/ml; **Tab:** 2 mg, 4 mg, 8 mg, 16 mg	**Adults: IM: Initial:** 5 mg IM. May repeat q6h. **Max:** 15 mg/d if ambulatory or 30 mg/d if hospitalized. **PO: Outpatients: Initial:** 4-8 mg tid. **Maint:** Reduce to min effective dose. **Inpatients:** 8-16 mg bid-qid. **Max:** 64 mg/d. **Peds: ≥12 yo:** Use lower limits of adult dose.	◙N ❋>
Thioridazine (Mellaril)	**Cnt:** 30 mg/ml, 100 mg/ ml; **Tab:** 10 mg, 15 mg, 25 mg, 50 mg, 100 mg, 150 mg, 200 mg	**Adults: Initial:** 50-100 mg tid. **Maint:** 200-800 mg/d given bid-qid. **Peds: Initial:** 0.5 mg/kg/d given in divided doses. **Max:** 3 mg/kg/d.	◙N ❋> QTc prolongation.

[30] Increased risk of death in elderly patients with dementia-related psychosis.

NAME	FORM/STRENGTH	DOSAGE	COMMENTS
Trifluoperazine	**Tab:** 1 mg, 2 mg, 5 mg, 10 mg	**Psychotic Disorders: Adults: Initial:** 2-5 mg bid. **Usual:** 15-20 mg/d. **Max:** 40 mg/d or more if needed. **Peds: 6-12 yo: Initial:** 1 mg qd-bid. Increase gradually until symptoms controlled. **Usual:** 15 mg/d. **Non-Psychotic Anxiety: Adults:** 1-2 mg bid. **Max:** 6 mg/d or >12 wks.	N v
THIOXANTHENE DERIVATIVES			
Thiothixene (Navane)	**Cap:** 1 mg, 2 mg, 5 mg, 10 mg, 20 mg	**Adults & Peds: ≥12 yo: Mild Condition: Initial:** 2 mg tid. **Titrate:** May increase to 15 mg/d. **Severe Condition: Initial:** 5 mg bid. **Usual:** 20-30 mg/d. **Max:** 60 mg/d.	N v

Bipolar Agents

NAME	FORM/STRENGTH	DOSAGE	COMMENTS
Aripiprazole (Abilify)	**Sol:** 1 mg/ml; **Tab:** 2 mg, 5 mg, 10 mg, 15 mg, 20 mg, 30 mg	**Bipolar Disorder: Acute Manic & Mixed Episodes: Adults: Initial:** 30 mg qd. **Titrate:** May decrease to 15 mg qd based on tolerability. Oral solution can be given on a mg-per-mg basis up to 25 mg. Patients receiving 30 mg tablets should receive 25 mg of the solution. Adjust dose w/ CYP3A4 inducers/inhibitors or w/ CYP2D6 inhibitors.	C v 30
Carbamazepine (Equetro)	**Cap,ER:** 100 mg, 200 mg, 300 mg	**Bipolar I Disorder: Acute Manic & Mixed Episodes: Adults: Initial:** 400 mg/d, given in divided doses, bid. **Titrate:** 200 mg/d. **Max:** 1600 mg/d.	D v

Divalproex Sodium (Depakote, Depakote ER)	**Tab,Delay:** 125 mg, 250 mg, 500 mg	**Bipolar Disorder: Manic Episodes: Depakote: Adults: Initial:** 750 mg in divided doses. **Titrate:** Increase rapidly to clinical effect. **Max:** 60 mg/kg/d. **Depakote ER: Adults: Initial:** 25 mg/kg/d. **Titrate:** Increase rapidly to clinical effect. **Max:** 60 mg/kg/d.	D v Hepatotoxic. Teratogenic. Pancreatitis.
Lamotrigine (Lamictal, Lamictal CD)	**Chewtab:** (CD) 2 mg, 5 mg, 25 mg; **Tab:** 25 mg, 100 mg, 150 mg, 200 mg	**Bipolar I Disorder: Maintenance: Adults: Patients Not Taking Carbamazepine (CBZ), Other Enzyme-Inducing Drugs (EIDs) or VPA: Weeks 1 & 2:** 25 mg/d. **Weeks 3 & 4:** 50 mg/d. **Week 5:** 100 mg/d. **Weeks 6 & 7:** 200 mg/d. **Patients taking VPA: Weeks 1 & 2:** 25 mg qod. **Weeks 3 & 4:** 25 mg/d. **Week 5:** 50 mg/d. **Weeks 6 & 7:** 100 mg/d. **Patients Taking CBZ (or other EIDs) & Not Taking VPA: Weeks 1 & 2:** 50 mg/d. **Weeks 3 & 4:** 100 mg/d (divided doses). **Week 5:** 200 mg/d (divided doses). **Week 6:** 300 mg/d (divided doses). **Week 7:** Up to 400 mg/d (divided doses). **After D/C of Psychotropic Dugs Excluding VPA, CBZ, or Other EIDs:** Maintain current dose. **After D/C of VPA & Current Lamotrigine Dose of 100 mg/d: Week 1:** 150 mg/d. **Week 2 & Onward:** 200 mg/d. **After D/C of CBZ or Other EIDs & Current Lamotrigine Dose of 400 mg/d: Week 1:** 400 mg/d. **Week 2:** 300 mg/d. **Week 3 & Onward:** 200 mg/d.	C v **H R** Serious rashes, Stevens-Johnson syndrome reported.

30 Increased risk of death in elderly patients with dementia-related psychosis.

NAME	FORM/STRENGTH	DOSAGE	COMMENTS
Lithium Carbonate (Eskalith, Eskalith CR)	**Cap:** 300 mg; **Tab,ER:** 450 mg	**Bipolar Disorder: Manic Episodes: Adults & Peds: ≥12 yo: Cap: Usual:** 1800 mg/d in divided doses given tid or qid. Desired serum levels of 1-1.5 mEq/L. **Long-Term Control: Cap:** 300 mg tid-qid. **Tab,ER**: 450 mg bid. Desired serum levels of 0.6-1.2 mEq/L.	◙N ❉v Lithium toxicity related to serum levels.
Lithium Citrate	**Syr:** 300 mg/5 ml	**Bipolar Disorder: Manic Episodes: Adults & Peds: ≥12 yo:** 600 mg tid, adjust to serum level 1-1.5 mEq/L. **Long Term Control:** 300 mg tid-qid, adjust to serum level 0.6-1.2 mEq/L.	◙D ❉v Lithium toxicity related to serum levels.
Olanzapine (Zyprexa, Zyprexa Zydis, Zyprexa IntraMuscular)	**Inj:** 10 mg; **Tab:** 2.5 mg, 5 mg, 7.5 mg, 10 mg, 15 mg, 20 mg; **Tab,Dissolve:** 5 mg, 10 mg, 15 mg, 20 mg	**Bipolar I Disorder: Acute Manic & Mixed Episodes: Adults: Monotherapy: PO: Initial:** 10-15 mg qd. **Combination Therapy w/ Lithium or Valproate: Initial:** 10 mg qd. **Range:** 5-20 mg/d. **Max:** 20 mg/d. **Titrate:** Adjust by 5 mg/d. **Max:** 20 mg/d. **Maintenance Monotherapy:** 5-20 mg/d. **Agitation Associated w/ Bipolar Mania: Inj: Initial:** 10 mg IM. **Range:** 2.5-10 mg IM. **Max:** 3 doses of 10 mg IM q2-4h. May initiate PO therapy when clinically appropriate.	◙C ❉v [30]
Olanzapine/Fluoxetine HCl (Symbyax)	**Cap:** 6-25 mg, 6-50 mg, 12-25 mg, 12-50 mg	**Bipolar Disorder: Depressive Episodes: Adults: Initial:** 6-25 mg qd in evening. **Range:** 6-25 mg to 12-50 mg. **Max:** 18-75 mg.	◙C ❉v [29, 30]

Quetiapine Fumarate (Seroquel)	**Tab:** 25 mg, 50 mg, 100 mg, 200 mg, 300 mg, 400 mg	**Bipolar I Disorder: Acute Manic Episodes: Adults: Monotherapy or Adjunct Therapy w/ Lithium or Divalproex: Initial:** 100 mg/d given bid on Day 1. **Titrate:** Increase to 400 mg/d given bid on Day 4 in increments of up to 100 mg/d given bid. Adjust doses up to 800 mg/d by Day 6 in increments of not greater than 200 mg/d. **Max:** 800 mg/d.	◙C ❋v **H** [30]
Risperidone (Risperdal, Risperdal M-Tab)	**Sol:** 1 mg/ml; **Tab:** 0.25 mg, 0.5 mg, 1 mg, 2 mg, 3 mg, 4 mg; **Tab,Dissolve:** 0.5 mg, 1 mg, 2 mg, 3 mg, 4 mg	**Bipolar I Disorder: Acute Manic & Mixed Episodes: Adults: Monotherapy or Adjunct Therapy w/ Lithium or Valproate: Initial:** 2-3 mg qd. **Titrate:** Increase by 1 mg qd. **Max:** 6 mg/d.	◙C ❋v **H R** [30]
Ziprasidone (Geodon)	**Cap:** 20 mg, 40 mg, 60 mg, 80 mg	**Bipolar Disorder: Acute Manic & Mixed Episodes: Adults: Initial:** 40 mg bid w/food. **Titrate:** Increase to 60-80 mg bid on 2nd day of treatment. **Maint:** 40-80 mg bid.	◙C ❋v [30]

Migraine Therapy

$5\text{-}HT_1$ AGONISTS

Almotriptan Malate (Axert)	**Tab:** 6.25 mg, 12.5 mg	**Acute Therapy: Adults: ≥18 yo: Initial:** 6.25 mg or 12.5 mg; may repeat after 2h. **Max:** 2 doses/24h.	◙C ❋> **H R**
Eletriptan HBr (Relpax)	**Tab:** 20 mg, 40 mg	**Acute Therapy: Adults: ≥18 yo: Initial:** 20 mg or 40 mg; may repeat after 2h. **Max:** 40 mg/dose or 80 mg/d.	◙C ❋> **H**

29 Antidepressants may increase the risk of suicidality in children and adolescents.
30 Increased risk of death in elderly patients with dementia-related psychosis.

NAME	FORM/STRENGTH	DOSAGE	COMMENTS
Frovatriptan Succinate (Frova)	**Tab:** 2.5 mg	**Acute Therapy: Adults: ≥18 yo: Initial:** 2.5 mg; may repeat after 2h. **Max:** 7.5 mg/d.	C >
Naratriptan HCl (Amerge)	**Tab:** 1 mg, 2.5 mg	**Acute Therapy: Adults: ≥18 yo: Initial:** 1 mg or 2.5 mg; may repeat once after 4h. **Max:** 5 mg/24h.	C > **H R**
Rizatriptan Benzoate (Maxalt, Maxalt-MLT)	**Tab:** 5 mg, 10 mg; **Tab,Dissolve (ODT):** 5 mg, 10 mg	**Acute Therapy: Adults: ≥18 yo: Initial:** 5 or 10 mg; may repeat q2h. **Max:** 30 mg/24h. Place ODT on tongue.	C > Adjust dose with propranolol.
Sumatriptan Succinate (Imitrex)	**Inj:** 6 mg/0.5 ml; **Nasal Spr:** 5 mg/spr, 20 mg/spr; **Tab:** 25 mg, 50 mg, 100 mg	**Acute Therapy: Adults: ≥18 yo: Initial: Inj:** 6 mg SC; may repeat in 1h. **Tab:** 25-100 mg PO; may repeat in 2h. **Nasal Spr:** 5 mg, 10 mg, or 20 mg; may repeat in 2h. **Max:** 12 mg/24h SC, 200 mg/24h PO; 40 mg/24h nasal spr,	C > **H** (Tab)
Zolmitriptan (Zomig, Zomig-ZMT)	**Nasal Spr:** 5 mg/spr; **Tab:** 2.5 mg, 5 mg; **Tab,Dissolve (ODT):** 2.5 mg, 5 mg	**Acute Therapy: Adults: ≥18 yo: Initial: PO:** 2.5 mg or lower; may repeat after 2 h. **Nasal Spr:** 5 mg; may repeat after 2 h. **Max:** 10 mg/24h. Place ODT on tongue.	C > **H**
ERGOT DERIVATIVES			
Caffeine/Ergot (Cafergot, Wigraine)	**Sup:** 100-2 mg; **Tab:** 100-1 mg	**Adults: Initial: Sup:** 1 sup PR at start of attack, then repeat after 1h if needed. **Max:** 2 sups/attack & 5 sups/wk. **Tab:** 2 tabs at start of attack, then 1 tab q30min. **Max:** 6 tabs/attack & 10 tabs/wk.	X v Life-threatening peripheral iscemia with sup & concomitant potent CYP450 3A4 inhibitors.

Dihydroergotamine (Migranal Nasal Spray, DHE 45)	**Inj:** 1 mg/ml; **Nasal Spr:** 0.5 mg/spr	**Adults: Initial: DHE 45:** 1 mg IV/IM/SC, repeat q1h prn up to a total dose of 3 mg IM/SC or 2 mg IV per 24h. **Max:** 6 ml/wk. **Migranal:** 1 spr per nostril, repeat in 15 min. **Max:** 6 spr/24h or 8 spr/wk.	◉X ✽v Life-threatening peripheral ischemia reported with potent CYP450 3A4 inhibitors.
NSAIDS			
Ibuprofen (Advil Migraine, Motrin Migraine)	**Cap:** (Advil) 200 mg; **Tab:** (Motrin) 200 mg	**Adults: Advil:** 400 mg w/ water. **Max:** 400 mg/d. **Motrin:** Take 200-400 mg w/ water. **Max:** 400 mg/d.	◉N ✽>
MISCELLANEOUS			
Caffeine/APAP/ASA (Excedrin Migraine)	**Tab:** 65-250-250 mg	**Adults:** 2 tabs w/ water. **Max:** 2 tabs/d.	◉N ✽>
Divalproex Sodium (Depakote, Depakote ER)	**Tab,Delay:** 125 mg, 250 mg, 500 mg; **Tab,ER:** 250 mg, 500 mg	**Prophylaxis: Depakote: Adults: ≥16 yo: Usual:** 250 mg bid. **Max:** 1000 mg/d. **Depakote ER: Adults: Initial:** 500 mg qd. **Maint:** 1000 mg/d.	◉D ✽v Hepatotoxic. Teratogenic. Pancreatitis.
Isometheptene/ Dichloralphenazone/APAP (Amidrine, Duradrin, Midrin)	**Cap:** 65-100-325 mg	**Adults:** 2 caps, then 1 cap q1h until relief. **Max:** 5 caps/12h.	◉N ✽>
Topiramate (Topamax)	**Cap:** 15 mg, 25 mg; **Tab:** 25 mg, 50 mg, 100 mg, 200 mg	**Migraine Prophylaxis: Titrate: Adults: Week 1:** 25 mg qpm. **Week 2:** 25 mg bid. **Week 3:** 25 mg qam & 50 mg qpm. **Week 4:** 50 mg bid. **Usual:** 50 mg bid.	◉C ✽> R

Muscle Relaxants

NAME	FORM/STRENGTH	DOSAGE	COMMENTS
Baclofen (Kemstro)	**Tab:** (Generic) 10 mg, 20 mg; **Tab (ODT):** (Kemstro) 10 mg, 20 mg	**Adults & Peds: ≥12 yo: Initial:** 5 mg tid x 3d. **Titrate:** Increase q3d by 5 mg tid. **Usual:** 40-80 mg/d. **Max:** 80 mg/d (20 mg qid).	N > **R**
Carisoprodol (Soma)	**Tab:** 350 mg	**Adults & Peds: ≥12 yo:** 350 mg tid & qhs.	N >
Carisoprodol/ASA (Soma Compound)	**Tab:** 200-325 mg	**Adults & Peds: ≥12 yo:** 1-2 tabs qid.	C v
Chlorzoxazone (Parafon Forte DSC)	**Tab:** 500 mg	**Adults: Usual:** 500 mg tid-qid. **Titrate:** May increase to 750 mg tid-qid.	N >
Cyclobenzaprine (Flexeril)	**Tab:** 5 mg, 10 mg	**Adults & Peds: ≥15 yo: Usual:** 5 mg tid. **Titrate:** May increase to 10 mg tid. Do not exceed 2-3 wks of therapy.	B > **H**
Dantrolene Sodium (Dantrium)	**Cap:** 25 mg, 50 mg, 100 mg, 200 mg	**Adults: Initial:** 25 mg qd x 7d. **Titrate:** Increase to 25 mg tid x 7d, then 50 mg tid x 7d, then 100 mg tid. **Max:** 100 mg qid. **Peds: ≥5 yo: Initial:** 0.5 mg/kg qd x 7d. **Titrate:** Increase to 0.5 mg/kg tid x 7d, then 1 mg/kg tid x 7d, then 2 mg/kg tid. **Max:** 100 mg qid.	N v **H** Hepatotoxicity.
Metaxalone (Skelaxin)	**Tab:** 800 mg	**Adults & Peds: >12 yo:** 800 mg tid-qid.	N v

Methocarbamol (Robaxin)	**Inj:** 100 mg/ml; **Tab:** 500 mg, 750 mg	**Adults: Tab: Initial:** (500 mg tab) 1.5 gm qid x 2-3d. **Maint:** 1 gm qid. **Initial:** (750 mg tab) 1.5 gm qid x 2-3d. **Maint:** 750 mg q4h or 1.5 gm tid. **Max:** 6 gm/d x 2-3d; 8 gm/d if severe. **IM/IV: Moderate Symptoms:** 1 gm.	C v
Orphenadrine Citrate (Norflex)	**Inj:** 30 mg/ml; **Tab,ER:** 100 mg	**Adults:** 100 mg PO bid or 60 mg IV/IM q12h.	C >
Orphenadrine/ASA/Caffeine (Norgesic, Norgesic Forte)	**Tab:** (Norgesic) 25-385-30 mg, (Norgesic Forte) 50-770-60 mg	**Adults: Norgesic:** 1-2 tabs tid-qid. **Norgesic Forte:** 1/2-1 tab tid-qid.	N >
Tizanidine HCl (Zanaflex)	**Cap:** 2 mg, 4 mg, 6 mg; **Tab:** 2 mg, 4 mg	**Adults: Initial:** 4 mg q6-8h.**Titrate:** Increase by 2-4 mg. **Usual:** 8 mg q6-8h. **Max:** 3 doses/24h or 36 mg/d.	C >

Obsessive-Compulsive Disorder

SSRIS

Fluoxetine (Prozac)	**Cap:** 10 mg, 20 mg, 40 mg; **Sol:** 20 mg/5 ml; **Tab:** 10 mg	**Adults: Initial:** 20 mg qam. **Maint:** 20-60 mg/d given qd or bid, am & noon. **Max:** 80 mg/d. **Peds: ≥7 yo: Adolescents & Higher-Wt Peds: Initial:** 10 mg/d. **Titrate:** Increase to 20 mg/d after 2 wks. Consider additional dose increases after several more wks if clinical improvement not observed. **Usual:** 20-60 mg/d. **Lower-Wt Peds: Initial:** 10 mg/d. **Titrate:** Consider additional dose increases after several wks if clinical improvement not observed. **Usual:** 20-30 mg/d. **Max:** 60 mg/d.	C v H [29]

[29] Antidepressants may increase the risk of suicidality in children and adolescents.

NAME	FORM/STRENGTH	DOSAGE	COMMENTS
Fluvoxamine	**Tab:** 25 mg, 50 mg, 100 mg	**Adults: Initial:** 50 mg qhs. **Titrate:** Increase by 50 mg q4-7d. **Maint:** 100-300 mg/d. **Max:** 300 mg/d. **8-17 yo: Initial:** 25 mg qhs. **Titrate:** Increase by 25 mg q4-7d. **Maint:** 50-200 mg/d. **Max: 8-11 yo:** 200 mg/d. **Adolescents:** 300 mg/d.	C v **H** [29]
Paroxetine HCl (Paxil)	**Susp:** 10 mg/5 ml; **Tab:** 10 mg, 20 mg, 30 mg, 40 mg	**Adults: Initial:** 20 mg qam. **Usual:** 40 mg/d. **Max:** 60 mg/d.	D > **H R** [29]
Paroxetine Mesylate (Pexeva)	**Tab:** 10 mg, 20 mg, 30 mg, 40 mg	**Adults: Initial:** 40 mg/d. **Max:** 60 mg/d.	C > **H R** [29]
Sertraline (Zoloft)	**Tab:** 25 mg, 50 mg, 100 mg; **Sol:** 20 mg/ml	**Initial: Adults & Peds: ≥13 yo:** 50 mg qd. **6-12 yo:** 25 mg qd. **Titrate:** Adjust wkly. **Max:** 200 mg/d.	C > **H** [29]

TRICYCLIC ANTIDEPRESSANTS

Clomipramine HCl (Anafranil)	**Cap:** 25 mg, 50 mg, 75 mg	**Adults: Initial:** 25 mg/d, increase to 100 mg/d within 1st 2 wks. **Titrate:** Increase over several wks. **Max:** 250 mg/d. May give qhs. **Peds: >10 yo: Initial:** 25 mg/d, increase to 3 mg/kg/d or 100 mg/d within 1st 2 wks. **Titrate:** Increase over several wks. **Max:** 3 mg/kg/d or 200 mg/d. May give qhs.	C v [29]

Miscellaneous

Dantrolene Sodium (Dantrium)	**Inj:** 20 mg	**Malignant Hyperthermia: Adults & Peds: Initial:** 1 mg/kg IV, until symptoms subside. **Max:** 10 mg/kg.	N > **H** Hepatotoxicity.

Etomidate (Amidate)	**Inj:** 2 mg/ml	**Adults & Peds: >10 yo:** 0.2-0.6 mg/kg IV. **Usual:** 0.3 mg/kg IV, over 30-60 sec.	◙C ❁>
Glatiramer (Copaxone)	**Inj:** 20 mg	**Relapsing-Remitting MS: Adults: ≥18 yo:** 20 mg SC qd.	◙B ❁>
Interferon beta-1a (Avonex)	**Inj:** 33 mcg	**Relapsing Forms of MS: Adults:** 30 mcg IM qwk.	◙C ❁v
Interferon beta-1a (Rebif)	**Inj:** 8.8 mcg/0.2 ml, 22 mcg/0.5 ml, 44 mcg/0.5 ml	**Relapsing Forms of MS: Adults: Initial:** 4.4 mcg or 8.8 mcg SC TIW. **Titrate:** Increase over a 4 wk period to 22 mcg or 44 mcg SC TIW. **Maint:** 22 mcg or 44 mcg SC TIW. **Leukopenia/Elevated LFTs:** Reduce dose by 20-50% until toxicity resolves. Administer dose at the same time qd (late afternoon, evening) on the same 3 days/wk at least 48h apart.	◙C ❁> **H**
Interferon beta-1b (Betaseron)	**Inj:** 0.3 mg	**Relapsing MS: Adults:** 0.25 mg SC qod.	◙C ❁v
Meprobamate/ASA (Equagesic)	**Tab:** 200-325 mg	**Musculoskeletal Disease: Adults & Peds: ≥12 yo: Usual:** 1-2 tabs tid-qid prn for pain w/ tension & anxiety.	◙N ❁>
Mitoxantrone (Novantrone)	**Inj:** 2 mg/ml	**Reduction of Neurologic Disability in MS: Adults:** 12 mg/m^2 q3mths.	◙D ❁v Bone marrow suppression. Myocardial toxicity. Secondary AML. [3]
Natalizumab (Tysabri)	**Inj:** 300 mg/15 ml	**Relapsing Forms of MS: Adults:** 300 mg IV q 4 wks.	◙C ❁>

3 Give only under supervision of a physician experienced with antineoplastics.
29 Antidepressants may increase the risk of suicidality in children and adolescents.

NAME	FORM/STRENGTH	DOSAGE	COMMENTS
Nimodipine (Nimotop)	**Cap:** 30 mg	**Subarachnoid Hemorrhage: Adults: Usual:** 60 mg q4h x 21d. Start within 96h of hemorrhage.	◙C ❁v **H**[58]
Sodium Oxybate CIII (Xyrem)	**Sol:** 500 mg/ml	**Adults & Peds ≥13 yo: Initial:** 2.25 g qhs, then 2.25 g 2.5-4 h later. **Titrate:** Increase by 0.75 g/dose q1-2wks. **Range:** 6-9 g/night. **Max:** 9 g/night. Take 1st dose at bedtime while in bed & 2nd dose while sitting in bed. Dilute each dose w/ 2 oz of water.	◙B ❁> **H**[54]

PULMONARY/RESPIRATORY

Asthma/COPD Preparations

ANTICHOLINERGICS

NAME	FORM/STRENGTH	DOSAGE	COMMENTS
Ipratropium Bromide (Atrovent, Atrovent HFA)	**Inhaler:** 0.018 mg/inh, (HFA) 0.017 mg/inh; **Sol,Neb:** 0.02%	**COPD: Adults & Peds: ≥12 yo: Inhaler/HFA Inhaler: Initial:** 2 inh qid. **Max:** 12 inh/24h. **Sol,Neb:** 1 vial (500 mcg/2.5 ml) nebulized tid-qid, separate by 6-8h.	◙B ❁>
Tiotropium Bromide (Spiriva)	**Cap,Inhalation:** 18 mcg	**COPD: Adults:** Inhale the contents of one cap qd, w/ HandiHaler device.	◙C ❁>

BRONCHODILATOR (BETA AGONISTS/ANTICHOLINERGICS)

NAME	FORM/STRENGTH	DOSAGE	COMMENTS
Albuterol Sulfate/ Ipratropium Bromide (Combivent)	**Inhaler:** 0.09-0.018 mg/inh	**COPD: Adults:** 2 inh qid. **Max:** 12 inh/24h.	◙C ❁v

BRONCHODILATOR COMBINATIONS

Albuterol Sulfate/Ipratropium Bromide (Duoneb)	**Sol:** 3-0.5 mg/3 ml	**Adults:** 3 ml qid via nebulizer. May give 2 additional doses/d if needed.	◙C ❊v
Fluticasone Propionate/ Salmeterol Xinafoate (Advair)	**Inhaler:** 100-50 mcg/inh, 250-50 mcg/inh, 500-50 mcg/inh	**Asthma: Adults & Peds: ≥12 yo:** 1 inh q12h; strength depends upon previous inhaled steroid therapy. **Max:** (500-50 mcg/inh) 1 inh bid. **4-11 yo: Symptomatic on Inhaled Steroid Therapy:** (100-50 mcg only) 1 inh q12h. **COPD: Adults:** (250-50 mcg only) 1 inh q12h.	◙C ❊> Asthma-related deaths reported.

BRONCHODILATORS (ALPHA/BETA AGONISTS)

Epinephrine (Adrenalin, Epipen, Epipen Jr)	**Inj:** (Adrenalin, Epipen) 1 mg/ml (1:1000), (Epipen Jr) 0.5 mg/ml (1:2000)	**Epipen/Epipen Jr: Anaphylaxis: Adults:** 0.3 mg IM. **Peds:** 0.15 mg or 0.3 mg (0.01 mg/kg) IM. May repeat if severe. **Adrenalin: Asthma/Allergy: Peds:** 0.01 mg/kg or 0.3 mg/m², up to 0.5 mg SC, repeat q4h if required.	◙C ❊>

54 Sodium oxybate is a GHB (gamma hydroxybutyrate), a known drug of abuse. Do not use with alcohol or other CNS depressants. Only available through Xyrem Success Program.

58 Do not administer IV or by other parenteral routes. Deaths and serious, life-threatening adverse events have occurred when contents of capsules have been injected parenterally.

NAME	FORM/STRENGTH	DOSAGE	COMMENTS
BRONCHODILATORS (BETA AGONISTS)			
Albuterol Sulfate (AccuNeb, ProAir HFA, Proventil HFA, Ventolin HFA)	(AccuNeb) **Sol,Neb:** 0.63 mg/3 ml, 1.25 mg/3 ml; (Generic) **Inhaler:** 0.09 mg/inh, (HFA) 0.09 mg/inh; **Sol, Neb:** 0.083%, 0.5%; (ProAir HFA) **Inhaler:** 0.09 mg/inh; (Proventil) **Inhaler:** 0.09 mg/inh, (HFA) 0.09 mg/inh; **Sol,Neb:** 0.083%, 0.5%; (Ventolin HFA) **Inhaler:** 0.09 mg/inh;	**Acute Bronchospasm/Asthma: AccuNeb: Peds: 6-12 yo w/ Severe Asthma or >40 kg or 11-12 yo: Initial:** 1.25 mg tid-qid. **2-12 yo:** 0.63 mg or 1.25 mg tid-qid via nebulizer. **ProAir HFA: Adults & Peds >12 yo:** 2 inh q4-6h or 1 inh q4h. **Proventil: Sol:** 2.5 mg tid-qid by nebulizer. **Proventil HFA/Ventolin HFA: Adults & Peds: ≥4 yo:** 2 inh q4-6h or 1 inh q4h. **Exercise-Induced Bronchospasm: Proventil Aerosol/ProAir HFA: Adults & Peds: ≥ 12 yo:** 2 inh 15 min before activity. **Proventil HFA/Ventolin HFA: Adults & Peds: ≥4 yo:** 2 inh 15-30 min before activity.	C v
Formoterol Fumarate (Foradil)	**Inhaler:** 12 mcg/inh	**Adults & Peds: ≥5 yo: Asthma/COPD:** 12 mcg q12h. **Max:** 24 mcg/d. **Exercise-Induced Bronchospasm:** 12 mcg 15 min prior to exercise. Do not give added dose if on q12h schedule. Give only by inhalation w/ Aerolizer Inhaler.	C >
Levalbuterol HCl (Xopenex, Xopenex HFA)	**Sol,Neb:** (Xopenex) 0.31 mg/3 ml, 0.63 mg/3 ml, 1.25 mg/3 ml; **HFA Inhaler:** (Xopenex HFA) 45 mcg/inh	**Adults & Peds: ≥12 yo: Sol,Neb: Bronchospasm: Initial:** 0.63 mg tid, q6-8h. **Severe Asthma:** 1.25 mg tid, q6-8h. **6-11 yo:** 0.31 mg tid. **Max:** 0.63 mg tid. Administer by neb. **≥4 yo: HFA Inhaler:** 90 mcg q4-6h or 45 mcg q4h may be suffcient.	C v

Metaproterenol Sulfate (Alupent)	(Alupent) **Inhaler:** 0.65 mg/inh; **Sol,Neb:** 0.6%; **Tab:** 10 mg; (Generic) **Sol,Neb:** 0.4%, 0.6%; **Syr:** 10 mg/5 ml; **Tab:** 10 mg, 20 mg	**Bronchospasm: Adults & Peds: ≥12 yo: Inhaler:** 2-3 inh q3-4h. **Max:** 12 inh/d. **Sol,Neb 0.4%, 0.6%:** 2.5 ml by IPPB tid-qid, up to q4h. **Syr/Tab: >9 yo or >60 lbs:** 20 mg tid-qid. **6-9 yo or <60 lbs:** 10 mg tid-qid. **Sol,Neb 5%: ≥12 yo: Neb/IPPB:** 0.2-0.3 ml (dilute in 2.5 ml saline) tid-qid. **Hand-bulb Neb:** 5-15 inh (undiluted) tid-qid. **6-12 yo: Neb:** 0.1-0.2 ml (dilute in 3 ml saline) by neb tid-qid.	◙C ❉>
Pirbuterol Acetate (Maxair, Maxair Autohaler)	**Autohaler:** 0.2 mg/inh **Inhaler:** 0.2 mg/inh	**Adults & Peds: ≥12 yo:** 1-2 inh q4-6h. **Max:** 12 inh/d.	◙C ❉>
Salmeterol Xinafoate (Serevent)	**Inhaler:** 21 mcg/inh; **Diskus:** 50 mcg	**Inhaler: ≥12 yo: Asthma/COPD:** 2 inh q12h. **EIB Prevention:** 2 inh 30-60 min before exercise. **Diskus: ≥4 yo: Asthma/COPD:** 1 inh q12h. **EIB Prevention:** 1 inh 30 min before exercise (do not give preventive doses if already on bid dose).	◙C ❉v Asthma-related deaths reported.
Terbutaline Sulfate (Brethine)	**Inj:** 1 mg/ml; **Tab:** 2.5 mg, 5 mg	**Adults & Peds: ≥15 yo: PO:** 5 mg tid. May reduce to 2.5 mg tid. **Max:** 15 mg/24h. **12-15 yo:** 2.5 mg tid. **Max:** 7.5 mg/24h. **Inj: ≥12 yo:** 0.25 mg SC into lateral deltoid area. May repeat within 15-30 min if no improvement. **Max:** 0.5 mg/4h.	◙B ❉>

NAME	FORM/STRENGTH	DOSAGE	COMMENTS
IGG1K MONOCLONAL ANTIBODY			
Omalizumab (Xolair)	**Inj:** 75 mg, 150 mg	**Adults & Peds: ≥12 yo:** 150-375 mg SC q2 or 4 wks based on body wt & pre-treatment serum total IgE level. **Max:** 150 mg/site. **30-90 kg & IgE ≥30-100 IU/ml:** 150 mg q4wks. **>90-150 kg & IgE ≥30-100 IU/ml or 30-90 kg & IgE >100-200 IU/ml or 30-60 kg & IgE >200-300 IU/ml:** 300 mg q4wks. **90-150 kg & IgE >100-200 IU/ml or >60-90 kg & IgE >200-300 IU/ml or 30-70 kg & IgE >300-400 IU/ml:** 225 mg q2wks. **>90-150 kg & IgE >200-300 IU/ml or >70-90 kg & IgE >300-400 IU/ml or 30-70 kg & IgE >400-500 IU/ml or 30-60 kg & IgE >500-600 IU/ml:** 300 mg q2wks. **>70-90 kg & IgE >400-500 IU/ml or >60-70 kg & IgE >500-600 IU/ml or 30-60 kg & IgE >600-700 I U/ml:** 375 mg q2wks.	◙B ❋>
INHALED CORTICOSTEROIDS			
Beclomethasone Dipropionate (Qvar)	**Inhaler:** 40 mcg/inh, 80 mcg/inh	**Adults & Adolesents: Previous Bronchodilator Only:** 40-80 mcg bid. **Max:** 320 mcg bid. **Previous Inhaled Corticosteroid Therapy:** 40-160 mcg bid. **Max:** 320 mcg bid. **5-11 yo: Previous Bronchodilator Only or Inhaled Corticosteroid:** 40 mcg bid. **Max:** 80 mcg bid. **Adults & Peds: ≥5 yo: Maint w/ Oral Corticosteroids:** May attempt gradual reduction of oral dose after 1 wk on inhaled therapy.	◙C ❋v

Budesonide (Pulmicort Respules, Pulmicort Turbuhaler)	**Respules:** 0.25 mg/2 ml; 0.5 mg/2 ml; **Turbuhaler:** 200 mcg/inh.	**Adults & Peds: ≥6 yo: Turbuhaler: Previous Bronchodilator Only/Inhaled Corticosteroid: Initial:** 200 mcg bid. (Mild-to-moderate asthma patients previously controlled on inhaled steroids may use 200-400 mcg qd). **Max:** 400 mcg bid. **Oral Corticosteroid: Max:** 400 mcg bid. **Respules: 1-8 yo: Previous Bronchodilator Only: Initial:** 0.5 mg qd or 0.25 mg bid. Administer via jet neb. **Max:** 0.5 mg/d. **Previous Inhaled Corticosteroid:** 0.5 mg qd or 0.25 mg bid. **Max:** 1 mg/d. **Previous Oral Corticosteroid:** 1 mg qd or 0.5 mg bid. **Max:** 1 mg/d. Gradually reduce PO corticosteroid after 1 wk of budesonide.	B > (Respules) B v (Turbuhaler)
Flunisolide (Aerobid, Aerobid-M)	**Inhaler:** 0.25 mg/inh	**Adults & Peds: ≥6 yo: Initial:** 2 inh bid. **Max: Adults:** 4 inh bid.	C >
Fluticasone Propionate (Flovent HFA)	**Inhaler:** 44 mcg/inh, 110 mcg/inh, 220 mcg/inh	**Adults & Peds: ≥12 yo: Previous Bronchodilator Only: Initial:** 88 mcg bid. **Max:** 440 mcg bid. **Previous Inhaled Corticosteroids: Initial:** 88-220 mcg bid. **Max:** 440 mcg bid. **Previous Oral Corticosteroids:** Initial: 440 mcg bid. **Max:** 880 mcg bid. **4-11 yo: Initial/Max:** 88 mcg bid. Reduce PO prednisone no faster than 2.5 mg/d wkly; begin at least 1 wk after start fluticasone.	C >
Mometasone Furoate (Asmanex)	**Inhaler:** 220 mcg/inh	**Adults & Peds: ≥12 yo: Previous Therapy w/ Bronchodilators Alone or Inhaled Corticosteroids: Initial:** 220 mcg qpm. **Max:** 440 mcg/d or 220 mcg bid. **Previous Therapy w/ Oral Corticosteroids: Initial:** 440 mcg bid. **Max:** 880 mcg/d. Titrate to lowest effective dose once asthma stability is achieved.	C >

NAME	FORM/STRENGTH	DOSAGE	COMMENTS
Triamcinolone Acetonide (Azmacort)	**Inhaler:** 100 mcg/inh	**Adults & Peds: >12 yo:** 2 inh tid-qid or 4 inh bid. **Severe Asthma: Initial:** 12-16 inh/d. **Max:** 16 inh/d. **6-12 yo:** 1-2 inh tid-qid or 2-4 inh bid. **Max:** 12 inh/d.	●C ❋>
LEUKOTRIENE MODIFIERS			
Montelukast Sodium (Singulair)	**Chewtab:** 4 mg, 5 mg; **Granules:** 4 mg/pkt; **Tab:** 10 mg	**Asthma: Adults & Peds: ≥15 yo:** 10 mg qpm. **6-14 yo:** 5 mg qpm. **2-5 yo: Chewtab/Granules:** 4 mg qpm. **12-23 mths: Granules:** 4 mg qpm.	●B ❋>
Zafirlukast (Accolate)	**Tab:** 10 mg, 20 mg	**Asthma: Adults & Peds: ≥12 yo:** 20 mg bid. **5-11 yo:** 10 mg bid. Administer 1h ac or 2h pc.	●B ❋v
Zileuton (Zyflo)	**Tab:** 600 mg	**Asthma: Adults & Peds: ≥12 yo:** 600 mg qid. w/ meals & hs.	●C ❋v **H**
MAST CELL STABILIZERS			
Cromolyn Sodium (Intal)	**Inhaler:** 0.8 mg/inh; **Sol,Neb:** 10 mg/ml	**Asthma: Inhaler: Adults & Peds: ≥5 yo: Usual/Max:** 2 inh qid. **Sol: ≥2 yo:** 20 mg qid via neb. **Acute Bronchospasm Prevention: Inhaler: ≥5 yo: Usual:** 2 inh 10-60 min before precipitant exposure. **Sol: ≥2 yo:** 20 mg via neb shortly before precipitant exposure.	●B ❋> **H R**
Nedocromil Sodium (Tilade)	**Inhaler:** 1.75 mg/inh	**Asthma: Adults & Peds: ≥ 6 yo:** 2 inh qid. May reduce to bid-tid once desired response observed.	●B ❋>

Aminophylline	**Inj:** 25 mg/ml; **Sol:** 105 mg/5 ml; **Tab:** 100 mg, 200 mg	**Chronic Treatment: Adults: Initial:** 16 mg/kg/24h PO or 400 mg/24h PO of theophylline given q6-8h. **Titrate:** Increase by 25% q3d as tolerated & adjust to 10-20 mg/ml. **Peds: 9 to <16 yo: Initial:** 6.3 mg/kg. **Maint:** 0.8 mg/kg/h. **1 to <9 yo: Initial:** 6.3 mg/kg. **Maint:** 1 mg/kg/h.	C v **H R**
Theophylline (Theo-24, Theolair)	**Cap,ER:** (Theo-24) 100 mg, 200 mg, 300 mg, 400 mg; **Tab:** (Theolair) 125 mg, 250 mg	**Theolair: Adults & Peds: ≥1 yo and >45 kg: Initial:** 300 mg/d divided q6-8h. **Titrate:** Increase to 400 mg/d divided q6-8h after 3d if tolerated, then to 600 mg/d divided q6-8h after 3 more days if needed & tolerated. **≥1 yo & <45 kg: Initial:** 12-14 mg/kg/d divided q4-6h. **Max:** 300 mg/d. **Titrate:** Increase to 16 mg/kg/d divided q4-h6 (**Max:** 400 mg/d) after 3d if tolerated, then increase to 20 mg/kg/d divided q4-6h (**Max:** 600mg/d) after 3 more days if needed & tolerated. **Theo-24: Adults & Peds: ≥12 yo & >45 kg: Initial:** 300-400 mg/d. **Titrate:** Increase to 400-600 mg/d after 3d if tolerated, then to >600 mg/d if needed & tolerated after 3 more days. **≥12 yo & <45 kg: Initial:** 12-14 mg/kg/d (**Max:** 300 mg/d). Increase to 16 mg/kg/d (**Max:** 400 mg/d) after 3d. May increase to 20 mg/kg/d (**Max:** 600 mg/d) if tolerated & needed after 3 more days.	C > **H R**

Miscellaneous

NAME	FORM/STRENGTH	DOSAGE	COMMENTS
Acetylcysteine (Mucomyst)	**Sol:** 10%, 20%	**Adults & Peds: Mucolytic: Nebulization (face mask, mouth piece, tracheostomy):** 1-10 ml of 20% or 2-10 ml of 10% q2-6h. **Usual:** 3-5 ml of 20% or 6-10 ml of 10% 3-4x/d. **Closed Tent or Croupette:** Up to 300 ml of 10% or 20%. **Direct Instillation:** 1-2 ml of 10% or 20% q1-4h. **Percutaneous Intratracheal Catheter:** 1-2 ml of 20% or 2-4 ml of 10% q1-4h. **Diagnostic Bronchograms:** Give before procedure. 2-3 doses of 1-2 ml of 20% or 2-4 ml of 10%.	◙B ❋>

UROLOGY

Benign Prostatic Hypertrophy

ALPHA$_1$ RECEPTOR BLOCKERS

NAME	FORM/STRENGTH	DOSAGE	COMMENTS
Alfuzosin HCl (Uroxatral)	**Tab,ER:** 10 mg	**Adults:** 10 mg immediately after the same meal qd.	◙B ❋v **H**
Doxazosin Mesylate (Cardura, Cardura XL)	**Tab:** 1 mg, 2 mg, 4 mg, 8 mg; **Tab,ER:** 4 mg, 8 mg	**Adults: Tab: Initial:** 1 mg qd in am or pm. **Titrate:** Increase q1-2wks. **Max:** 8 mg/d. **Tab,ER: Initial:** 4 mg qd w/ breakfast. **Titrate:** May increase to 8 mg after 3-4 wks. **Max:** 8 mg. Swallow whole; do not chew, divide, cut, or crush.	◙C ❋> (Tab) ❋v (Tab,ER)
Tamsulosin HCl (Flomax)	**Cap:** 0.4 mg	**Adults:** 0.4 mg qd, 1/2h after same meal each day. If fail to respond after 2-4 wks, may increase to 0.8 mg qd. If therapy is interrupted for several days, restart w/ 0.4 mg qd.	◙B ❋v

Terazosin (Hytrin)	**Cap:** 1 mg, 2 mg, 5 mg, 10 mg	**Adults: Initial:** 1 mg qhs. **Titrate:** Increase stepwise to 10 mg qd. **Max:** 20 mg.	C >

ALPHA-REDUCTASE INHIBITORS

Dutasteride (Avodart)	**Cap:** 0.5 mg	**Adults:** 0.5 mg qd.	X v
Finasteride (Proscar)	**Tab:** 5 mg	**Adults: Monotherapy/Concomitant Doxazosin:** 5 mg qd.	X v

Enuresis Management

Desmopressin Acetate (DDAVP)	**Nasal Spr:** 10 mcg/spr; **Rhinal Tube:** 0.01%; **Tab:** 0.1 mg, 0.2 mg	**Adults & Peds: ≥6 yo: Tab: Initial:** 0.2 mg PO qhs. **Titrate:** May increase up to 0.6 mg. **Max:** Up to 6 mths. **Spray/Tube: Initial:** 20 mcg intranasally qhs. **Titrate:** Decrease to 10 mcg or increase up to 40 mcg if needed. **Max:** 4-8 wks. Administer 1/2 dose per nostril.	B >
Flavoxate HCl (Urispas)	**Tab:** 100 mg	**Adults & Peds: ≥12 yo:** 100-200 mg tid-qid. Reduce dose w/ improvement.	B >

Erectile Dysfunction

ALPHA$_2$ RECEPTOR BLOCKERS

Yohimbine HCl (Aphrodyne)	**Tab:** 5.4 mg	**Adults: Usual:** 5.4 mg tid up to 10 wks. If side effects occur, decrease to 1/2 tab tid, then gradually increase back to usual dose.	N > **R** Do not use in pregnancy.

NAME	FORM/STRENGTH	DOSAGE	COMMENTS
PHOSPHODIESTERASE TYPE 5 INHIBITOR			
Sildenafil Citrate (Viagra)	**Tab:** 25 mg, 50 mg, 100 mg	**Adults: Usual:** 50 mg qd 1h (range 0.5-4 h) before sexual activity. **Titrate:** May decrease to 25 mg qd or increase to 100 mg qd. **Max:** 100 mg qd. **Concomitant CYP450 3A4 Inhibitors: Initial:** 25 mg qd. **Concomitant Ritonavir: Max:** 25 mg q48h.	●B ❀v **H R** CI with nitrates.
Tadalafil (Cialis)	**Tab:** 5 mg, 10 mg, 20 mg	**Adults: Initial:** 10 mg prior to sexual activity at frequency of up to once daily. **Titrate:** May decrease to 5 mg or increase to 20 mg based on response. **With Potent CYP3A4 inhibitors (eg, ketoconazole, itraconazole, ritonavir): Max:** 10 mg/72 h.	●B ❀v **H R** CI with nitrates.
Vardenafil HCl (Levitra)	**Tab:** 2.5 mg, 5 mg, 10 mg, 20 mg	**Adults: Initial:** 10 mg 60 min prior to sexual activity at frequency of up to once daily. **Titrate:** May decrease to 5 mg or increase to max of 20 mg based on response. **Elderly: ≥65 yrs: Initial:** 5 mg. **Concomitant Ritonavir: Max:** 2.5 mg/72 h. **Concomitant Indinavir, Ketoconazole 400 mg daily/Itraconazole 400 mg daily: Max:** 2.5 mg/24 h. **Concomitant Ketoconazole 200 mg daily/Itraconazole 200 mg daily/Erythromycin: Max:** 5 mg/24 h.	●B ❀v **H** CI with nitrates or nitric oxide donors.

Alprostadil (Caverject, Caverject Impulse, Edex, MUSE Urethral Suppository)	**Inj:** 5 mcg, 10 mcg, 10 mcg/ml, 20 mcg, 20 mcg/ml, 40 mcg; **Sup, Urethral:** 125 mcg, 250 mcg, 500 mcg, 1000 mcg	**Adults: Muse: Transurethral: Initial:** 125-250 mcg. **Titrate:** Increase as necessary to achieve erection. **Max:** 2 sup/24 h. **Caverject, Edex: Intracavernosal: Vasculogenic/Psychogenic/Mixed Etiology: Initial:** 2.5 mcg. **Partial Response:** Increase by 2.5 mcg, then by 5-10 mcg until desired response. **No Response:** Increase by 5 mcg, then by 5-10 mcg until desired response. **Neurogenic Etiology (Spinal Cord Injury): Initial:** 1.25 mcg. **Partial/No Response:** May give 2nd dose of 2.5 mcg, 3rd dose of 5 mcg, then may increase by 5 mcg until desired response. **Max:** 60 mcg/dose. Reduce dose if erection >1h. Give no more than TIW; allow 24 h between doses. If no initial response, may give next higher dose within 1h. If partial response, give next higher dose after 24 h.	▣C ❃v

Urinary Acidifiers

Dibasic Sodium Phosphate/Monobasic Potassium Phosphate/Monobasic Sodium Phosphate (K-Phos Neutral)	**Tab:** 250 mg phos/ 298 mg sodium (13 mEq)/ 45 mg potassium (1.1 mEq)	**Adults:** 1-2 tabs qid. **Peds: >4 yo:**1 tab qid. Take w/ meals & hs w/ full glass of water.	▣C ❃>

NAME	FORM/STRENGTH	DOSAGE	COMMENTS
Potassium Acid Phosphate (K-Phos Original)	**Tab:** 500 mg (114 mg phosphorus/144 mg potassium [3.7 mEq])	**Adults:** Dissolve 2 tabs in 6-8 oz of water & drink qid, w/ meals & qhs.	C >
Sodium Phosphate/ Dipotassium Phosphate/ Disodium Phosphate (Uro-KP-Neutral)	**Tab:** 258 mg phos/ 49.4 mg potassium/ 262.4 mg sodium	**Adults:** 1-2 tabs qid w/full glass of water.	C >

Urinary Alkalinizers

Potassium Citrate (Urocit-K)	**Tab,ER:** 5 mEq, 10 mEq	**Adults: Severe Hypocitraturia (Urinary Citrate <150 mg/d):** 20 mEq tid or 15 mEq qid w/ meals. **Mild/Moderate Hypocitraturia (Urinary Citrate ≥150 mg/d:** 10 mEq tid. **Max:** 100 mEq/d.	C >
Potassium Citrate/Sodium Citrate/Citric Acid (Polycitra)	**Syr:** 550-500-334 mg/ 5 ml	**Adults:** 15-30 ml qid pc & qhs; dilute w/ water. **Peds:** 5-15 ml qid pc & qhs; dilute w/ water.	N >
Sodium Bicarbonate	**Tab:** 325 mg, 650 mg	**Adults:** 325 mg-2 gm up to qid. **Max: <60 yo:** 15 gm/d. **≥60 yo:** 8 gm/d.	N >
Sodium Citrate/Citric Acid (Bicitra, Oracit)	**Sol:** (Bicitra) 500-334 mg/5 ml; (Oracit) 490-640 mg/5 ml	**Adults:** Dilute 10-30 ml in 30-90 ml water & drink pc & qhs. **Peds: ≥2 yo:** Dilute 5-15 ml in 30-90 ml water & drink pc & qhs.	N >

Urinary Retention

PARASYMPATHETIC STIMULANTS

Bethanechol (Urecholine)	**Tab:** 5 mg, 10 mg, 25 mg, 50 mg;	**Adults: Initial:** 5-10 mg. **Titrate:** May repeat q1h until satisfactory response or 50 mg given. **Usual:** 10-50 mg tid-qid. **Max:** 200 mg/d.	C v

Urinary Tract Antispasmodics

PARASYMPATHOLYTICS

Darifenacin (Enablex)	**Tab,ER:** 7.5 mg, 15 mg	**Overactive Bladder: Adults: Initial:** 7.5 mg qd w/ liquid. **Max:** 15 mg qd. **Hepatic Dysfunction/ Concomitant CYP3A4 Inhibitors:** Do not exceed 7.5 mg/d.	C > H
Hyoscyamine Sulfate (Cystospaz)	**Tab:** 0.15 mg	**Adults:** 0.15-0.3 mg qid prn.	C >
Hyoscyamine Sulfate (Levbid, Levsin, Levsinex, NuLev)	(Levbid) **Tab,ER:** 0.375 mg; (Levsin) **Drops:** 0.125 mg/ml; **Eli:** 0.125 mg/5 ml; **Inj:** 0.5 mg/ml; **Tab:** 0.125 mg; **Tab,SL:** 0.125 mg; (Levsinex) **Cap,ER:** 0.375 mg; (NuLev) **Tab,Dissolve (ODT):** 0.125 mg	**Adults & Peds: ≥12 yo: Drops/Eli/ODT/Tab/Tab,SL:** 0.125-0.25 mg q4h or prn. **Max:** 1.5 mg/24h. **Cap, Tab,ER:** 0.375-0.75 mg q12h; or 1 cap q8h. **Max:** 1.5 mg/24h. **2 to <12 yo: ODT/Tab/Tab,SL:** 0.0625-0.125 mg q4h or prn. **Max:** 0.75 mg/24h. **Eli:** Give q4h or prn. **10 kg:** 1.25 ml. **20 kg:** 2.5 ml. **40 kg:** 3.75 ml. **50 kg:** 5 ml. **Max:** 30 ml/24h. **Drops:** 0.25-1 ml q4h or prn. **Max:** 6 ml/24h. **<2 yo: Drops:** Give q4h or prn. **3.4 kg:** 4 gtts. **Max:** 24 gtts/24h. **5 kg:** 5 gtts. **Max:** 30 gtts/24h. **7 kg:** 6 gtts. **Max:** 36 gtts/24h. **10 kg:** 8 gtts. **Max:** 48 gtts/24h.	C >
Oxybutynin Chloride (Ditropan, Ditropan XL)	**Syr:** 5 mg/5 ml; **Tab:** 5 mg; **Tab,ER:** 5 mg, 10 mg, 15 mg	**Overactive Bladder: Adults: Tab/Syr:** 5 mg bid-tid. **Max:** 5 mg qid. **Tab,ER: Initial:** 5 or 10 mg qd. **Titrate:** May increase qwk by 5 mg. **Max:** 30 mg/d. **Peds: >5 yo: Tab/Syr:** 5 mg bid. **Max:** 5 mg tid. **Detrusor Overactivity: Peds: ≥6 yo: Tab,ER: Initial:** 5 mg qd. **Titrate:** May increase qwk by 5 mg. **Max:** 20 mg/d.	B >

NAME	FORM/STRENGTH	DOSAGE	COMMENTS
Oxybutynin (Oxytrol)	**Patch:** 36 mg (3.9 mg/d)	**Overactive Bladder: Adults:** 3.9 mg/d 2x/wk (q3-4d). Apply to abdomen, hip, or buttock.	●B ❁>
Solifenacin Succinate (VESIcare)	**Tab:** 5 mg, 10 mg	**Overactive Bladder: Adults:** 5 mg qd. **Max:** 10 mg qd.	●C ❁> **H R**
Tolterodine (Detrol, Detrol LA)	**Cap,ER** 2 mg, 4 mg; **Tab:** 1 mg, 2 mg	**Overactive Bladder: Adults: Cap,ER:** 4 mg qd. May decrease to 2 mg qd depending on response & tolerability. **Tab: Initial:** 2 mg bid. **Maint:** 1-2 mg bid.	●C ❁v **H R**
Trospium Chloride (Sanctura)	**Tab:** 20 mg	**Overactive Bladder: Adults:** 20 mg bid. Take at least 1 h before meals or on an empty stomach.	●C ❁> **R**

INDEX

H

I

P